CLINICAL HEMORHEOLOGY

CLINICAL HEMORHEOLOGY

Applications in Cardiovascular and Hematological Disease, Diabetes, Surgery and Gynecology

edited by

S. CHIEN

Department of Physiology, College of Surgeons and Physicians
Columbia University, New York, U.S.A.

J. DORMANDY

Department of Surgery, St. James' and St. George's Hospital
London, U.K.

E. ERNST and A. MATRAI

Hemorheology Research Unit, University Clinic
Munich, F.R.G.

1987 **MARTINUS NIJHOFF PUBLISHERS**
a member of the KLUWER ACADEMIC PUBLISHERS GROUP
DORDRECHT / BOSTON / LANCASTER

Distributors

for the United States and Canada: Kluwer Academic Publishers, P.O. Box 358, Accord Station, Hingham, MA 02018-0358, USA
for the UK and Ireland: Kluwer Academic Publishers, MTP Press Limited, Falcon House, Queen Square, Lancaster LA1 1RN, UK
for all other countries: Kluwer Academic Publishers Group, Distribution Center, P.O. Box 322, 3300 AH Dordrecht, The Netherlands

Library of Congress Cataloging in Publication Data

Clinical hemorheology.

Includes bibliographies and index.
1. Blood--Circulation, Disorders of.
2. Hemodynamics. 3. Rheology (Biology) 4. Blood flow.
5. Blood hyperviscosity syndrome. I. Chien, Shu.
II. Title: Hemorheology. [DNLM: 1. Blood Circulation.
2. Blood Vessels. 3. Rheology. WG 106 C6415]
RC636.C55 1986 616.1 86-8337

ISBN-13: 978-94-010-8404-8 e-ISBN-13: 978-94-009-4285-1
DOI: 10.1007/978-94-009-4285-1

Copyright

Contents

Preface

The task the editors have set themselves is to survey the field of clinical hemorheology from basic principles to up-to-date research. It is only in a new science like this that it is possible to span the whole field in a book of this size.

Hemorheology, as a new approach to the study and management of a wide range of circulatory diseases, is now beginning to appear with increasing frequency in general as well as specialized medical journals. Hemorheology is also just beginning to creep into the undergraduate medical curriculum. Therefore, the majority of graduate doctors are unequipped to assess the place of hemorheology in the overall framework of circulatory physiology and pathology or to assess its relevance to their everyday practice. It is hoped that this book will fill this gap.

The approach of the book is interdisciplinary. The first part deals with basic principles of blood flow, circulation and hemorheology. It has been written with the general doctor in mind, who has no special knowledge of hemodynamics and rheological concepts, terminology or methodology. To maintain the emphasis on practical clinical applications, all the chapters in the second part of the book have been written by clinical specialists practicing in the individual areas of disease. The book is so designed that clinicians may be able to read the relevant chapters in the second part of the book in isolation, using the basic science aspects contained in the first part of the book as reference chapters.

Because hemorheology is a new science, its precise place in clinical medicine and surgery is still controversial. With the help of this book readers will be able to assess for themselves the evidence available at the moment, as well as the rapidly expanding new clinical literature of the applications of hemorheology.

S. Chien
J. Dormandy
E. Ernst
A. Matrai

1
Introduction: On the way to modern clinical hemorheology

Alfred L. Copley
Laboratory of Biorheology, Polytechnic University, Brooklyn, NY 11201, United States of America

Clinical hemorheology embraces one of the main areas in the practice of medicine, and goes back to ancient times [1]. Modern clinical hemorheology is practiced in different fields of medicine and surgery, as dealt with in this book and indicated in its subtitle.

It may be considered rather extraneous to acquaint the Reader with certain personal memories in this introduction, but the development of modern clinical hemorheology is to some extent associated with them. I began my career in the biomedical sciences in 1932 on the purification of thrombin in Würzburg at the Institute of Physiology under the direction of Edgar Wöhlisch who, at that time, was the leading authority on blood coagulation in Germany. He assigned to me, a medical student in the sixth semester, the teaching of blood clotting and its disorders to my fellow students in the fourth and fifth semesters. What I could not understand and explain to them was the phenomenon of a markedly prolonged coagulation time and a normal bleeding time in hemophilia and, vice versa, a normal coagulation time and prolonged bleeding time in thrombocytopenic purpura. Wöhlisch could not explain these apparently paradoxic findings and merely thought that the platelets may have something to do with them.

In 1939, ten years after rheology was founded as an organized science in Washington D.C., I pursued my clinical hemorheological studies at the Hixon Laboratory of Medical Research at the University of Kansas Medical School. During this time, I studied hemophiliacs and my first report on thixotropy of hemophilic and heparinized blood was published two years later [2]. During my stay at this Institute, Lalich and I attacked the problem of bleeding time in normal subjects and hemophilic patients with a new method, which we developed [3,4], without changes in hemodynamic pressure. We found that bleeding into physiological saline at 37°C, after infliction of a wound in the end phalanx of a finger, resulted in a free flow of blood [3]. The Copley-Lalich bleeding time is a truly clinical hemorheological test which has not yet been widely used. In connection with this test, we developed the "clot resistance" test [3], named more adequately later "wound thrombus resistance" [4], made several minutes following the bleeding time by the application of a cuff-pressure below the systolic pressure. Recurrence of bleeding from the wound inflicted for the bleeding time may thus be provoked. We found that the bleeding time measures the initiation of in vivo hemostasis while wound thrombus resistance, its maintenance [4]. In making the bleeding tests we observed several other phenomena which we described, including the seepage into saline of a whitish flow, named "lymph time" [3]. These in vivo hemorheological phenomena still need further exploration.

As in normal subjects, the Copley-Lalich bleeding time was found to be within 3 minutes in hemophiliacs [5]. However, the wound thrombus resistance was always impaired in hemophiliacs which explains the recurrence of bleeding even from small wounds [4]. Lalich and Copley [6] described an extra vivum clinical hemorheological test which measures clot firmness in special viscometer tubes, to which pressure is applied. Clot firmness was found markedly reduced with blood from hemophilic patients [6].

Two other in vivo clinical hemorheological tests, employing negative pressures, developed later, measure capillary or vascular fragility by petechial counts and detect capillary hemorrhagic diathesis with the so-called "ecchymosis test" [4,7,21].

During my stay at the Hixon Laboratory, we made studies on viscosity, yield value, thixotropy, dilatancy and age-hardening of blood, secured with different anticoagulants, from healthy human subjects. A modified falling ball or so-called "rolling ball" viscometer, used at different shearing stresses, permitted the determination of flow properties of blood systems [8]. These studies, which were among the first reported on the anomalous flow properties of blood, were published by Copley, Krchma and Whitney in 1942. This communication in the Journal of General Physiology was particularly welcomed by rheologists in different countries, and created an impact that ultimately led to biorheology as an organized life science.

In 1943, I was asked by the British Society of Rheology to act as chairman of a Symposium on the Application of Rheology in Medical Science, held in Oxford in 1944, which I could not attend because of the war. Several years later, I was invited to give a Plenary Lecture on "Rheological Problems in Biology" at the First International Congress on Rheology, held in Scheveningen, Holland in 1948. There, I introduced the term "biorheology" in a survey [9], the first of its kind, of biorheological, including hemorheological, observations and studies. I stated that "I am convinced that rheology will play a very important role in the biological sciences including medicine of tomorrow. As observations on the flow of blood helped initiate the science of rheology, it is my belief that from continued observations on other properties of this very special part of life, namely blood, and of blood constituents, a combination of the sciences of rheology and biology is bound to serve the well-being of our species" [9].

The term "hemorheology" was introduced for the rheology of blood and of the blood vessel wall in a lecture before the Society of Rheology at the 25th

Anniversary Meeting of the American Institute of Physics, held in Chicago in 1951. At that time, I defined hemorheology as being "concerned with deformation and flow properties of cellular and plasmatic components of blood in macroscopic, microscopic, and submicroscopic dimensions, and with the rheological properties of vessel structure with which blood comes in direct contact" [10]. Although I have done experimental research in different areas of the biomedical sciences, hemorheology became my main interest.

Modern clinical hemorheology is based on theoretical and experimental hemorheology as well as on clinical findings. Theoretical hemorheology is subdivided into two areas; one deals with theoretical rheological aspects, the other with mechanisms of physiological or patho-physiological processes pertaining to phenomena and findings in experimental and clinical hemorheology.

A strong impetus to the organization of modern hemorheology was given at a conference which I initiated, entitled "Flow of Blood in Relation to the Vessel Wall", held in 1958 at Charing Cross Hospital Medical School of the University of London, and organized with the physicist George W. Scott Blair of the Physics Department, National Institute for Research in Dairying, University of Reading. The success of this meeting indicated the need for further actvities and drew the attention of the Faraday Society. Subsequent discussions between F.J.W. Roughton, FRS of Cambridge University, R.G. Macfarlane, FRS of the Radcliffe Infirmary, Oxford, G.W. Scott Blair and myself led to an Informal Discussion, entitled "Flow Properties of Blood and Other Biological Systems", convened jointly by the Colloid and Biophysics Committee of the Faraday Society and the British Society of Rheology. It was locally promoted by R.G. Macfarlane and held at the University Laboratory of Physiology, Oxford in September 1959 [11].

The great success of the conference in Oxford in 1959 came to the attention of Robert Maxwell, publisher of Pergamon Press, who encouraged the publication of an international journal, founded by A.L. Copley and G.W. Scott Blair, and named BIORHEOLOGY – AN INTERNATIONAL JOURNAL. It began as a quarterly publication in 1962 and since 1974 is published bimonthly. In 1972, it became the official journal of the International Society of Biorheology.

In 1962, I was asked by R.S. Marvin of the National Bureau of Standards, Washington, D.C., co-chairman of the Fourth International Congress on Rheology, held in August 1963 at Brown University, Providence, R.I., U.S.A., to organize a session on biorheology. This happened just prior to a journey to Europe where I found enthusiastic support. Moreover, I was fortunate to secure financial support for more than thirty participants from many countries. Instead of one session at the Congress, as originally proposed, we had eleven sessions, comprising the Symposium on Biorheology [12] and, in addition, three lectures before the entire Congress. These presentations on hemorheology and other branches of biorheology contributed more than any previous meetings to the establishment of biorheology as an organized science. I dedicated the Symposium volume to one of its participants, my friend Robin Fåhraeus as "Pioneer and Nestor of Contemporary Hemorheology".

In 1965, I thought the time was ripe to have an International Conference on Hemorheology, which I organized together with G. Bugliarello, A.C. Burton, L.E. Gelin, M. Joly, H. Hartert, S. Oka, G.W. Scott Blair, A. Silberberg, R.E. Wells and R.L. Whitmore in July 1966 at the University of Iceland under its auspices in Reykjavik. At this conference the International Society of Hemorheology was founded and I was elected its first President. A number of papers on clinical hemorheology were reported and Robin Fåhraeus became the first Poiseuille Awardee of the new Society [13].

The Second International Conference of the International Society of Hemorheology, with Helmut Hartert as Chairman, took place at the University of Heidelberg under its auspices in 1969. At this conference it was decided that the International Society of Hemorheology should be extended to include all other fields of biorheology and was renamed "The International Society of Biorheology". Soon after, the Society became an Affiliated Commission of the International Union of Pure and Applied Biophysics.

The First International Congress of Biorheology was held, in association with the VI. International Congress on Rheology, at Lyon, France in 1972. Prior to the Congress at Lyon, our Society was represented at the IV. International Congress of Biophysics, held at Moscow University, USSR, with a special "Symposium on Biorheology" [23].

The Second, Third, Fourth and Fifth International Congresses of Biorheology took place in 1975 in Rehovot, Israel at the Weizmann Institute of Science; in 1978 in La Jolla at the University of California/San Diego; in 1981 in Tokyo at Jikei University; and in 1983 in Baden-Baden, F.R. Germany under the auspices of the University of Freiburg i.Br. The Sixth International Congress of Biorheology took place in 1986 in Vancouver, B.C., Canada. The Proceedings of all International Congresses of Biorheology were published in BIORHEOLOGY. Many communications dealt with clinical hemorheology, presented as plenary lectures, symposia, papers and exhibitions.

Clinical hemorheology is practiced more and more by many physicians, surgeons and biomedical scientists in many countries. Laboratories of biorheology including clinical hemorheology, and even departments become increasingly available in medical schools, universities, research institutions, hospitals and blood transfusion centers all over the globe.

The marked increase of original contributions to clinical hemorheology necessitated a journal of clinical investigations to serve as an aid in the practice in many fields of medicine. I founded this journal, named CLINICAL HEMORHEOLOGY, and asked Siegfried Witte to join me as Co-Editor-in-Chief. It began publication as a bimonthly journal in 1981. Its aims are to acquaint physicians and surgeons with clinical hemorheology and to advance hemorheological diagnostic, therapeutic and prophylactic approaches toward better medical care. Leading investigators in clinical hemorheology from many countries serve as Editors. The new journal is a Companion Journal of BIORHEOLOGY.

Communications dealing with clinical hemorheology are published since 1981 in CLINICAL HEMORHEOLOGY, while those on theoretical and experimental hemorheology appear in BIORHEOLOGY.

The dissemination of knowledge regarding hemorheology occurred in several ways. A number of lectures, sessions and symposia were jointly organized by the International Society of Biorheology with the International Congress of Hematology, the International Congress of the International Union of Physiological Sciences, and the International Congress of Biophysics, among others.

The advancement of clinical hemorheology was not limited to the activities of international or national biomedical societies or groups. The "United States-Japan Cooperative Seminar on Hemorheology and Thrombosis", which I initiated, was organized with Shosuke Okamoto as United States and Japan Coordinators and held at Kobe, Japan in 1975 in association with the National Science Foundation of the United States and the Japan Society for the Promotion of Science [14]. A Symposium on Biorheology, initiated by Ching-Rong Huang and organized by him and A.L. Copley, took place in New York at the annual meeting of the American Institute of Chemical Engineers in 1977 [15]. The New York Academy of Sciences held in 1982 in New York an international conference, which I initiated, entitled "Surface Phenomena in Hemorheology. Their Theoretical, Experimental and Clinical Aspects", organized by A.L. Copley and G.V.F. Seaman [16].

At the International Congress on Blood Transfusion, held in Tokyo in 1960, I was invited to give a Special Lecture on Hemorheology, co-authored by G.W. Scott Blair. This lecture stimulated research studies on hemorheology, including clinical hemorheology, in Japan and later led to the foundation of the Japan Society of Biorheology [24]. Thereafter, other national societies or groups were founded. They are the French Society of Biorheology (Société de Biorhéologie de Langue Française), the German Society of Clinical Hemorheology, the Italian Society of Hemorheology, the Forum of Clinical Hemorheology of the Royal Society of Medicine (England), the Portuguese Society of Hemorheology, the French Working Group on Red Blood Cell Filtration (Groupe de Travail sur la Filtration Erythrocytaire), and others. Some of these organizations have more than three hundred members. A recent appeal by American and Canadian biorheologists for the foundation of an American Society of Biorheology had enthusiastic response and led in April 1985 to a meeting at Anaheim, California, where a steering committee, chaired by Shu Chien, was formed for this binational society.

Of particular interest is the establishment of the European Conference on Clinical Hemorheology, first held at Nancy, France in 1979, organized by J.F. Stoltz and P. Drouin [17]. Since that time, this Conference is held every two years in different countries and, beginning with the Second Conference, its Proceedings are published in CLINICAL HEMORHEOLOGY. The Second Conference took place in 1981 in London, chaired by John Dormandy, under the auspices of the

Royal Society of Medicine. The Third Conference, chaired by Holger Schmid-Schönbein and H. Rieger, was held, in part together with the Fourth International Congress of Biorheology, in Baden-Baden, F.R. Germany. The Fourth Conference, chaired by Tullio Di Perri, took place in Siena, Italy in 1985, while the Fifth Conference was held in Bordeaux, France and chaired by M.R. Boisseau.

The publication of books pertaining to hemorheology and clinical hemorheology is steadily increasing and with them the awareness of the significance of what they are intended to convey.

The teaching of biorheology and of clinical hemorheology in universities, medical schools and research institutions is on the increase. Thus far, the first Chair of Biorheology was instituted in 1980 at the Weizmann Institute of Science, Rehovot, Israel and given to Alex Silberberg. It may be expected that clinical hemorheology will become an important subject in the curriculum of medical schools.

This brings me to what, I believe, will constitute an expanded scope of clinical hemorheology. From my physiological studies of bleeding and in vivo hemostasis, made about forty-five years ago, I was fully aware that the blood and the vessel wall constitute one entity. Because of this recognition I did not limit in 1951 the definition of hemorheology to the rheology of blood, but included that of the vessel wall. In 1960, I emphasized the existence of this entity, and in 1981 proposed for it the name "vessel-blood organ" [18]. This highly sophisticated organ, penetrating all other organs, contains, in both its portions, tissues of highly diverse structures with numerous functions and a great variety of constituents. The boundary of the two portions of this organ is an endo-endothelial lining [19], proposed to consist of fibrin and fibrinogenin (i.e. fibrinogen clotted without thrombin participation). Fibrin(ogenin) is considered to surround the endothelial cells and to be one of the main constituents of the basement membrane. Accordingly, fibrin(ogenin) is thought to play a crucial role in transcapillary transport [20]. Its proposed physiological presence provides a bridge between the two portions of the vessel-blood organ [25].

Recently I emphasized [1] that modern clinical hemorheology will need to be extended to include the rheology of the interstitial spaces and their contents, the parenchymal cells, the lymph channels or lymphatics, and its walls. For this extension of hemorheology I introduced the term "parahemorheology". In my appraisal, this field will play a growing role in clinical hemorheology [26].

The Editors of this book invited me to write its Introduction with emphasis on the history of clinical hemorheology as a background to the subject. Advancement of knowledge of the vessel-blood organ is expected to widen the scope of clinical hemorheology. This volume is the result of concerted great efforts by the Editors and Authors to communicate to the Readers the present status and scope of this clinical branch of the science of biorheology. The learned contributions by the Authors of this book serve as an introduction to the expanding role of clinical hemorheology towards better medical care and the maintenance of health.

Alfred L. Copley
New York, N.Y.

References

1. Copley A.L. 1985: History of clinical hemorheology. Plenary Lecture, 4. Europ. Conf. Clin. Hemorheol., Siena. Clin. Hemorheol. 5, 765-812.
2. Copley A.L. 1941: The phenomenon of thixotropy in hemophilic and heparinized blood. Science 94, 543-544.
3. Copley A.L., Lalich J.J. 1942: Bleeding time, lymph time, and clot resistance in man. J. Clin. Invest. 21, 145-152.
4. Copley A.L. 1974: Bleeding time, other in vivo hemostasis tests and the arrest of hemorrhage. Thromb. Res. 4, 1-23.
5. Copley A.L., Lalich J.J. 1942: The influence of blood transfusion and injections of bursa pastoris (Shepherd's Purse) extract on the clot resistance in two hemophiliacs. Am. J. Med. Sci. 204, 665-670.
6. Lalich J.J., Copley A.L. 1942: A study of clot firmness in viscometer tubes. Proc. Soc. Exp. Biol. Med. 51, 232-235.
7. Copley A.L., Kozam G. 1951: Capillary fragility and the ecchymosis test in man. J. Appl. Physiol. 4, 311-327.
8. Copley A.L., Krchma L.C., Whitney M.E. 1942: Humoral rheology I. Viscosity studies and anomalous flow properties of human blood systems with heparin and other anticoagulants. J. Gen. Physiol. 26, 49-64.
9. Copley A.L. 1949: Rheological problems in biology. In: Proceedings of the International Congress on Rheology, Holland, 1948. J.M. Burgers et al. (eds.) Amsterdam: North-Holland Publ. Co. Part I, 47-61, Part III, 8-11.
10. Copley A.L. 1952: The rheology of blood. A survey. J. Colloid. Sci. 7, 223-233.
11. Copley A.L., Stainsby G. (eds.) 1960: Flow properties of blood and other biological systems, Oxford, 1959. London-New York: Pergamon Press, 464 pp.
12. Copley A.L. (ed.) 1965: Symposium on Biorheology. Proc. 4. International Congr. on Rheology, Brown University, Providence, R.I. 1963. Part 4, New York: Interscience Publ. – John Wiley and Sons, 645 pp.
13. Copley A.L. (ed.) 1968: Hemorheology. Proc. 1. Internat. Conf., Reykjavik, Iceland, 1966. Oxford – New York: Pergamon Press, 869 pp.
14. Copley A.L., Okamoto S. (eds.) 1975: Hemorheology and thrombosis. Proc. United States-Japan Cooperative Seminar, Kobe, Japan. New York-Oxford, Pergamon Press, 1976, 440 pp.; Thromb. Res., suppl. II, 1976.
15. Huang C.-R., Copley A.L. (eds.) 1978: Biorheology. New York, American Institute of Chemical Engineers (AICHE Symposium Series, Number 182, volume 74), 141 pp.
16. Copley A.L., Seaman G.V.F. (eds.) 1983: Surface phenomena in hemorheology. Their Theoretical, Experimental and Clinical Aspects, Ann. N.Y. Acad. Sciences, 416, 761 pp.
17. Stoltz J.F., Drouin P. (eds.) 1980: Hemorheology and diseases. Nancy, 1979, Paris: Doin Éditeurs, 709 pp.
18. Copley A.L. 1982: The future of biorheology. Biorheol. 19, 47-69, 1982.
19. Copley A.L. (ed.) 1983: The Endo-endothelial fibrin lining. Symposium of the XII. European

Conference on Microcirculation, Jerusalem 1982. Oxford – New York, Pergamon Press, 1983, second printing, 1984, 160 pp.; Thromb. Res., Suppl. V, 160 pp.;

20. Copley A.L. 1984: The endoendothelial fibrin lining as the crucial barrier and the role of fibrin(ogenin) gels in controlling transcapillary transport. Biorheol. 21, 135-153, 1984.
21. Copley A.L. 1948: The ecchymosis test for capillary hemorrhagic diathesis. Science 107, 201-202.
22. Lee E.H., Copley A.L. (eds.) 1965: Proc. 4th Internat. Congr. on Rheology, Brown University, Providence, R.I. 1963. Part I, New York: Interscience Publ. John Wiley and Sons, 383 pp.
23. Copley A.L. 1973: Biorheology as an organized science: A brief survey. In: IV. International Biophysics Congress, Moscow 1972. Vol. IV Symposial Papers. Pushchino, Academy of Sciences of USSR, pp. 409-411.
24. Copley A.L. 1981: Hemorheology in Japan: A brief history. Clin. Hemorheol. 3, 323-325.
25. Copley, A.L. 1986: Endoendothelial fibrin(ogenin) lining: The interface between the two portions of the vessel-blood organ. In: Seno, S., Copley, A.L. Hamashima, Y., Venkatachalan, M.A. (eds.) Glomerular dysfunction and biopathology of vascular wall. Tokyo - New York - London, Academic Press, in press.
26. Copley, A.L. 1986: Hemorheological and parahemorheological aspects of the vessel-blood organ affecting ischemia. In: Hartmann, A. and Kuschinsky, W. (eds.) Cerebral ischemia and hemorheology. Berlin - Heidelberg - New York, Springer, in press.

2
Biophysics

A. Matrai *, R.B. Whittington ° and R. Skalak +
** Clinic for physical Medicine, University of Munich, 8000 Munich, Ziemssenstr. 1.,Federal Republic of Germany, and Department of Nuclear Medicine, University Medical School, Pecs, Hungary*
° Institute of Medical and Dental Bioengineering, Royal Liverpool Hospital, Liverpool, and Department of Haematology, King's College Hospital, London, United Kingdom
+ Bioengineering Institute, Columbia University, New York, United States of America

2.1. Basic concepts

Any physician interested in the field of clinical hemorheology may expect to encounter certain characteristic physical phenomena and their associated terminology. This chapter gives a brief survey of the biophysical terminology and definitions most often used in hemorheology.

2.1.1. Rheology

The science of mechanics deals in general with the motions and deformations of material bodies under the action of applied forces. Rheology (flow-study) is a branch of mechanics concerned with deformation and flow properties of various materials under mechanical forces.

When any material body is subjected to external forces, its shape and/or size will change. Any such change involves relative displacement of material points within the body and is described, in general, as deformation. A body is said to flow if the deformation increases (or decreases) continuously with time.

The main categories of materials usually studied in rheology are solids, fluids, and viscoelastic materials which show a combination of fluid and solid behavior. A solid is a material which can sustain forces with a fixed deformation (like a steel spring). Usually solids are linearly elastic: here the deformation is proportional to the applied force; but the original shape is recovered when the force is removed. A plastic solid, however, does not regain its original shape when released. There remains a permanent deformation.

A fluid (viscous material) continuously deforms (i.e. flows) as long as any unbalanced forces are applied to it. The term fluid embraces both the liquid and gaseous states. A viscous fluid is called Newtonian or linear if the flow rate is proportional to the force applied (like gases and many liquids, such as water, oil, mercury, etc.). Nonlinear liquids are also of importance in rheology. The materials of interest may be either homogeneous or heterogeneous (containing more than one phase) like suspensions and emulsions. Suspensions ordinarily consist of solid particles dispersed in a homogeneous liquid in which they are insoluble; emulsions are formed by the dispersion of liquid droplets in a homogeneous liquid with which they are immiscible. Blood is a non-Newtonian (or nonlinear) mixture. Here the principal suspended phase is neither liquid nor solid, but a collection of liquid droplets each enclosed in a solid, elastic envelope. Therefore blood does not fall in any simple category, although it shows some similarities to emulsions.

Another phenomenon of interest in rheology is the behavior of the interfaces between different phases. Fascinating rheological and biochemical phenomena can occur at interfaces, not attributable to the bulk properties of the materials, and which play important roles in life processes.

The basic concepts expressed above are given quantitative definition in the subsequent paragraphs. For this purpose, some vocabulary of stress and strain is introduced next.

2.1.2. Stress, strain and strain rate

One can intuitively expect that a force will deform a large body less than a smaller body subjected to the same force. Experiment shows that the degree of deformation (strain) depends on the force applied per unit area (stress). Hence the stress τ (Greek tau) is defined as the force per unit area, i.e.,

$$\tau = F/A \qquad \text{Unit N/m}^2 \tag{1}$$

where F is the force acting on the area A. Since the force F may in general have components perpendicular and parallel to the surface, the stress components are also so identified: Shear stress τ is the force per unit area acting parallel (or tangential) to the area A. Normal stress N is the force per unit area acting perpendicularly (or normally) to the area A. Normal stresses are further described as tensile or compressive stresses depending on whether they tend to extend or to compress the body. Pressure is the compressive stress in a fluid. By considering the equilibrium of an infinitesimally-small volume of a fluid at rest, it may easily be shown that the pressure-intensity at any point must be the same in all directions. When the fluid is in motion, however, this is no longer true, and a pressure-gradient is established in the direction of motion. It is axiomatic that in a Newtonian liquid at rest, no shearing-force exists; but a fluid in motion can have both pressure and shear stresses at any point. The units of stress-component and pressure are indicated in Table 2.1. Shear, tensile, and compressive stresses are illustrated in Fig. 2.1b, 2.1c and 2.1d respectively.

Table 2.1. Units of stress and pressure.

Quantity	Units		Ratio of units (b)/(a)
	(a) cgs	(b) S.I.	
Area (A)	cm^2	m^2	10^4
Force (F)	dyne	Newton = N	10^5
Stress (τ)	dyne/cm^2	Pascal = N/m^2	10
Pressure (p)	dyne/cm^2	Pascal = N/m^2	10

The strain in a body is a measure of the degree of deformation. Many different strain-measures are used. Different strain components are associated with the different stress components as indicated in Fig. 2.1. Shear stress and shear strain (Fig. 2.1b) are most commonly of interest in hemorheology. In a shear deformation, the layers of material move in parallel planes in a progressive manner, from bottom to top in Fig. 2.1 b. The shear strain γ (Greek gamma) is change in the angle (originally 90°) of the element shown, i.e.,

$$\gamma = \frac{\Delta x}{\Delta y} \qquad \text{Unit: m/m} \tag{2}$$

where Δx is the distance the uppermost layer has moved relative to the bottom layer and Δy is the (constant) height of the element. A familiar example of a large shear deformation is the cutting action of scissors or shears which concentrate the deformation in a narrow zone and cause rupture of the material in shear.

Corresponding to tensile or compressive stresses, the extensional or compressive strain ϵ (Greek epsilon) is defined as the change in length produced by the stress divided by the initial length, i.e.,

$$\epsilon = \frac{\Delta L}{L_0} \qquad \text{Unit: m/m} \tag{3}$$

where ΔL is the change in length and L_0 is initial length (Fig. 2.1c, 2.1d). The change in length is $\Delta L = (L_1 - L_0)$, where L_1 is the final length.

The extensional strains (or normal strains) and the shear strains in various directions at a point form a set called the strain tensor. Similarly, the stress components form a set called the stress tensor. The properties and relations of such tensors are of interest in general problems of rheology (see Fung, 1981), but only simple shear will be discussed extensively here as this is adequate for most hemorheological questions.

In the continuing deformation which constitutes flow, the strain rate (or shear rate) is defined as the shear deformation in unit time. Following Newton's

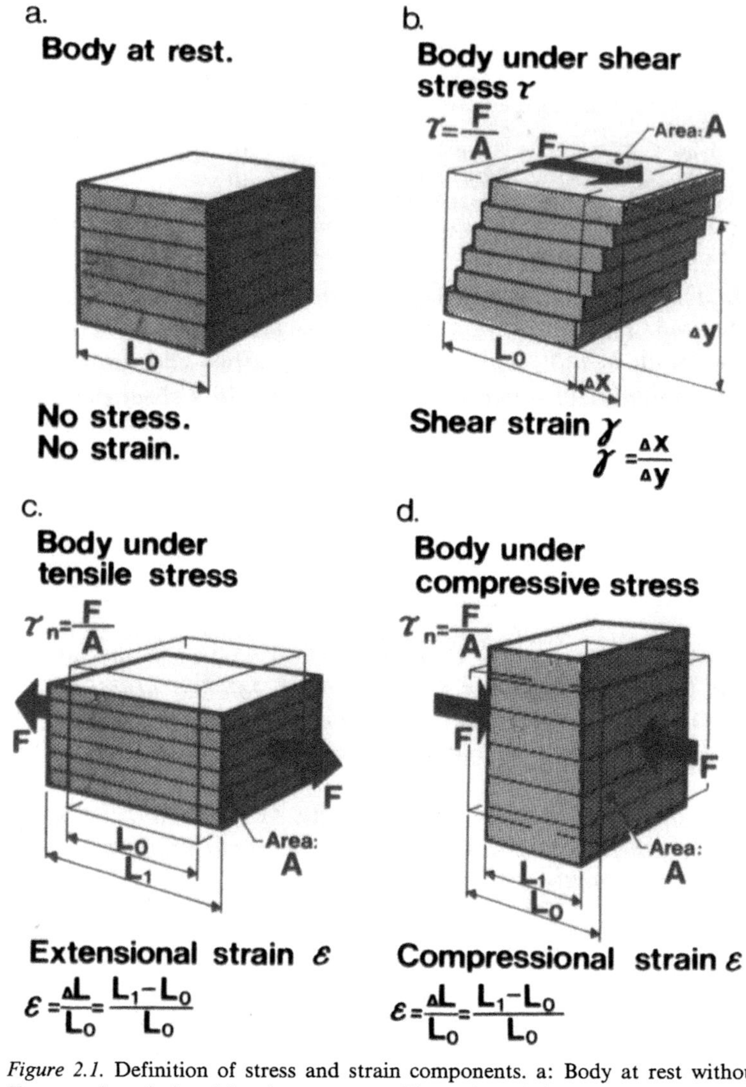

Figure 2.1. Definition of stress and strain components. a: Body at rest without stress or strain. b: Shear strain γ induced by shear stress τ. The action of the tangential (shear) force F is to cause a shift of each plane a distance x which varies linearly with the height y. The shear strain γ is defined by $\gamma = \Delta x / \Delta y$. c: Extensional strain ϵ induced by tensile stress τ_n. The tensile force F produces a length L_1 of the element which is greater than the initial length L_0. By definition $\epsilon = (L_1 - L_0)/ L_0$. d: Compressive strain ϵ induced by compressive stress τ_n. The compressive force F reduces the length of the element to L_1 which is less than the initial length L_0. By definition $\epsilon = (L_1 - L_0)/L_0$. Note compressive strains are negative numbers by this definition.

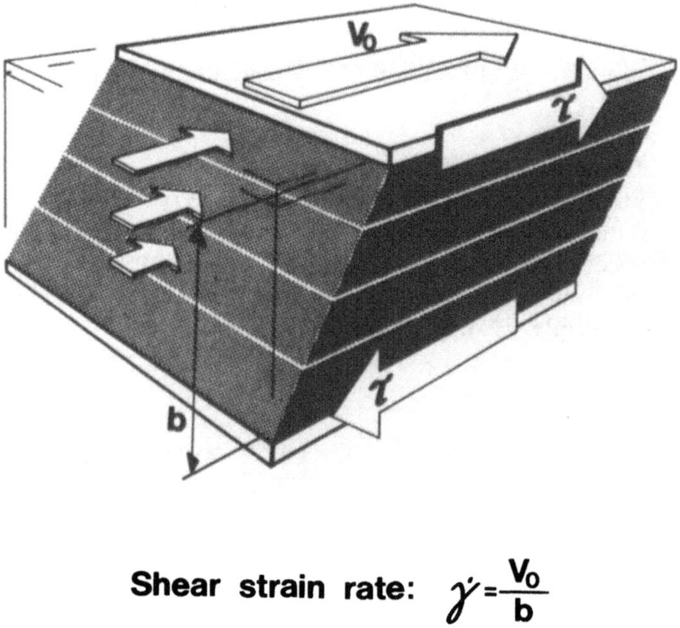

Figure 2.2. Steady shear strain rate of a fluid between two parallel plates. The spacing between plates is b and the relative velocity of the upper plate is V_0, parallel to the lower fixed plate. The shear strain rate is $\dot{\gamma} = V_0/b$ (unit: s^{-1}).

"dot-notation" (introduced in 1671), the symbol $\dot{\gamma}$ is commonly used for shear rate, or time-rate of change of shear-strain (another, frequently used symbol is D). If $\Delta\gamma$ be the change in strain which occurs in time Δt, then

$$\dot{\gamma} = \Delta\gamma/\Delta t = d\gamma/dt \text{ as} \Delta t \to 0 \qquad \text{Unit: s}^{-1} \tag{4}$$

Thus the form $d\gamma/dt$ indicates the infinitesimal limit of $\Delta\gamma/\Delta t$, and is called the time-differential of γ. Shear rate has the dimensions s^{-1} (inverse seconds). The strain itself (γ or ϵ) is dimensionless.

In a plane shear flow, the shear rate is equal to the velocity gradient. In Fig. 2.2, the upper plate is assumed to be moving at velocity V_0 parallel to the fixed lower plate. Then the velocity gradient or shear rate is

$$\dot{\gamma} = \Delta V/\Delta y = V_0/b \tag{5}$$

where $\Delta V = V_0 - V$ is the difference in velocity and Δy the separation of the plates. Strain rate $\dot{\epsilon}$ may also be defined for extensional and compressional strains as $(d\epsilon/dt)$, but will not be used herein.

2.1.3. Elastic solid and viscous fluid

The relation of stress to strain or to strain-rate in a body depends on the physical properties of the material.
A solid body is said to be elastic if
A: the strain is a function of the stress and
B: the body recovers its initial shape when the stress is removed.

Under these conditions, the energy imparted to the body during deformation is stored in it and is recovered when the stress is removed. The relation of stress to strain in an elastic material may be nonlinear in general: but usually stress is proportional to strain. For example, in simple shear (Fig. 2.1b)

$$\tau = G\gamma \tag{6}$$

where G is the shear modulus of the material and τ and γ are the shear stress and shear strain. In simple tension or compression (Fig. 2.1c, 2.1d), the linear elastic relation is

$$\tau_n = E\epsilon \tag{7}$$

where E is the elastic modulus for direct stress, usually called "Young's modulus". τ_n is the normal (or direct) stress and ϵ is the extensional strain. E is named in honor of Thomas Young, a London physician who defined the elastic modulus E in connection with testing arterial walls, circa 1809.

The two equations 6 and 7 are special cases of more general relations describing elastic materials [1]. The two elastic moduli G and E are different, G being less than E.

A viscous fluid is defined as one in which the rate of shear strain is a function of the shear stress. This implies that, if the shear stress is not zero, the fluid continues to deform. It follows that
A: the total deformation is dependent on the duration of the applied stress,
B: there is no recovery of shape when the stress is removed, and
C: all of the energy imparted (work done) during deformation is dissipated as heat.

A linear viscous fluid is called *Newtonian* and is defined by the proportionality of shear rate to shear stress, Fig. 2.2:

$$\tau = \eta\dot{\gamma} \tag{8}$$

where η (Greek eta) is called the viscosity. The symbol μ (Greek mu) is also often used for viscosity. In non-Newtonian liquids the relation of stress to strain rate is nonlinear. The classification of such liquids is discussed in the next section.

The term "viscous" derives from the Latin name of the parasitic plant misletoe (viscum album), whose white berries contain a very sticky, viscous juice which serves to attach the seeds to branches, where they germinate and take root.

2.1.4. Classification of viscous liquids

Different flow behaviors can be described on the basis of flow curves which are plots of shear stresses (τ) against shear rates ($\dot{\gamma}$) derived from experiments or theory in simple shear as in Fig. 2.2. For a Newtonian liquid, the flow curve is a straight line through the origin (Fig. 2.3a). The slope of the line is a measure of the viscosity of the liquid. From equation (8) the viscosity η is:

$$\eta = \tau/\dot{\gamma} = \tan \alpha \qquad \text{Unit: Ns/m}^2 \tag{9}$$

Some units of η are shown in Table 2.2. The basic units of viscosity indicated, namely, the *Pascal-second* and *Poise*, are too large for convenience in hemorheology. The *milli-Pascal-second* (mPas) or *centipoise* (cP) are interchangeable units of convenient size, each being equal to 0.001 Ns/m^2.

The Poise is named after the French physician J.L.M. Poiseuille whose careful experiments in the mid-nineteenth century established the first accurate relation for the flow of water, alcohol and mercury through glass capillaries, including the variation with temperature. His interest was, in fact, hemorheological, concerning capillary flow. He empirically derived the correct form of the relationship of flow rate to pressure drop and capillary diameter and length. It is ironical that the adoption of S.I. units has led to the honoring of the wrong man in relation to viscosity (Pascal instead of Poiseuille).

The fluidity ϕ (Greek phi) is defined as the reciprocal of the viscosity η ($\phi = 1/\eta$). A solid has zero fluidity. Newtonian liquids have a fluidity and a viscosity which depend on temperature but are independent of variations in shear rate, shear stress or pressure.

A non-Newtonian liquid does not exhibit the simple straight-line flow curve of Fig. 2.3a. Some examples of significance in hemorheology are shown in Fig. 2.3b and discussed below.

Table 2.2. Units of viscosity (η).

	cgs	S.I.
Name	Poise	Pascal-second
Symbol	P	Pas
Units	dyne sec/cm^2	Newton sec/m^2
Relation of viscosity units	1 P = 0.1 Pas	1 Pas = 10 P

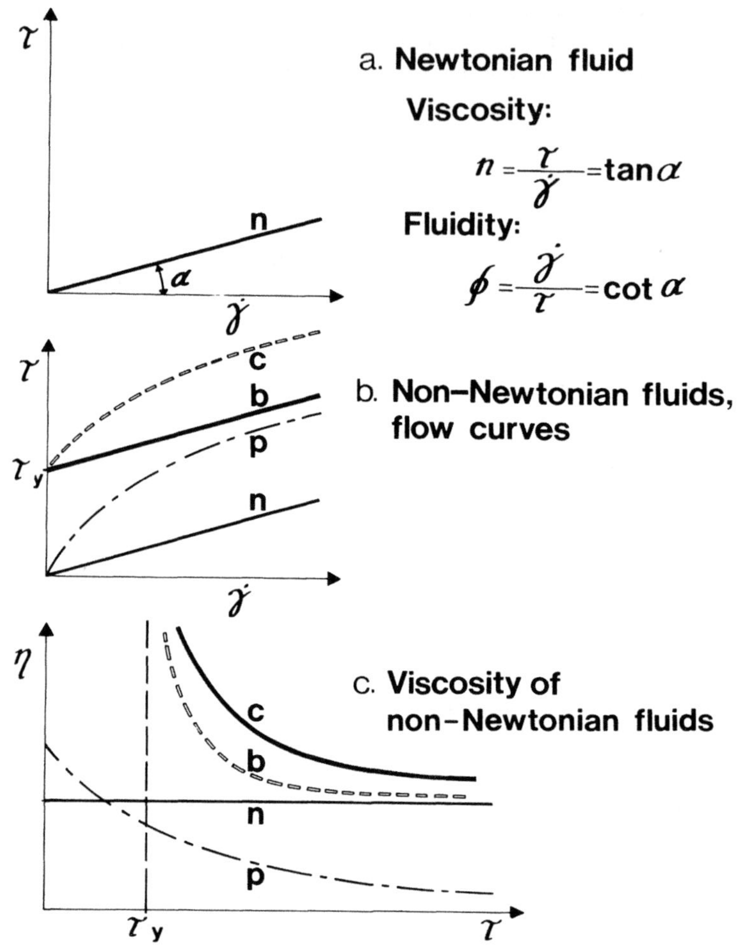

Figure 2.3. Classification of some common fluid models. a: Newtonian fluid. The flow curve of the Newtonian fluid is a straight line the slope of which is a measure of the viscosity. b: Flow curves of the Newtonian fluid (n), Bingham plastic (b), Casson fluid (c) and a pseudoplastic (p). The Bingham plastic and the Casson fluid have a finite yield stress τ_y. c: Viscosity of non-Newtonian fluids in Fig. 2.3b are shown as a function of the shear stress τ. The curves (n,b,c,p) indicate the viscosity curves for Newtonian fluid, Bingham plastic, Casson fluid and pseudoplastic, respectively.

It is of interest to define plastic behavior first; plastics are not, strictly speaking, liquids. They behave like solids at low stresses and exhibit some liquid behavior at high stresses. The classic Bingham plastic is illustrated by curve (b) in Fig. 2.3b. The flow curve is a straight line which starts at a finite shear stress value, τ_y, which is the yield stress of the plastic. Below the yield stress the response of the plastic is entirely elastic and not shown in Fig. 2.3b. When a stress above the yield point is applied the plastic responds with a continuous deformation like a liquid according to the flow curve shown. The flow curve above the yield point may also be a curved line as shown by the curve (c) in Fig. 2.3b. An example is the Casson model originally introduced to describe the flow behavior of paint. It has also been applied to blood. The question, as to whether blood has a yield stress or not, has been much debated and is still uncertain. It may depend on the circumstances involved, and is in any case a very small value, if not zero. The curve (p) illustrates pseudoplastic behavior. The flow curve starts at the origin and is concave downward. It resembles plastic behavior but has no finite yield stress.

Non-Newtonian liquids may also be described by means of a plot of the viscosity vs. shear stress as shown in Fig. 2.3c, or by a plot of the viscosity vs. shear rate (not shown). The viscosity at any point of a flow curve, such as those shown in Fig. 2.3b, is defined by using the equation 9. For a Newtonian liquid this results in the constant viscosity shown by the curve (n) in Fig. 2.3c. The curves (b,c,p) in Fig. 2.3c show the viscosities which pertain to Bingham, Casson, and pseudoplastic materials, respectively.

The classification of non-Newtonian liquids based on their flow curves may be incomplete for several reasons. The flow curves show only the steady-state behavior in a limited range of shear stresses. Elastic behavior before yielding is not shown, and there may be an elastic component to the response during transient flow which is not indicated. Further, the flow behavior of many non-Newtonian liquids depends also on the shearing history of the materials. In other words, the liquid properties may also be time-dependent. A typical kind of time dependence is *thixotropy*.

A thixotropic liquid has a high viscosity when first sheared, starting from rest. The continuous shearing results in a decreasing viscosity as time progresses. The phenomenon is repeatable after the liquid is allowed to remain at rest for some time (Fig. 2.4). Thixotropy is usually a result of the partial destruction, by shearing, of the internal structure. While at rest, this internal structure may build up again, restoring the initial properties. This phenomenon is also referred to as *structural viscosity*.

2.1.5. Viscoelasticity

A more complete characterization of general non-Newtonian behavior can be expressed in terms of viscoelasticity. A viscoelastic body has some characteristics of a solid and some behavior similar to that of a liquid. Viscoelastic materials may be termed viscoelastic solids or viscoelastic liquids, depending on whether their behavior resembles more nearly solids or liquids. For example, a sponge filled with a viscous oil may represent a viscoelastic solid. If the surface of the sponge is sealed so the oil cannot run out of it, the sponge will appear to be an

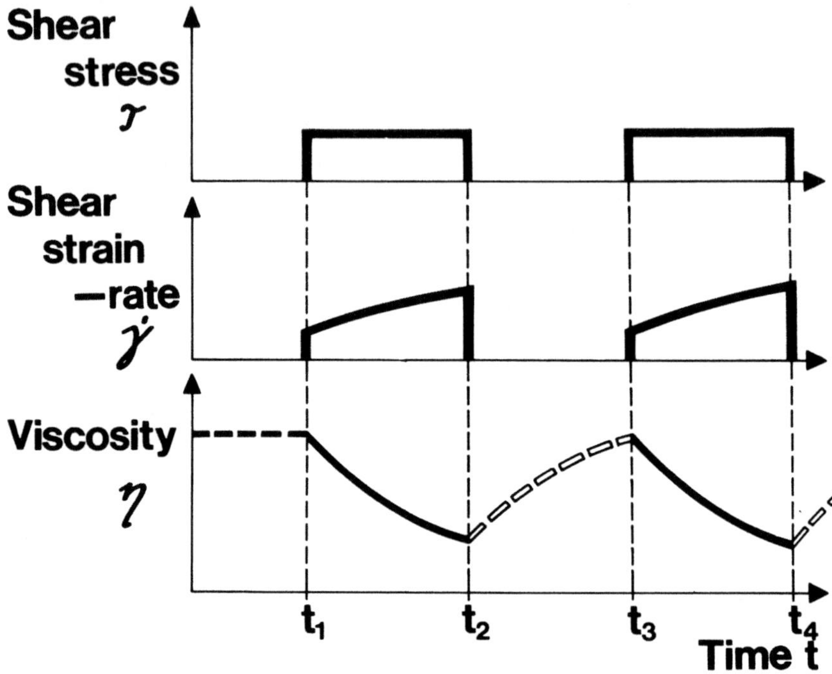

Figure 2.4. Response of a thixotropic fluid to intermittent shear stress. When a step change in shear stress is applied, the shearing of the sample results in progressive degradation of the internal structure of the fluid and the viscosity decreases in time. When the shear stress is removed the internal structure reverts to its original form. The dotted portions of the viscosity curves show the initial viscosity that would be observed if a shear stress were suddenly applied.

elastic solid under very slow deformation. However, if it is subject to high frequency oscillations in shear, the test results will appear to be nearly fluid. A viscoelastic liquid may consist of separate elastic particles suspended in a viscous liquid, like red blood cells in plasma. In this case a test at low shear rates will give results as for a fluid. But at sufficiently high frequencies, there may be some elastic behavior due to the deformation of the elastic particles in suspension.

In general, a viscoelastic body is assumed to have some internal elastic structure which is capable of storing energy when deformed, and which results in recovery of the original shape of the body (recoil), at least to some extent, after the stress is removed. In the general concept of a viscoelastic body, the elastic structure coexists throughout the body with the viscous component, which manifests itself in various ways. The viscous component may slow down the response of the elastic part, so that deformation is gradual and recoil is also slowed or incomplete. Further, the viscous component can result in energy dissipation during any deformation of the material.

The theory of linear viscoelastic materials is conveniently summarized by regarding the stress as being due to two independent components at the same time. One part of the stress is considered to be elastic, i.e. proportional to the strain, γ, and a second viscous component is assumed to be proportional to the rate of deformation or strain rate, $\dot{\gamma}$. When a material is tested in simple shearing motion, the mechanical properties of the material are characterized by two moduli. One is the elastic modulus (η'' = eta double prime), which is like the shear modulus of a purely elastic material. The second property is a viscosity (η' = eta prime) or loss modulus which is associated with the fluid-like behavior. This vocabulary can be made quantitative by considering small sinusoidal oscillations of the shear strain. For example, consider the shear strain γ to be a sinusoidal function of time given by:

$$\gamma = \gamma_0 \sin \omega t \tag{10}$$

where γ_0 is a constant representing the maximum value of the shear strain, ω is the circular frequency (radians/second), and t is time. The shear stress required to produce the oscillatory strain of equation (10) will be in general given by:

$$\tau = \eta''\gamma + \eta'\dot{\gamma} \tag{11}$$

where $\dot{\gamma}$ is the rate of shear-strain, found by differentiating γ with respect to t, so that:

$$\dot{\gamma} = \omega\gamma_0 \cos \omega t \tag{12}$$

Substituting equations (10) and (12) into equation (11) gives the shear stress as:

$$\tau = \gamma_0(\eta'' \sin \omega t + \omega\eta' \cos \omega t) \tag{13}$$

Equations 10 and 13 may be considered to give formal definitions of η' and η''. They are material properties required to make equation 13 hold true. In general, the moduli η' and η'' are functions of frequency. This is normally to be expected, even if the viscoelastic model is linear. If the moduli η' and η'' also vary with amplitude of the motion γ_0, then the material is said to exhibit nonlinear viscoelasticity. The application of viscoelastic models to blood and other suspensions and emulsions can be difficult, since the elastic component of the stress may not be associated with a stable elastic structure. The elasticity observed in blood may be due to the formation of rouleaux, which may be destroyed by a sufficient increase in the amplitude of motion. This may cause the blood to exhibit nonlinear viscoelasticity and/or thixotropy. The viscosity of a viscoelastic liquid is less ambiguous. Usually the viscosity at a fixed, steady shear-rate is a definite and reproducible property. The steady-shear viscosity of a viscoelastic liquid is not directly equal to the viscoelastic coefficient η', but can be related to it [2,3].

2.1.6. Surface rheology

The properties of biomembranes and surface-adsorbed macromolecular layers are important aspects of biorheology and will probably gain in importance in the future. Monomolecular and oligomolecular layers of macromolecules can have fascinating properties (e.g. extremely viscous or elastic behavior), from which molecular interactions can be inferred. The mechanics of these thin layers at air-liquid or liquid-liquid interfaces can be studied by surface rheological methods [4,5,6].

In surface rheology one usually considers the thin layer at an interface to be modelled as a surface of zero thickness. The macroscopic properties of interest are usually those for the interface as a whole. This approach avoids consideration of the thickness of the interface layer, which is difficult to define and to measure. In the theoretical, two-dimensional system, shear strain and shear rate are defined as in ordinary (bulk) rheology. The definitions of γ, $\dot{\gamma}$, and ϵ in Fig. 2.1 and 2.2 apply, as if the membrane in question were the front face of the elements shown. But the stress components in a surface of a membrane are defined with different dimensions as compared to the bulk case, because of the zero thickness assumption. The surface shear stress (τ_s) in a membrane is defined as the shearing force, F, divided by the length, L, of the edge (Fig. 2.5a)

$$\tau_s = F/L \qquad \text{Unit: N/m} \tag{14}$$

Similarly, the normal stress τ_{ns} in a surface is defined as the tensile force in the membrane divided by the length of the edge over which it acts:

$$\tau_{ns} = F_n/L \qquad \text{Unit: N/m} \tag{15}$$

The units of τ_s and τ_{ns} are the same as those of surface tension (N/m). In fact, the usual surface tension σ_0 (Greek sigma) on any interface of a liquid and a gas is an example of surface stress in which the shear stress τ_s is zero and the normal stress τ_{ns} is equal in all directions in the surface and is exactly σ_0. It represents a potential energy per unit area of surface (N/m).

For small deformations, an elastic shear modulus can be defined for a surface, analogous to Equation 6:

$$\tau_s = G_s\gamma \tag{16}$$

where G_s is a surface shear modulus having units of N/m.

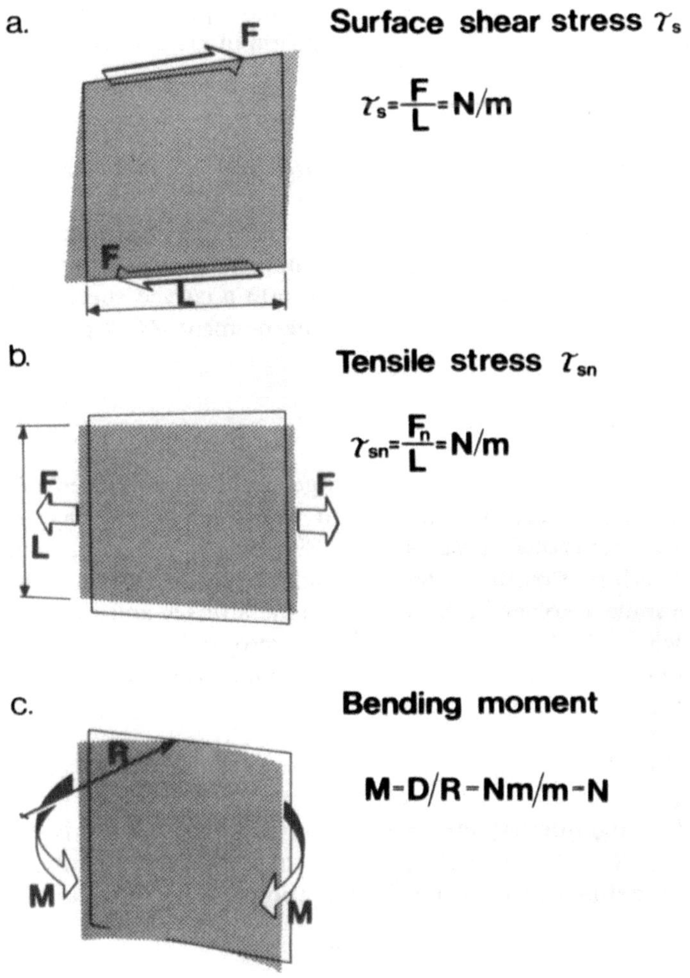

Figure 2.5. Definitions of the stresses τ_s, τ_{sn} and the bending moment M in a membrane. D is a bending stiffness and R is a radius of curvature.

An extensional modulus may also be defined for simple tension, as in Equation 7:

$$\tau_{ns} = E_s \epsilon \tag{17}$$

where E_s is an elastic modulus (N/m) analogous to Young's modulus.

For a membrane it is useful to introduce an area modulus or area compressibility. The normal stress τ_{ns} for an isotropic expansion of area is defined by

$$\tau_{ns} = \sigma_0 + K\Delta A/A \tag{18}$$

where σ_0 is the initial surface tension, A is the initial area and ΔA is the change in surface area; K is the areal elastic modulus (N/m).

Membranes also have bending stiffness, which is an elastic resistance to changes in curvature. As shown in Fig. 2.5c, a bending moment (Nm/m) per unit length is required to bend an originally flat membrane into a curved sheet with radius of curvature R. For linearly elastic behavior the moment M is proportional to the curvature:

$$M = B/R \qquad \text{Unit: Nm/m} = \text{N} \tag{19}$$

B is the bending stiffness which has units of Nm. In general the curvatures and bending moments in different directions at a point in a membrane may be different and form a two-dimensional tensor system. Similarly, the tensions and shears in the membrane form another two-dimensional tensor system. The equilibrium of the membrane involves both the membrane stresses and bending moments. In the case where the bending moments are zero and the tension is only the isotropic surface tension, the equations of equilibrium reduce to Laplace's law

$$p_i - p_0 = \sigma_0(1/R_1 + 1/R_2) \tag{20}$$

where p_i and p_0 represent the internal and external pressure of a cell, σ_0 is the surface tension, and R_1, R_2 are the principal radii of curvature. Finally, a surface viscosity may be defined analogously to Equation 9. Here the surface viscosity η_s is defined by

$$\eta_s = \tau_s/\dot{\gamma} \qquad \text{Unit: Ns/m} \tag{21}$$

where $\dot{\gamma}$ is the shear strain rate produced by the surface shear stress τ_s.

2.2. Viscometry

A viscometer is a device in which a sample fluid is subjected to a prescribed stress field, the resulting flow being measured (controlled shear stress methods); or alternatively, a prescribed flow is induced, and the required shear stress is measured (controlled shear rate methods). Usually, in applying theoretical solutions to viscometry, it is assumed that the flow is steady and streamline. In practice, precautions must be taken to ensure these conditions. In addition, successful viscometry requires careful control of the temperature of the sample and vigilance in avoidance of air bubbles, clots, sedimented cells, surface tension effects or other artifacts.

2.2.1. Laminar and turbulent flow

In slow viscous flow between parallel plates, the liquid particles move in parallel planes or sheets (laminae). Therefore, such a flow is referred to as laminar flow. The same term is often loosely applied to any form of streamline flow. However, there is an important distinction: in truly laminar flow (between parallel plates), the shear-rate ($\dot{\gamma}$) is synonymous with the transverse velocity-gradient (dv/dy). But in the rotating-cylinder viscometer, for example, the streamline paths are concentric and $\dot{\gamma} \neq dv/dr$. In steady, streamline flow the liquid elements move along permanent paths (paths fixed in space) which may be rendered visible by the injection of thin streams of dye. These dyed paths are not necessarily linear or parallel: they may be curved, non-uniform, convergent or divergent – though the latter case is intrinsically unstable. The only essentials are that the streamlines be smooth and permanent, not changing with time. In unsteady streamline flow the velocities at any point may be time-dependent, but the streamlines remain visible and identifiable, even though their form may change with time. In contrast to laminar flow, turbulent flow has no steady or smooth streamlines, but rather the flow is chaotic with a random component of velocity superimposed on the mean flow. The presence of turbulence in a flow has dramatic effects on the diffusion of dissolved or suspended matter and on the stress field or pressure drop.

Observations of pressure head loss during the flow of water in pipes had, over centuries, accumulated two contradictory bodies of evidence. Some data showed that the loss of pressure was strictly proportional to the speed of flow as in Poiseuille's experiments [7]. Other data implied that the pressure drop was proportional to the square of the flow velocity. In 1884, in a paper delivered to the Royal Institution, entitled "On the two manners of motion of water", Professor Osborne Reynolds showed that both sets of data were correct, depending on the state of flow. On the one hand, laminar flow was proportional to the pressure drop as reported by Poiseuille. On the other hand, in turbulent flow, the pressure drop was approximately proportional to the square of the mean velocity. Reynolds first gave a criterion as to whether a flow would be laminar or turbulent. He identified streamlines in laminar flow by injections of dye. The dyed streamlines would be perfectly steady at low velocities. Then as the flow rate was increased, the streamlines waved about somewhat, stable but disturbed. Finally at a certain flow rate, the dye would suddenly diffuse into a cloud, the initial smooth pattern of flow being destroyed. This was the onset of turbulence.

Reynolds showed that the streamlines were stable provided that the parameter *Re* did not exceed a certain critical number. *Re* is given by

$$Re = \bar{v}D\frac{\rho}{\eta} \tag{22}$$

where $\bar{v}$ is the mean velocity in the pipe, D is the pipe diameter, ρ (Greek rho) is the density of the fluid and η (Greek eta) is the viscosity. The parameter *Re* is dimensionless and is called the *Reynolds number* in honour of Osborne Reynolds. The units of $\bar{v}$, ρ, D and η must be in a consistent system in computing R_e. For example: in S.I. units they are m/s, kg/m^3, m, Pascal-sec, respectively; or in cgs units cm/s, g/cm^3, cm, Poise, respectively.

When the Reynolds number of a flow in a straight pipe of circular cross-section is greater than 2000, turbulent flow usually results. At higher Reynolds numbers, laminar flow may be achieved with very carefully controlled experimental conditions, but it is unstable. When the Reynolds number is less than 100, the flow will usually be strictly laminar. For Reynolds numbers between 100 and 2000, some turbulence may be present, depending on entrance conditions, unsteadiness, bends or other disturbances of the flow. In laminar flow, the pressure drop and energy loss are directly dependent on the shear stresses which are linearily related to the flow rate. In turbulent flow, the flow resistance is augmented by inertial effects, which are proportional to the square of the velocity, although the ultimate dissipation of energy is dependent on the viscosity of the fluid. These effects are quantitatively dependent on the surface-roughness of the tube.

2.2.2. Temperature control

The viscosity of most liquids decreases as temperature increases. The viscosities of blood and plasma depend strongly on temperature. Consequently, precise control of the sample temperature is necessary to detect changes in viscosity reliably. The variation of blood (and plasma) viscosity with temperature is not the same as that of water. There are considerable individual variations in this respect [8,9]. It is preferable to carry out measurements for clinical studies at body temperature. For the sake of comparability with published data by different authors, recording and reporting the temperature at which tests were carried out is a *sine qua non*, including the experimental variation of sample temperatures.

2.2.3. Steady-flow viscometers

There are several types of viscometers, some of which are used (or are intended for use) by clinical hemorheologists. Several of the more common instruments are discussed in this chapter.

In steady-flow viscometers, the fluid motion is assumed to be stationary with no change of flow rate or velocity field during the measuring procedure. Many viscometers are intended for use with steady flow so that shear rates are constant in each test. By running several tests at different shear rates, the complete flow behavior of the test fluid can be discerned.

2.2.4. *Tube viscometers*

A steady tube-flow can be produced by a constant pressure difference, Δp, between two points a distance, L, apart along a tube as shown in Fig. 2.6a. The quotient, $\Delta p/L$, is the *pressure gradient*. As a consequence of the tube geometry, there is a specific profile of shear stress in the tube flow (Fig. 2.6b) for any homogeneous liquid, whether the flow is streamline or turbulent. The shear stress is zero at the tube axis and increases linearly with the distance from the axis, reaching its greatest value, τ_w, at the tube wall. The shear stress at any distance (r) from the tube axis is given by:

$$\tau_r = \frac{\Delta pr}{2L} \tag{23}$$

The shear stress at the tube wall, τ_w, is calculated by replacing r with the tube radius, R, in Equation 23. When the shear stress and the viscosity are known, the shear rate can be computed. The viscosity at any shear rate is defined by Equation 9, even if the fluid is non-Newtonian. Thus the shear rate at distance r from the tube axis is:

$$\dot{\gamma}_r = \tau_r/\eta \tag{24}$$

where the viscosity η may be a function of τ or $\dot{\gamma}$. In any case, the shear rate is also zero on the axis of the tube, and reaches its greatest value at the wall. Newtonian fluids give rise to shear rate profiles which are straight lines through the origin $r=0$, $\dot{\gamma}=0$ (curve n in Fig. 2.6c). A non-Newtonian pseudoplastic liquid shows a non-linear shear rate profile also passing through the origin (curve p in Fig. 2.6c). The shear rate in fluids with a yield stress, such as the hypothetical Bingham plastic, remains zero for some distance from the tube axis until the shear stress reaches the yield stress. The central core of the fluid in the tube moves at uniform velocity without being sheared. This phenomenon is referred to as *plug flow* of the central core. In some cases the plug flow may occupy most of the cross section. In venules after a period of stasis, a mass of red blood cells may accumulate, subsequently moving as a plug when the flow is first restored.

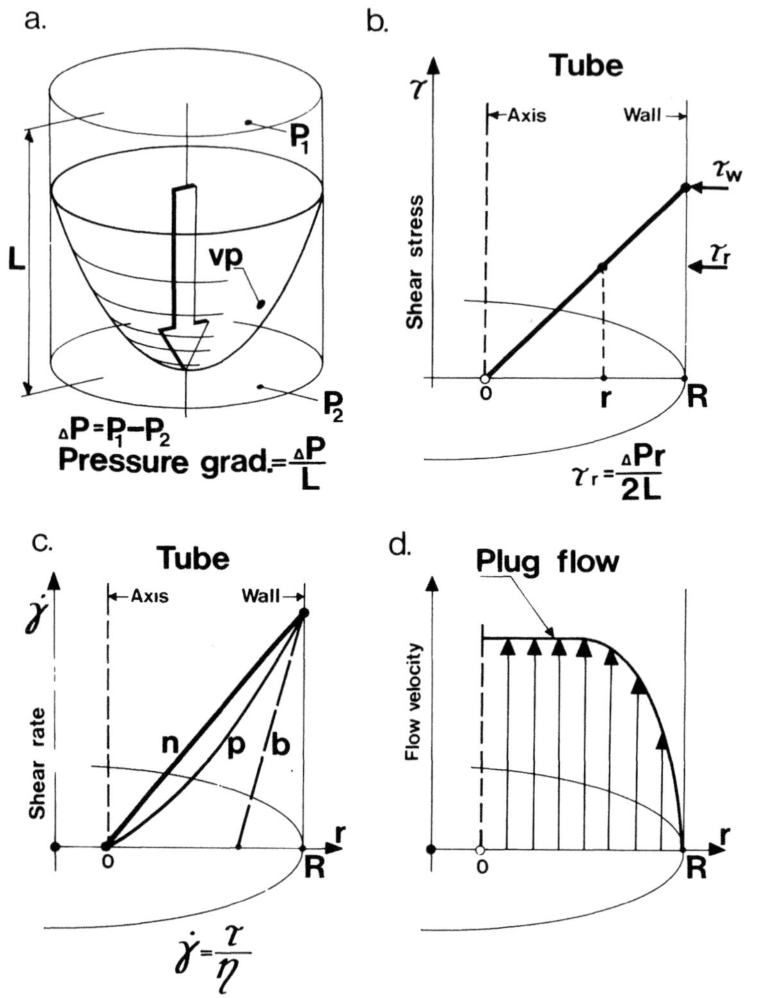

Figure 2.6. Tube flow. a: Pressure gradient in a tube is defined as $\Delta p/L$; where Δp is the drop of pressure in a distance L. In a horizontal tube filled with Newtonian fluid there is no pressure-gradient without flow, and there can be no flow without pressure-gradient. The flow velocity in the tube varies as shown by the velocity profile (v_p). The velocity is zero at the tube wall, and maximum at the tube axis.

b: Shear stress is zero at the tube axis and increases linearly with the distance (r) from the tube axis, reaching its greatest value (τ_w) at the tube wall.

c: Shear rate in the tube varies with radius (r) depending on the shear stress, and on the flow properties of the particular fluid. e.g. n = Newtonian; p = pseudoplastic; b = Bingham plastic

d: Contribution of different fluid-layers to flow-resistance depends on their distance from the flow axis and the flow properties of the fluid. The curve shown is for a Bingham fluid which has a core of plug flow. For a Newtonian fluid the plug radius is zero, but 1/3 of the flow-resistance depends on the marginal layer of 1/10 tube radius thickeness. This phenomenon is of particular importance in the flow of suspensions; it can also cause significant errors in tube viscometry (carry-over). One can also show, that the contribution of the central half of the cross section to the total flow-resistance is very little, although it carries a large fraction of the total discharge. The rheological properties of the fluid travelling in the central core are of relatively less significance to the viscous resistance.

For Newtonian fluids, the viscosity can be calculated directly from the tube dimensions, flow rate and the pressure drop, using the Hagen-Poiseuille equation:

$$\eta = \frac{R^4 \pi \Delta p}{8LQ} \tag{25}$$

where Δp is the pressure head, R and L are the internal radius of the tube and the length over which Δp occurs, and Q is the volumetric flow rate. Equation 25 is applicable only to steady, streamline flow of Newtonian liquids in straight cylindrical tubes, with negligible end-effects. To avoid end-effects the length L over which pressure is measured, should be well away from the ends of the tube (for details see ref. 10). Uniform streamline tube flows of Newtonian fluids follow Equation 25 and are often referred to as *Poiseuille-flow*. If Δp and Q are measured for a non-Newtonian liquid in a tube viscometer, and Equation 25 is used to compute a viscosity, the result is called the *apparent viscosity*, η_a. This is the viscosity of a Newtonian fluid, which would have the same flow rate Q when flowing under the same pressure head. In a non-Newtonian fluid the viscosity varies across the tube cross section, because the shear stress varies; so the apparent viscosity is representative of the average viscosity of the fluid, rather then being equal to the viscosity of the non-Newtonian fluid at a particular shear rate. However, it is possible to determine the flow curve of non-Newtonian liquids using tube viscometers by measuring the apparent viscosities at several pressure heads and applying the *Rabinowitch-Mooney equation* [11]. There are such tube viscometers, designed particularly to study blood rheology [12-15]. Detailed theory of tube viscometry is given in [16] and [17].

There are two phenomena of particular importance in clinical viscometry using tube viscometers, viz. *carry over* and *meniscus resistance*.

After making a measurement, a thin layer of the liquid measured is always retained on the tube wall, unless the tube is carefully washed and dried. This residual layer is known as *carry-over*. It can significantly influence the result of the next test. As the Hagen-Poiseuille equation shows, the flow rate Q in a tube is proportional to the 4th power of the tube radius R. If the radius of the tube is reduced from R to $0.9R$, the flow due to the same pressure gradient will be reduced by the factor $(0.9)^4 = 0.66$ or about 2/3. This is equivalent to saying that about 1/3 of the viscous resistance resides in the layer occupying the outermost 1/10 of the radius. Thus a thin layer of contamination can significantly affect flow rate. The effect will show time-dependency, if the *carry-over* layer is miscible with the new sample, and is gradually washed out.

The resistance associated with air-liquid interfaces in narrow tubes can absorb a significant proportion of the pressure head applied [18,19]. A retreating meniscus leaves a thin liquid film on the tube wall. Here the *meniscus resistance* depends on the surface tension of the fluid-air interface and on the reciprocal of the internal radius of the tube. For example, in the case of blood or plasma, the retreating meniscus in tubes of 0.8 and 0.3 mm internal radii cause pressure-head losses of about 100 and 250 Pa (1 and 2.5 cm water column), respectively. An advancing meniscus in a tube with wet walls has an opposite effect of the same magnitude. It tends to pull the fluid into the tube. In contrast to a wet tube, the effect of an advancing meniscus of a dry tube of non-wettable material is quite unpredictable.

Some commercially available tube viscometers

Harkness viscometer. Manufacturer: Coulter Electronics, High Street South, Dunstable, Bedfordshire LU6 3HT, U.K. This is one of the most frequently-used machines. A mercury column, 50 mm high, drives the fluid through a narrow glass tube (internal diameter: 0.38 mm; length: 200 mm) between two reservoirs. The flow rate is measured by detecting the displacement of the mercury [20]. Sample volume: 0.5–2.5 ml. In experienced hands 1 ml volume is enough to take triplicate readings within a coefficient of variation of 0.5 %. Advantages: the whole measuring procedure is visible, so the user can easily recognize tube blockage. Calibration is possible by water or any other calibration fluid. Several independent users have published results (e.g.: 21-24). Temperature control is achieved by water bath. Weak points include tube blockage and that the first reading on a fresh sample is subject to carry-over; the mechanical timer has a relatively short life time (2000 to 3000 tests); cleaning and replacing the mercury-filled manometer tube is awkward, and may require service personnel. Price US$ 3000.

Luckham Clinical Viscometer. Manufacturer: Luckham Ltd. (Victoria Gardens, Burgess Hill, West Sussex, RHIS 9QN, U.K.). This machine was designed to overcome some disadvantages of the Coulter-Harkness viscometer. The flow time of the sample (0.5 ml) is measured by optical detection of the trailing meniscus in a flowmeter tube, connected to a coiled stainless steel tube (internal diameter: 0.5 mm; length: 1000 mm). The pressure head is set to a level, such that the flow time equals sample viscosity in mPas units. This device decreases carry-over effects by flushing the tube with the sample before the test. The coefficient of variation is similar to that of the Harkness viscometer [25]. Temperature control: the tube is immersed in an oil filled chamber, maintained at preset temperature by an electric heater and tap water cooler. The sample entering the tube is at ambient temperature. Price US$ 3000.

Industrial tube viscometers
Many laboratory glassware suppliers sell simple and inexpensive (US$ 30-50) glass-tube viscometers widely used in industry. Some of these (micro-Ubbelohde, micro-Ostwald) are designed to measure small volumes (1–2 ml), and can be

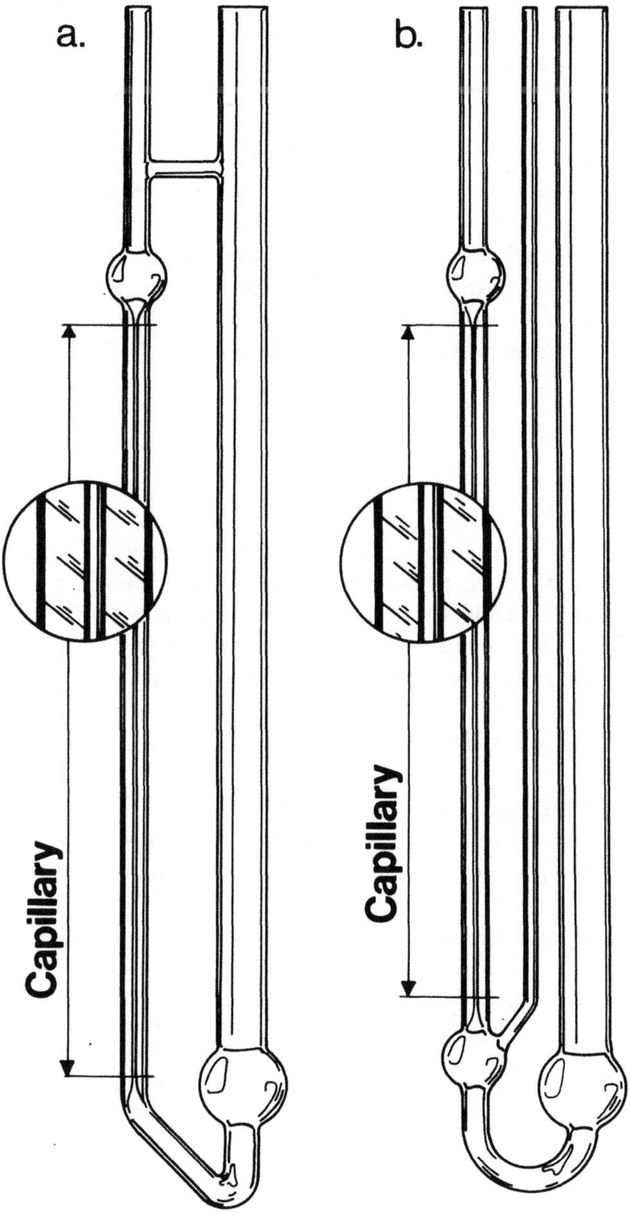

Figure 2.7. Simple glass tube viscometers.
a: micro-Ostwald viscometer, sample volume: 2–3 ml.
b: micro-Ubbelohde viscometer, sample volume: 1–3 ml.
Internal diameter of the glass capillary should be between 0.32–0.40 mm for plasma testing.

useful for hemorheologists (Fig. 2.7). Such glassware in an appropriate water bath, with the use of a good stopwatch, can result in measurements as accurate as any of the special-purpose instruments. There are also automated versions of the industrial viscometers, sold for US$ 1000-3000; but they usually require a larger test fluid sample (5–15 ml).

For the viscometers shown in Fig. 2.7, the ratio of the flow times of two liquids is proportional to the ratio of their kinematic viscosities. Because the driving force of the flow is the hydrostatic pressure generated by the sample in a vertical tube, the flow time is proportional to η/ρ. This quotient (*viscosity divided by density*) is defined as *kinematic viscosity* (unit: cm^2/s) and is usually denoted by the symbol ν (Greek nu). After measuring the flow times of a calibration fluid (t_1) and the sample (t_2), the relative viscosity, η_r, of the sample fluid can be calculated as follows:

$$\eta_r = \frac{t_2}{t_1}\frac{\rho_1}{\rho_2} \tag{26}$$

where ρ_1 (Greek rho) and ρ_2 are the densities of the calibration and sample fluids, respectively. The density of blood plasma varies with its protein content between 1020–1032 kg/m^3. The red cells are denser (1093 kg/m^3), because they contain more protein [26,27]. The density of blood (ρ_B in kg/m^3) can be calculated from hematocrit (Hct in 1/l) or hemoglobin (Hb in g/l):

$$\rho_B = 1026 + Hb/5 \text{ or } \rho_B = 1026 + 67Hct \tag{27}$$

The error of the approximate formulas 27 is less than 0.5%.

Viscosities and kinematic viscosities of water at different temperatures are shown in Table 2.3. Using these data, one can estimate the viscosities that would

Table 2.3. Viscosity (η, mPas) and kinematic viscosity (ν, cm^2/s) of water at different temperatures (T, °C).

1	η	ν	1	η	ν
0	1.7921	1.7924	28	0.836	0.839
4	1.5674	1.5674	29	0.818	0.821
10	1.3077	1.3081	30	0.801	0.803
20	1.005	1.007	31	0.784	0.788
21	0.981	0.983	32	0.768	0.772
22	0.958	0.960	33	0.752	0.756
23	0.936	0.938	34	0.737	0.741
24	0.914	0.916	35	0.723	0.727
25	0.894	0.897	36	0.709	0.713
26	0.874	0.877	37	0.695	0.700
27	0.855	0.858	38	0.681	0.686

be measured at different temperatures. If A is the viscosity measured at 25°C, the approximation for the viscosity of the same sample at 37°C, B will be

$$B = A\frac{W(37)}{W(25)} = \frac{A}{1.286} \tag{28}$$

where $W(37)$ and $W(25)$ are the viscosities of water at 37 and 25°C, respectively. Viscosity of plasma samples containing paraproteins or cryoglobulins may have different temperature dependence, resulting in faulty calculated viscosities with more than 50% error (9), if using Equation 28.

2.2.5. Rotational viscometers

In a rotational viscometer the fluid sample is sheared in a narrow gap between two surfaces, usually one rotating and the other stationary. Two frequently used geometries are the cone-and-plate (Fig. 2.8b) or two coaxial cylinders (*Couette viscometer*; Fig. 2.8c). In coaxial-cylinder systems the inner cylinder is often referred to as the *bob*, and the external one as the *cup*. In such systems, the shear rate is determined by geometrical dimensions and by the speed of rotation. The shear stress is calculated from the torque and from the geometrical dimensions. *Torque* is the product of a rotating force and the distance of its action from the centre of rotation (Fig. 2.8a). The same torque can be the result of a large force acting near to the centre of rotation, or of a small force acting far from the centre of rotation. The uniformity of the shear field depends on the *internal radius/gap width* ratio: e.g. if this ratio is 10, there is a 20% variation of the shear stress in the gap (Fig. 2.8d). Obviously, the shear rate in the gap follows the inhomogeneity of the shear stress, and so does the viscosity of a non-Newtonian fluid. In a cone-plate system a more uniform shear-field results because the gap width proportionally increases with the radius.

Sources of error in coaxial viscometry
Temperature control is more complicated than in tube viscometry, because there are more parts involved and the measuring head has to be disassembled and cleaned before each test. If the measuring head is connected to thermally uncontrolled components, there may be temperature-gradients within the measuring system, particularly if the head is metallic. Then the temperature of the sample may be rather different from that of the water circulating in the jacket. Miniaturised thermocuple or thermistor units are suitable for frequent monitoring of the sample when actually in the cup.

The construction of rotational viscometers allows measurements at low shear, but there may be some additional artifacts of significance when blood is measured at low speeds.

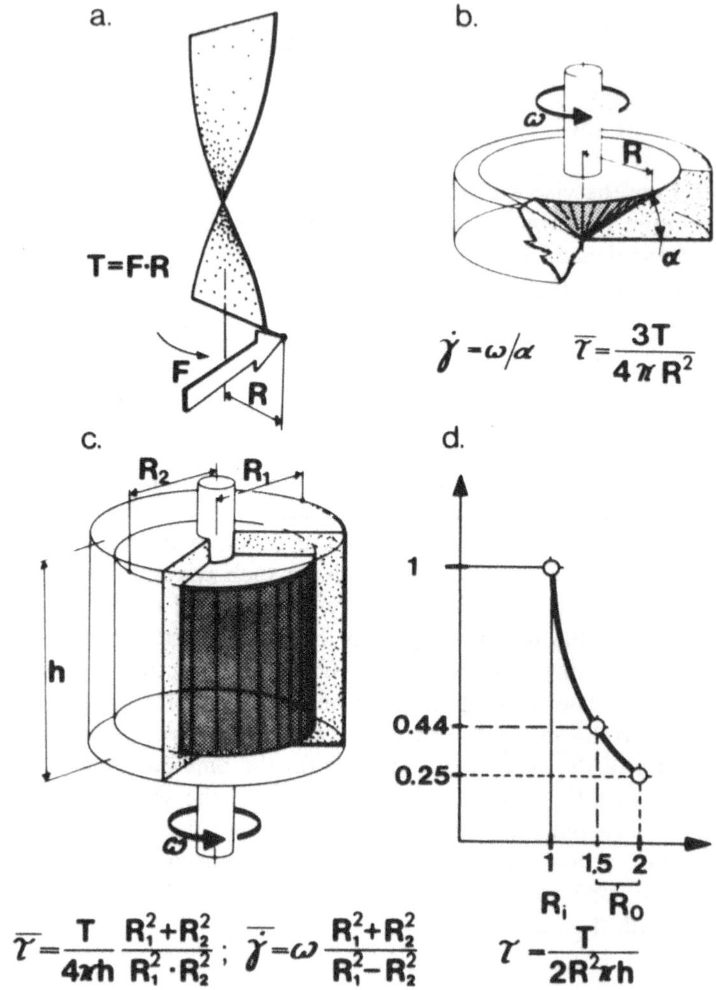

Figure 2.8. Rotational viscometry. $\bar{\tau}$ and $\bar{\dot{\gamma}}$ are the average shear stress and shear rate in the gap. The circular frequency ω (radians/sec) is defined by $\omega = 2\pi f$, where f is the frequency of rotation (cycles/sec).

a: Torque (T) is defined as the product FR, where the force F is applied at a radius R from the axis of rotation.

b: Shear stress and shear rate in cone-and-plate viscometer.

c: Shear stress and shear rate in coaxial cylinder viscometer.

d: The shear stress between coaxial cylinders (vertical axis) varies with radius (horizontal axis). The inhomogeneity of the shear field in the gap (curve) depends on the diameters of the internal and external cylinders.

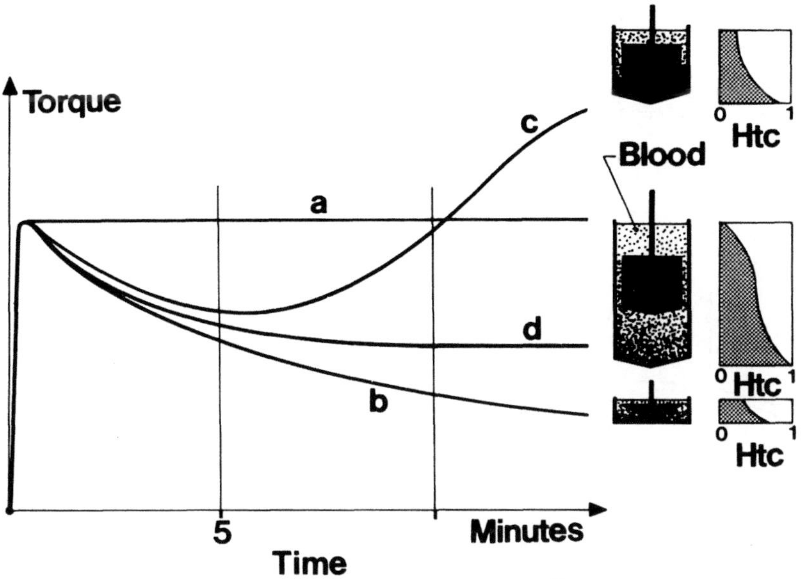

Figure 2.9. Aggregation and sedimentation in viscometry. Time-dependent changes in the blood sample placed in the viscometer result in artifactual changes of viscosity-readings at constant shear. Torque at constant rotational speed is plotted against time in three measuring systems. The small graphs on the right of each curve illustrate the assumed variation of red cell concentration (Htc) in the sheared zone of the sample.
a: Homogeneous liquid with no time-dependence (e.g. calibration fluid).
b: Blood sheared in a cone-and-plate system. Progressive aggregation and sedimentation builds up a cell-free layer under the cone, decreasing the measured viscosity with time.
c: Blood sheared in conicylindric system. The initial decrease of the torque (caused by aggregation or phase separation) is later compensated by the effect of sedimentation: although there is some decrease of viscosity in the top layer of the sample, the settled red cell mass at the bottom of the sample is of disproportionately high viscosity, causing net increase of torque.
d: Blood is sheared in a system similar to *B*, but with large sample-spaces above and under the bob. This arrangement eliminates most of the red-cell concentration changes within the sheared zone of the sample. This curve shows that the initially progressive aggregation reaches a steady state after some time, if sheared continuously.

Phase separation is the change of the suspension-homogeneity before or during the test; due to aggregation and sedimentation of blood cells. This can result in separation into cell-free and cell-rich zones. Thereafter most of the shearing occurs in the cell-poor zones of the sample, which have low viscosity, resulting in spurious, low readings. In contrast to this, sedimentation of the cells can fill the lower part of the gap with a concentrated cell suspension of high viscosity, resulting in spurious, high readings (Fig. 2.9).

Surface tension: if the contact between the liquid surface and the measuring-head is not uniform along the periphery, the bob can be pulled in different directions during rotation, resulting in apparent torque changes.

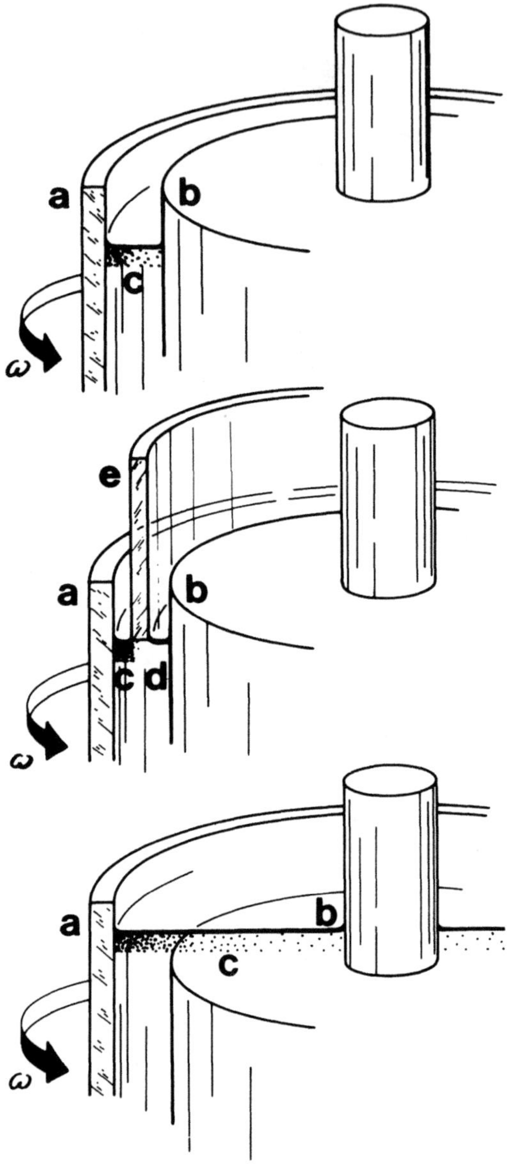

Figure 2.10. Surface film and guard ring. A viscous (or viscoelastic) surface film of adsorbed proteins builds up at the air-blood (and also at an oil-blood) interface. *a*: rotating-part of the measuring head; *b*: sensor-part of the measuring head; *c*: sheared surface-film; *d*: unsheared surface-film; *e*: guard ring.
Top: The surface film transmits an additional drag between the steady and rotating parts of the viscometer, increasing the measured torque.
Middle: A fixed guard ring immersed in the surface absorbs the drag caused by the surface film. There is no movement between the guard ring and the sensor part of the viscometer: this segment of the surface layer is not sheared.
Bottom: Providing a large liquid surface broken by a narrow shaft of the sensor also diminishes surface-film effects.

Viscous or viscoelastic *surface films* of adsorbed proteins have been described at blood-air and plasma-air interfaces [28,29]. Such layers may be time dependent [6], and cause a torque in addition to the one caused by the viscosity of the sample. This can significantly increase the reading when the torque originating from viscous drag of the liquid is small, as when measuring plasma or blood at low shear rates. The spurious torque resulting from such films is proportional to the square of the internal radius of the air-liquid interface. This artifact can be avoided by installing a guard-ring [30,31]. This is a stationary ring immersed in the sample surface, to absorb torque transmitted by the surface film (Fig. 2.10b). A guard ring cannot be applied to viscometers which measure the torque on the rotating bob. A less laborious, but also effective, way to eliminate this artifact is by using a large air-liquid interface broken only by a central shaft of small radius (Fig. 2.10c).

In rotational viscometers with wider gaps (> 2mm), non-laminar (unstable or turbulent) flow can occur when measuring plasma viscosity at high shear rates.

Range of reliability

In most rotational viscometers a wide range of shear rates or stresses can be selected; but in many instruments, the extremes of this range are of insufficient accuracy. To evaluate one's own instrument, the *torque/angular velocity* quotients for a Newtonian test-liquid can be calculated and plotted throughout the measuring range. The useful measuring range of the instrument is shown by the horizontal segment of this plot. The useful measuring range varies with the viscosity. In most cases there is an upper limit of shear stress or shear rate, caused by instability of the flow, and a lower limit due to torque originating from other sources than the viscosity of the sample, or due to insufficient resolution of the torque-measuring system. The useful range is wider for more viscous liquids, because higher torque improves readings at low shear stresses, and also lowers the Reynolds number and increases flow stability at high shear stresses.

Some commercially available rotational viscometers

Wells-Brookfield Micro Viscometer. This was an early commercial viscometer designed for hemorheologists [32], and is currently manufactured by Brookfield Engineering Laboratories Inc. (240 Cushing Str. Stoughton, Massachusetts 02072, USA). This machine utilizes a cone-and-plate measuring head requiring 1 ml of sample fluid. The cone is coupled by a spring to a motor, whose rotational speed can be pre-set to a range of frequencies. The strain of the spring is proportional to the torque exerted on the sample and can be read directly on a calibrated scale. The latest model has a digital display. The cone-and-plate system is sensitive to sedimentation of blood, resulting in poor reproducibility of the results at low shear-rates ($< 23\ s^{-1}$). Surface film artifacts can be also significant at low torques, because of the large diameter of the cone. This may be responsible for the erroneously high plasma-viscosity results sometimes measured with this machine at low shear rates. The useful measuring-range is above 23 s^{-1}. The whole measuring-head is incorporated in a water jacket which provides the best thermostatic control among the rotational viscometers discussed here. There are numerous publications of hemorheological applications (24,33-38). Price US$ 4000.

Contraves LS-30. Manufacturer: Contraves AG, Schaffhauserstr. 580, Zürich, CH-8052, Switzerland. This is the latest, improved version of earlier models, such as LS-2 and LS-100 [39].

The working principle is similar to the one applied first to viscometry by Gilinson et al. [40]. The outer cylinder (cup) rotates at preset frequencies covering shear rates from 10^{-3} to 10^{2} s^{-1}. The torque required to keep the internal cylinder (bob) in steady position against the drag of the fluid is measured by a sensitive (10^{-10} Nm) opto-electromagnetic feedback circuit. The LS-30 has an outstanding sensitivity not matched by any other viscometer discussed here. However, it is also very sensitive to alignment changes. It has to be placed on a vibration-free, solid-stone table. The alignment of the machine has to be checked frequently, since the bob is suspended on a 30 cm-long torsion wire, and is kept in the centered position by its weight only. This weak centering can result in erroneous readings at the highest rotation speeds, especially if the viscosity of the sample is high (>5 mPas). Temperature control: the rotating metal jacket supporting the cup can be perfused from a thermostatically controlled water bath.

The construction of LS-30 (manual lifting and lowering of the bob) allows the application of a simple and convenient method of controlling the shear history of the sample [41], providing excellent reproducibility of results at shear rates as low as 0.1 s^{-1}. In earlier models this is not possible, because of the difficult centering of the magnetized measuring head. More recently, the measuring head is made of antimagnetic steel. Measuring range: according to the authors' experience, the LS-30 (using the measuring head No. 1, volume = 1ml) can be conveniently used for blood viscosity tests at rotational steps between 10-29 (0.3–94.5 s^{-1}). The bob often swings out at speed 30 (shear rate 128 s^{-1}); but the machine has performed satisfactorily at speed 29. Because of the operational principle, the attainment of a given shear stress requires the displacement of the bob by a proportionate angle. Consequently, the sample has to be sheared for a time before the steady-state torque is reached. The time taken by this process at speeds below step 10 ($\dot{\gamma} = 0.1$ s^{-1}) is usually longer than 20 s, allowing progressive changes in the sample (aggregation and sedimentation), and making difficult the interpretation of the results. Therefore the use of speeds less than step 10 is of little advantage in this machine. There are many hemorheological studies using this equipment [24,36-38,42-45]. Price of the basic version: US$ 20 000.

Haake Rotovisco. The manufacturer (Haake Messtechnik, Dieselstr. 6, D-7500 Karlsruhe 41, FRG) has a wide range of viscometers. The model RV100-CV100 combination is used by biorheologists. The working principle of this machine is similar to the one used by the LS-30: the cup rotates at selected frequencies and the torque is measured on the stationary bob. The important difference is in the suspension of the bob, which is kept in a central position by an air-bearing system, reducing sensitivity to vibration and to alignment-changes. The measuring head also has a guard ring. Although the air bearing has very little friction, the sensitivity of such systems is considerably less then with a torsional wire suspension. The special compressor required to feed the air bearing is supplied with the machine. The sample volume for blood-viscosity studies depends on the geometry, and is 3.5 ml for the most sensitive system. The useful measuring range is from 1 s^{-1} to 300 s^{-1}. The viscometer does not display the results, but they have to be read from the graphs drawn by the built-in plotter. Temperature control is maintained by water circulating system. Hemorheological references: 37, 46, 47. Price of the basic version is US$ 20 000.

Carri-med CSS Rheometer. This shear-stress-controlled viscometer is manufactured in England (Carri-med Ltd., Vincent Lane, Dorking, Surrey RH4 3Y1, U. K.). It gained a considerable popularity among rheologists because of the advantageous measuring principle. The instrument features a bob suspended from an air-bearing rotated by an electromagnetic drive of constant torque (selected by the user). The resulting displacement or angular velocity is measured. This system enables one to measure yield stress [48] in pathological blood and at high hematocrits. The required sample volume is 3.5 ml and the shear stress measuring range is 0.02–1000 Pa. The lower limit is similar to that of the Haake machine. But blood tests are less relevant at shear stresses above 10 Pa (i.e. at shear rates above approximately 2000 s^{-1}), because of possibility of non-laminar flow between the coaxial cylinders. At low shear stresses (< 0.05 Pa) surface artifacts can be significant. The machine displays angular velocity (or optionally, angular displacement, at low speeds). Viscosity values are calculated from the preset torque by dividing it by the measured angular velocity and multiplying by a system constant. Temperature control is achieved by an electronic heater or water circulator (optional). The Carri-Med-CSS can use any compressed air source (at a pressure of 0.3 MPa = 3 atmospheres, or more), because of the separate air filter and pressure regulating unit supplied with the machine. Hemorheological references: 24, 38, 43, 49. Price of the basic unit: US$ 10 000.

Falling ball viscometer

Höppler has designed the first falling ball viscometer [50] in Karlsruhe, at Haake Messtechnik. The *Bloodtester* is a recent adaptation of this method, designed for clinical blood and plasma viscometry. The sample is filled in a precision-cut glass syringe, together with a disposable gold-plated iron sphere. Then the syringe is placed into the machine, where a rotating magnet lifts the sphere to the top of the syringe. Thereafter the sphere is released, and the falling time between two photosensors is measured and displayed. There are two syringe sizes supplied: 60 μl for microtests, and 300 μl for more accurate measurements. Coefficients of variation for plasma viscosity tests are 1.8% and 0.9%, respectively. Apparent viscosity of whole blood can be also measured by this machine, but it is difficult to determine the shear field between the falling ball and cylinder wall. Price: US$ 3000.

2.2.6. Oscillatory flow methods

Some rotational viscometers can produce steady, unsteady or oscillatory flow. Usually, for steady flow, the moving cylinder is rotated at a constant, selected speed or torque. For unsteady flow, the instrument may make excursions in velocity (or torque); the speed of rotation being gradually increased from rest to a maximal rate, and then returned to rest. The whole manoeuvre is carried out in a predetermined time. This unsteady flow procedure may be designated as the "excursive" or "ramp" method.

Oscillatory flow is a periodic shear-deformation, usually a sinusoidal function of time. Similar techniques can be applied to tube viscometry. Oscillatory-flow tests are used in clinical hemorheology to study viscoelastic properties of whole blood usually at frequencies of 0.1 to about 3 Hz. The viscous and elastic properties of the sample are computed from the measured amplitude of shear stress and its phase lag relative to shear rate, using equations 10-13, discussed earlier in this chapter. There are theoretical advantages in using such systems for non-Newtonian liquids:

A: Continuous shearing might eliminate some clinically-relevant properties of blood, but these properties might be measurable in oscillatory tests.

B: Unsteady flow, although much less regular than the above simple sinusoidal motion, does occur in vivo, generally superimposed upon a steady flow.

The sine-wave applied as a pattern of deformation in oscillatory tests, has some special characteristics. Its time-rate-of-change is an identical sine-wave shifted by 90° (1/4 cycle). The sum of two sine waves is always a third sine, whose peak lies between the two added peaks. Consequently, in oscillatory flow, the deformation and rate of deformation (rate of shear) are separated in phase by 90°, although following the same pattern. If the sheared sample is purely viscous, the shear stress will be in phase with the deformation rate. If the sample is purely elastic, there will be a 90° shift between shear rate and shear stress; but the stress will be in phase with the deformation. Intermediate values of the phase shift (Fig. 2.11) are characteristic of the relative degree of viscous and elastic properties when both are present together. In the middle of a sinusoidal cycle of deformation (at 0°, 180° and 360°), the sample is sheared at maximal rate, but the actual deformation is zero (see Fig. 2.11). Any shear stress present at this moment can only be attributed to viscous properties of the sample as modeled by Equation 11. At the maximal amplitude of the deformation (90° or 270°), the shear deformation has its maximum, whereas the rate of shear is zero (the direction of shearing

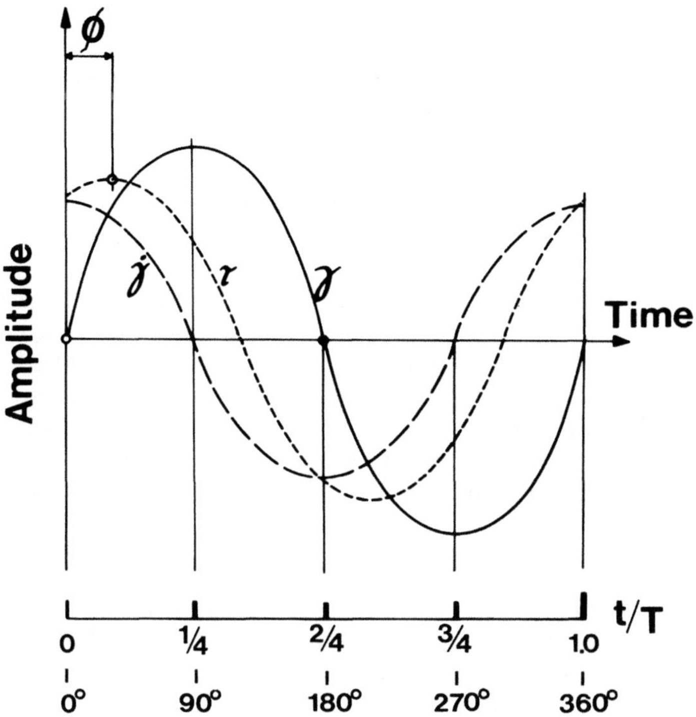

$$\eta' = \frac{\tau_{max}}{\gamma_{max}} \cos\phi$$

$$\eta'' = \frac{\tau_{max}}{\dot{\gamma}_{max}} \sin\phi$$

Figure 2.11. Principles of oscillatory viscometry. The variations of shear stress τ, shear deformation γ and shear rate $\dot{\gamma}$ are all sinusoidal in time, but have different phases. The phase of $\dot{\gamma}$ is always 90° ahead of γ but the phase of τ depends on the fluid properties.

is just changing). Any stress present at this moment is stored in the sample, indicating its elasticity. In other words: the shear stress in oscillatory motion is always the sum of viscous and elastic components, but one can find such points on the time scale, where either the viscous or the elastic component is momentarily zero, and the shear stress is actually generated by one of the two components only. The calculation of the two components η' and η'' (loss modulus and storage modulus) defined in Equation 11 is simple, but there are considerable technical difficulties in measuring the necessary amplitudes and phase shifts. Furthermore some significant cautions related to such tests must be kept in mind:

A: Application of the theory requires linearity of both elastic and viscous components in regard to amplitude of deformation used. Any non-linearity in the properties of the material tested (thixotropy, particle orientation, desaggregation) can appear as spurious elasticity in such tests.

B: Acceleration of the liquid subjected to sinusoidal oscillations is in phase with the deformation. Consequently, any effects of inertia of the liquid or measuring system-components may appear as a spurious elastic component of the fluid. Correction of this artifact can be rather complicated, depending on the instrument design.

The viscous component derived by oscillatory methods is equivalent to the viscosity measured in viscometers applying steady flow only, if the elastic component is negligible (i.e., if the fluid studied is Newtonian). In other fluids, the deformation-related (elastic) component always contributes to the viscosity measured by steady flow tests, especially at low shear. Consequently, results derived by oscillatory tests cannot be replaced or verified by steady flow methods. Calibration fluids of standard viscoelastic properties are not readily available.

Commercially-available oscillating viscometers
Contraves, *Haake and Carrimed* all have oscillatory versions of their instruments available. The evaluation of the results is possible from plotted curves, but it is easier with the computerized versions of these instruments, the appropriate software provided. The prices of these oscillatory systems are about twice those of the basic versions.

Oscillating Capillary Rheometer and Density Meter. This is a tube viscometer with oscillating flow mode, originally described by Thurston [51], manufactured by A. Paar K.G., (Kaertnerstr. 322, A-8054 Graz, Austria). Using a sample volume of 1.5 ml, this equipment determines and plots the viscous and elastic components of viscoelasticity as a function of shear rate in the range of 0.2–200 s^{-1}, applying a standard operating frequency of 2 Hz. The machine also measures plasma viscosity, hematocrit and blood density. This equipment has been applied in some clinical studies (e.g. 52). Price: US$ 20 000.

2.3. Other techniques quantifying blood rheology

Besides viscometry, there are several other methods adopted in clinical hemorheology to study some particular aspects of blood rheology. Among these, optical aggregometry and blood filtration are discussed here.

2.3.1. Optical aggregometry

Aggregation of platelets and leucocytes is usually studied after addition of aggregating agents, evoking very strong attractive forces between these particles.

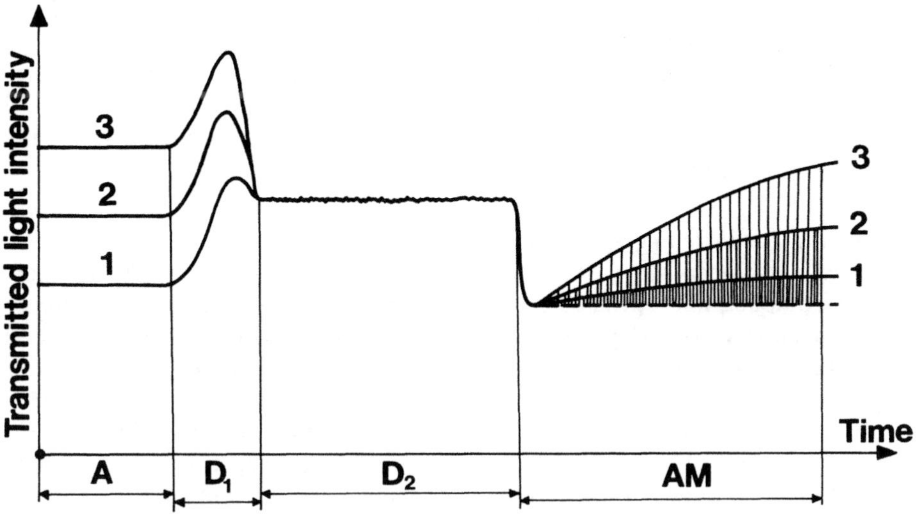

Figure 2.12. Measuring-principle of an optical blood-aggregometer. Transmitted light is plotted as a function of time, recorded from the analog output of the Myrenne aggregometer. Three samples are shown, (aggregometer readings in brackets): 1) low aggregability (4.7); 2) medium aggregability (13.6); 3) high aggregability (37.2). The light transmission curve has 4 phases in each measuring cycle: *A*: aggregated blood in stasis; *D*1: desaggregating transient, with an overshoot probably due to orientation of red cell aggregates; *D*2: desaggregated blood during intensive shearing at 600 s^{-1} shear rate; *AM*: aggregation process after rotation has stopped. Aggregation is measured in the first 10 seconds of the *AM* phase, as the area under the light transmission curves (shaded fields).

During such tests the suspensions are sheared, by mixing the sample with a magnetic bar at constant rate to prevent development of inhomogeneity. In such systems, the quantificaion of shear is difficult, because the resulting shear rate and shear stress depend not only on the rate of rotation, but also on the shape and size of the magnetic bar and vessel. Furthermore, the shear field in these systems is extremely heterogeneous: there is a high shear zone between the magnetic bar and the bottom of the vessel, and a low shear zone at the top of the sample. There are smaller forces involved in the aggregation of red cells, therefore optical methods assessing red cell aggregation utilize low shear rates or stasis [56,57].

Fig. 2.12 shows a pattern of light transmission, as detected by the Myrenne aggregometer, and also the evaluation of this signal as a red cell aggregation parameter. Optical aggregometry has the advantage of being a direct measure of the process seen by the researcher under the microscope. However, the parameters derived from the optical signal are only indirectly related to the aggregating forces. These forces are in fact causing the phenomenon, and they are more directly measured by viscometric methods (see Chapter 3). Red-cell aggregation has also been studied by detecting the presence of doublets and triplets of red cells in a diluted suspension with a cell-counting method [58,59].

The calibration of optical aggregometers is difficult, since suspension standards of specified aggregation properties are not available. Therefore different normal and pathological values might be reported by scientists even using the same make of equipment.

Commercially available aggregometer

The Myrenne aggregometer (Myrenne GmbH, Steffensgasse 9, D-5106 Roetgen, FRG) is a compact, microprocessor-controlled device. It consists of a flat perspex cone and a closely spaced plastic plate. For hemorheological testing, 20 μl of anticoagulated whole blood is placed between the cone and plate. The sample is disaggregated by shearing at 600 s^{-1} for 10 seconds, and the change of infrared light absorption is converted into an aggregation parameter (see Fig. 2.12). A more recent version of this machine can also measure aggregation at a low shear rate, in addition to the usual measurements during stasis. One test takes about 30 seconds. This method has a coefficient of variation for repeated tests on the same sample of about 5%. Successive samples from the same blood show more variation (8%). Hemorheological references: 59-62. Price US$ 4,000.

2.3.2. Blood filtration

The deformability of red cells has been observed as long ago as the early microscopic studies of Loewenhook, (cited by 36). The quantitation of red-cell deformability has been attempted by various blood-filtration methods. The narrow channels in different filters have similar diameters to those of the capillaries in the microcirculation. Hence, from the behavior of blood in filtration systems, some information can be inferred about its flow properties in small blood vessels. Blood-filtration or red cell filtration tests have been used in hematology [63-66], in physiology [67-68], and gained popularity in the 1970's [69-71] in clinical medicine. There is abundant literature on blood filtration methodology and clinical results (see reviews 72-74). This section summarizes the methods available for clinical research, and discusses their background.

Principles of filtration tests

In all blood-filtration methods, a pressure head drives the cell suspension through a filter, and flow properties are calculated from the pressure-flow data [75]. The value of pressure head in the filtration systems is most important, because it determines flow conditions (shear stress) in the filter (Fig. 2.13). Technical details (suction, or positive hydrostatic pressure, constant flow or gravity-driven flow) are less important than the pressure drop across the filter.

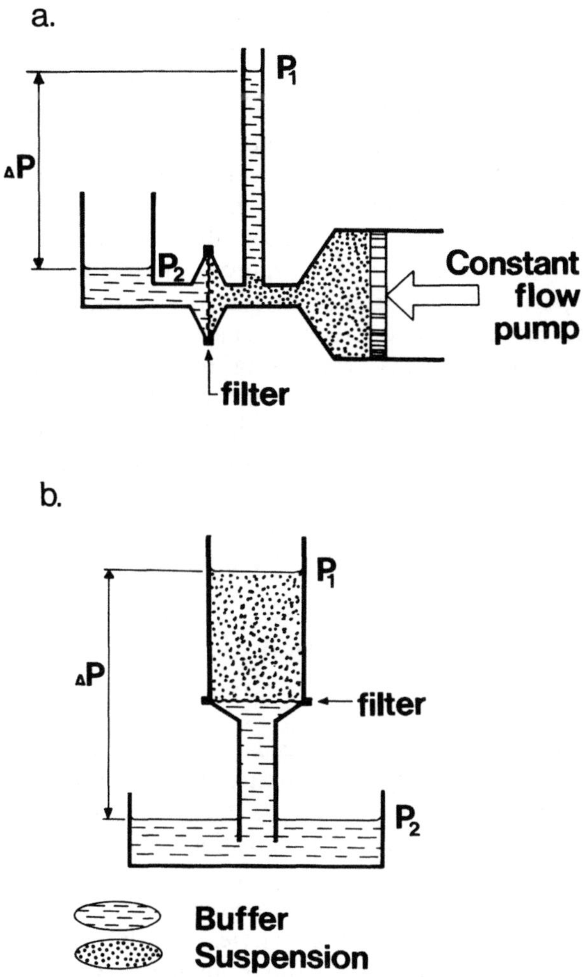

Figure 2.13. Filtration pressure. In a filtration system, pressure head is defined as the pressure difference between the upstream and downstream sides of the filter. Pressure loss in other parts of the system is supposed to be negligible. *a*: constant flow system; *b*: variable pressure head – variable flow system. p_1 and p_2 are upstream and downstream pressures, respectively.

Blood filtration methods are sometimes classified according to the mechanical system controlling the pressure head: constant flow, constant pressure or variable pressure and variable flow methods. In the variable pressure – variable flow methods the weight of the suspension usually provides the pressure head which therefore decreases as the suspension is filtered.

There are different filter types utilized in blood filtration tests [76]. Some have irregular networks of channels (filter paper, silver filters), and some have more-regular, but still not uniform channels (Nuclepore filters). The individual filters from the same source are not necessarily all uniform, and the conductance of each filter should be calibrated before testing suspensions. A convenient way to do this is by measuring the flow of the suspending medium alone through the filter, before testing the suspension itself. Flow of air through the filter can also be used to measure conductance of dry filters [76]. The earlier reported large test-to-test variations of blood filterability measurements (e.g. 73) were probably not entirely caused by filter differences. Imperfect design of filter chamber (e.g. trapped air bubbles) also have may contributed to the variations observed.

Suspension hematocrit is of particular importance in filtration tests. Techniques applying lower cell concentrations (hematocrit < 0.15) are probably more sensitive to individual cell properties, whereas tests using hematocrit above 0.20–0.25, are probably more influenced by cell-cell interactions. These higher hematocrits may result in a layer of cells collecting on the upstream face of the filter. The hematocrit of a suspension prepared for filtration has to be measured more accurately than for hematological purposes, and preferably kept constant, if individual cell parameters are to be calculated from the filtration test.

There are several factors which determine the suspension flow rate in a blood filtration system:

A: the flow properties of the suspending medium
B: the flow properties of the red cells travelling through the filter
C: the change of filter-conductance by reversible or irreversible blockage of some pores.

The influence of blood components other than red cells can be significant [77]. Effects of plasma viscosity variations can be largely eliminated by calibrating the filter at each test with the suspending medium. The presence of leukocytes, thrombocytes or other particles can be associated with progressive filter blockage, and other factors can also contribute (see Fig. 14). To minimize effects of leukocytes, most authors remove the buffy coat after centrifuging heparinized blood [78,79]. This method removes 90–98% of the leucokytes, and 90–95% of the platelets. Others use washed red cell suspension with residual platelets and leukocytes less then 2–3% of the native blood. The most efficient removal of leukocytes (95–99%) and platelets (> 99%) is possible by Imugard cotton wool filtration [80,81]. It has been also shown, that leukocytes and thrombocytes in EDTA anticoagulated blood, pass the Nuclepore filters more easily, than those in heparin anticoagulated blood [82-84]. Furthermore, there is a considerable difference between the filter-passage time of different leukocyte subpopulations [85,86]. It is now recommended, that whatever procedures are used, a white cell count should be made. Leukocyte counts as low as $50/\mu l$ can significantly affect filtration results [87].

Filter blockage is probably the most important phenomenon in blood filtration. When using a cell suspension of 0.05 hematocrit, there are about 5×10^5 red cells in one μl. In most RCF tests the first reading (flow rate or pressure

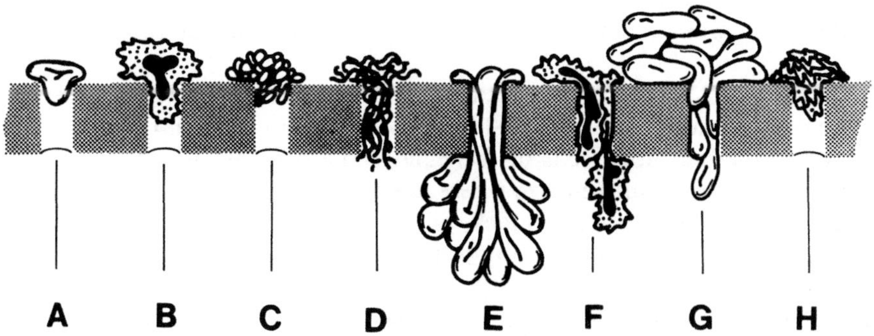

Figure 2.14. Filter blockage. Filter pores can be blocked by different particles and cell debris, even if the filtrate is a washed red cell suspension. *A*: rigid red cells; *B*: rigid leukocytes; *C*: platelet aggregates; *D*: protein flocculates; *E*: "grape clusters" built up of red cells; *F*: adhesive leukocytes; *G*: sedimented red cells; *H*: microclots. Microscopic air bubbles can also block pores (not shown in this figure). Pore blockage can be permanent, or transient. In most cases, pores can be unclogged by higher pressure or reverse flow.

head) is taken after 0.5–1 ml suspension has been already filtered. Considering a Nuclepore filter (13 mm diameter) with about $2–3 \times 10^5$ pores in the effective filtration area, one can calculate that on average 1000–2000 red cells have negotiated each pore at this time. Therefore a small fraction of rigid red cells (e.g. 1/1000) can completely block the filter at this stage. If there are only 25 rigid cells/μl (= 0.005%) retained in the pores, the result can still be a flow-rate decrease of 10%.

The filter-blocking is frequently considered as an artifact in RCF tests. However, those particles blocking the filter (these may be stiff red cells, leukocytes, platelet aggregates, etc. as shown in Fig. 2.14) might also block capillaries in the microcirculation, contributing to pathological processes.

Quantifying filter-blockage is possible in most filtration tests, if filter-conductance (flow rate/pressure head) can be determined as a function of the volume filtered. The fall in filter-conductance is directly proportional to the fraction of pores blocked. Fig. 2.15 shows how one can apply this to different methods. The clogging of the filter is to be related to the volume filtered, since the number of blocking particles arriving at the filter depends on the volume filtered.

In the ideal case of permanently blocking particles, the filter-conductance versus filtered-volume plot is a straight line, with its slope ($\cot\alpha$) giving the concentration of clogging particles (C_c)

$$C_c = N_0 \cot \alpha \tag{29}$$

where N_0 is the number of pores at the beginning of filtration and $\cot\alpha$ is the fractional decrease of filter-conductance after filtering 1 ml suspension. However, in real cases, the filter conductance versus filtered-volume plot is only initially a straight line. It becomes a curve, after filtering a suspension, for the following reasons:

A: Pore-blocking is not permanent, but it reflects rather a prolonged transit time. Leukocytes may take 100–1000 times as long to pass through a filter compared to the red blood cells or the bulk of the suspension.

B: The pores are of non-uniform size (there are also pore doublets and triplets), larger pores have less chance to block, and then for a shorter time.

C: In constant-flow systems, unblocking of the pores is facilitated by the gradual increase of the pressure head.

Therefore, the analysis of pressure curves in such systems is more complicated [88], and requires pressure curves of good resolution to separate effects of different components (red cells, leukocytes, etc.).

Red-cell-deformability indices can be derived from the filtration rate of the suspending medium, initial filtration rate, hematocrit of the suspension, and the corresponding pressure drops.

It has been shown, that average red cell transit time can be calculated from blood filtration tests [89]. The most frequently adopted parameter X to express red cell deformability based on filtration tests is

$$X = 1 + \frac{(F_m/F_s - 1)}{Hct} \tag{30}$$

where Hct is the hematocrit, F_m and F_s are the filtration rates of suspending medium and suspension (assuming it to contain only red cells), respectively under the same pressure head. Different groups have used this or very similar equations [23,79,88,90,91], giving different names to the parameter X. The parameter X can be regarded as the apparent viscosity of the cells relative to that of the suspending medium. If one finds, for red blood cells, that $X = 9$, it means that in the particular mechanical system, the viscosity of a red cell appears to be 9 times higher than the viscosity of the suspending medium.

It is also possible to replace hematocrit with red cell count (RCC) in the above equation. This might be preferable, since red cell counts can be measured more accurately than hematocrit (when using cell-counters), particularly in the diluted suspensions used in filtration tests. In this case define the parameter X' by

$$X' = MCV + \frac{(F_m/F_s - 1)}{RCC} \tag{31}$$

the parameter X' can be regarded as the volume of suspending medium retained because of the passage of one red cell through the filter (MCV is the mean red cell volume). Thus, $X' = 900 \times 10^{-9}$ μl means, that the presence of red cells delays the filtration so that, on the average, one red cell is responsible for retaining 900×10^{-9} μl (= 900 mμ^3) of suspending medium (in addition to its own volume) on the upstream side of the filter (this may be regarded as an apparent *red cell volume increment* [95]).

Another version of this red cell deformability parameter is

$$\beta = 1 + \frac{(F_m/F_s - 1)}{Hct} V \tag{32}$$

The parameter β (Greek beta) can be regarded as the factor by which a cell increases the resistance of one pore compared to the flow of suspending medium alone. In other words, the volumetric flow rate is β times slower in a pore whilst a red cell is flowing through it [88]. If a constant-flow technique is used, the resistance factor β may be computed by the equation

$$\beta = 1 + (p_i/p_0 - 1)\frac{V}{Hct} \tag{33}$$

where p_i is the initial pressure measured for the suspension and p_0 is the pressure measured for suspending fluid only, at the same flow rate [88]. V is the volume ratio of one red cell to the volume of one pore and Hct is the fractional hematocrit in the suspension. When the suspension contains both red and white cells, it is very important to measure p_i within one or two seconds (depending on the flow rate) of the start of flow, if an index of red cell deformability is desired, uncontaminated by white cell effects, which cause a rise in pressure at later times.

Blood filtration equipment

The *Filtrometer MF* 4 is a microprocessor-controlled device [93], adopting a variable pressure and variable flow rate system. In this instrument, there is a linear decrease of pressure head from 300 to 0 Pa during a test. The filtered volume (1 ml) is recorded as a function of time, and blood filtration parameters are calculated from this curve. The designers of this equipment did not aim at measuring the initial filtration rate, and interpret the test as polymicroviscometry. Manufacturer: Myrenne GmbH. Steffensgasse 9, D-5106 Roetgen, West Germany. Price US$ 4,000.

The *Hemorheometre* was the first filtration machine designed to avoid filter clogging effects [79,94], by determining the initial filtration rate. It measures the flow time of 60 μl of suspension (0.05–0.10 hematocrit) through a horizontal filter, driven by a decreasing pressure head (500 to 400 Pa). This machine has been used by several research groups [81,83,95]. The initial filtration rate measured by this device, is affected by a subpopulation of rigid cells (e.g. leukocytes or sickle cells), if their concentration is above 100/μl [74,92]. Manufacturer: I.M.H. 2, allee du Jardin de la Cure, 95470 Saint-Witz, France. Price US$ 3,000.

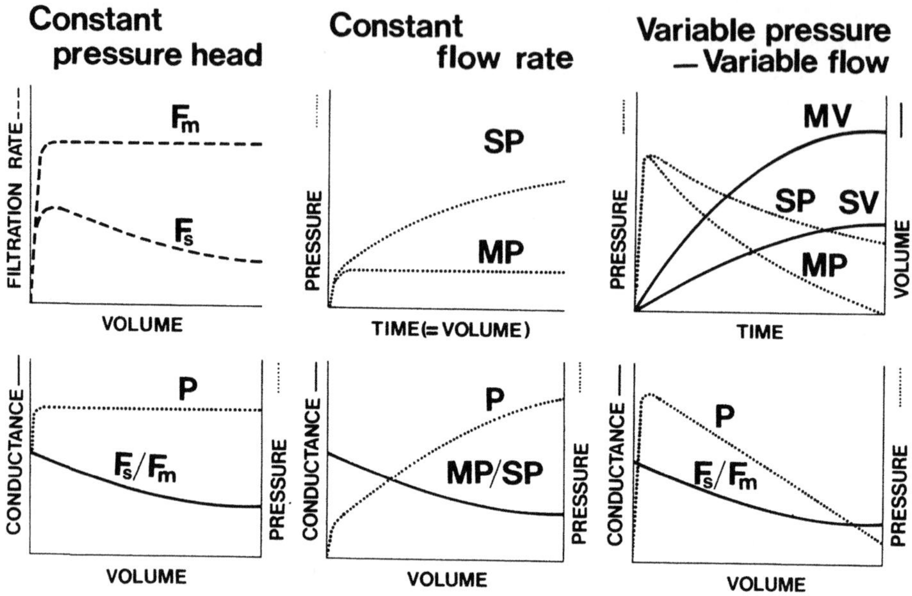

Figure 2.15. Analysis of filtration curves. The quantifying of filter blockage is required for the assessment of red cell deformability in filtration systems. This can be achieved in most blood filtration tests, as shown for all three types of blood filtration methods.

Top left: In a constant pressure head system the filtration rates of the suspension (S) and of the suspending medium (M) are measured as functions of volume filtered.

Bottom left: The relative conductance of the filter (ratio S/M), as plotted against the volume filtered, shows the extent of progressive filter clogging. From this curve, the initial S/M ratio can be calculated by extrapolation to zero volume ($t = 0$). Pressure head (p) remains constant throughout the test.

Top centre: in constant flow systems, pressures generated by the constant flow pump are plotted against the volume filtered, both for the suspending medium (MP) and suspension (SP).

Bottom centre: filter conductance is calculated by the ratio of the pressure heads at any volume filtered (MP/SP). The filter conductance is measured in such systems at gradually increasing pressure heads (p), resulting in possible unclogging of the filter. Initial MP/SP ratio can be extrapolated to $t = 0$ from this curve.

Top right: in a variable pressure head – variable flow rate system the changing pressure heads (MP,SP) and filtered volumes (MV, SV) of suspending medium and suspension are recorded as functions of time. This results in curves which are difficult to analyse. However, in most systems the pressure head decreases as a linear function of volume filtered, therefore plotting filtration rates against filtered volumes simplifies the picture.

Bottom right: filter conductance can be calculated as the ratio of filtration rates of suspending medium ($Fm = \Delta MV/\Delta t$) and suspension ($Fs = \Delta SV/\Delta t$) measured at respective filtered volumes ($=$ identical pressure heads). In such systems filter conductance (Fs/Fm) is determined under a continuously decreasing pressure head (p), resulting in more progressive filter blockage, as compared to constant pressure head systems. The initial Fs/Fm ratio can be calculated by extrapolating the curve to $t = 0$.

The *St. George's Filtrometer* applies constant pressure head and vertically positioned filter [95]. In this microcomputer-controlled equipment, the filtration rate is measured in three subsequent steps (23 μl each) at the beginning of the filtration. This procedure allows quantification of initial filter clogging, and extrapolation to the initial filtration rate. Filtration of 1 ml suspension is also possible, to measure low concentrations of filter-blocking particles. Using this machine, initial filtration rate and clogging rate can be measured, even if pore clogging is present. Manufacturer: Carri-Med Ltd., Vincent Lane, Dorking, Surrey RH4 3Y1, England. Price US$ 4,000.

The *SEFAM Erythrometer* [96] is a microcomputer-controlled, automatized instrument, applying the constant flow principle. It measures first the constant pressure generated when buffer is filtered (PI). Thereafter cell suspension (hematocrit = 0.005) is filtered (5 ml/min flow rate), resulting in a gradual build-up of pressure head. The final pressure after 3 minutes (PF) is recorded. Deformability index is calculated as the ratio PF/PI. This machine cannot measure initial filtration rate necessary to calculate red cell deformability parameters. Manufacturer: SEFAM, B.P. 511, 54008 Nancy Cedex, France. Price US$ 4,000.

2.4. Rheology of normal blood

The flow properties of blood are determined by hematocrit, plasma viscosity, red cell aggregation and deformability [34,36,97-99]. The rheology of a normal subject's blood varies with shear stress (or shear rate), and is mainly determined by plasma viscosity and hematocrit at high shear rates. Red cell aggregability plays a significant role in low shear flow. In normal concentrations, white blood cells have very little effect on bulk viscosity, which is in sharp contrast to the major effects they can have in the microcirculation, or in filtration tests. Chapter 2 discusses red cell aggregation and deformability in detail.

2.4.1. Shear dependence

Fig. 2.16 illustrates the flow of blood under steady flow conditions, and shows the reduction in viscosity following a rise in shear-stress or in shear-rate. The straight lines are for two Newtonian liquids, water (W), and an oil of 10 mPas viscosity (X). On such a plot, all Newtonian liquids give straight lines through the origin. Their slope is equal to the viscosity. Since shear rate is in s^{-1}, then if shear stress is in mPa, the slope is in mPas, and is the viscosity in these units. The flow-curve of blood (B) becomes increasingly linear as the stress increases, but it is seen to descend more steeply as the origin is approached. Thus the viscosity and the degree of shear sensitivity (non-Newtonian behavior) both increase as the shear stress is reduced. The flow curve of blood will intersect the line for oil at a

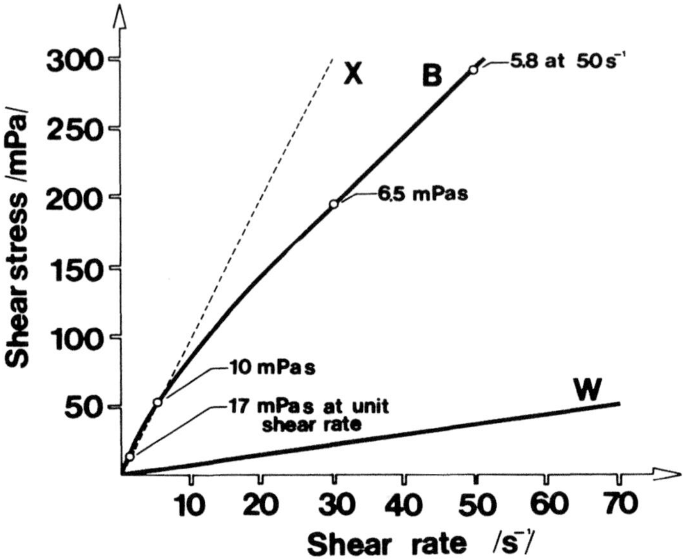

Figure 2.16. Flow curve for a normal blood at 37°C. Hematocrit = 0.40, plasma viscosity = 1.30 mPas. Straight lines are for Newtonian liquids, water (*W*) and an oil of 10 mPas viscosity (*X*).

finite value of stress. At shear stresses lower than this point, the blood will be more viscous than the oil. In the example shown, the intersection is at about 51 mPa (shear rate about 5.1 s^{-1}). At 1 s^{-1} shear rate, the viscosity has risen to about 17 mPas. That the curve (*B*) is convex upwards is of general and indeed fundamental interest: it signifies that the rheologic response of whole blood to increasing shear is a fall in viscosity (reduced *shear stress/shear rate* ratio). This property must be common to all systems depending for life upon the circulation of deformable corpuscles. It is difficult to visualise a conservative system in which the non-Newtonianism worked in the opposite direction: an increase in cardiac effort meeting with an increase in viscosity.

In clinical hemorheological literature, the blood viscosity (ratio $\tau/\dot{\gamma}$) is frequently used to display the rheological properties of blood [100]. Viscosity can be plotted as a function of shear stress (Fig. 2.17a), or of shear rate (Fig. 2.17b). The latter presentation may be misleading, because it disproportionally extends the low shear part of the curve. In fact, there is probably little significance in debating blood viscosity at shear rates under 0.1 s^{-1}, since it represents virtually no flow in most circumstances: what is significant is the shear stress required to re-establish flow after stasis. It has not yet been rigorously established how realistic viscosities at shear rates of less than 1 s^{-1} may be. In any event, at an order of magnitude lower, virtually no flow is taking place in small vessels, as the following calculation shows.

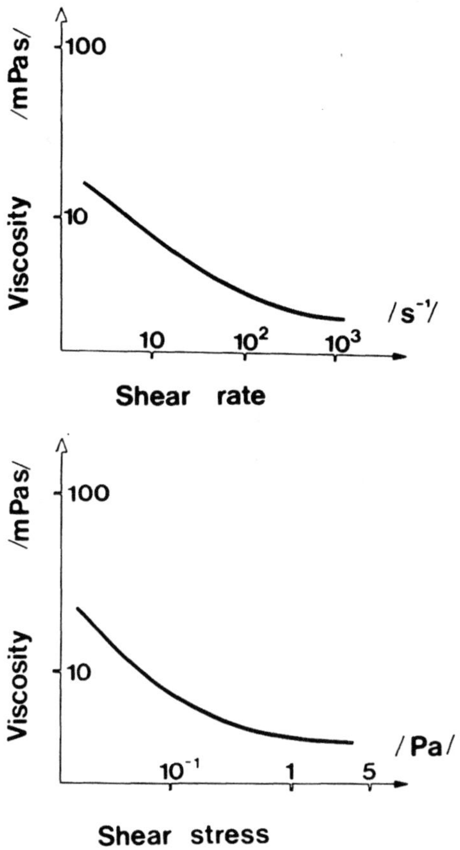

Figure 2.17. Viscosity of a normal blood sample. Anticoagulation with heparin, measuring temperature 37°C, hematocrit 0.44, and plasma viscosity 1.17 mPas.
Upper plot: viscosity as a function of shear rate
Lower plot: viscosity as a function of shear stress

In streamline flow of a Newtonian liquid in a circular tube, the ratio *mean velocity/tube radius* is equal to $\dot{\gamma}_w/4$, where $\dot{\gamma}_w$ is the rate of shear at the wall of the tube. Hence $\dot{\gamma}_w = 0.1\ s^{-1}$ represents flow rates of 0.0125 mm/s (0.75 mm/min) and 0.125 μ/s (7.5 μ/min) in tubes of 1 mm and 10 μm diameter, respectively. These are physiologically-insignificant velocities. The degree of approximation involved in applying this calculation to blood, depends upon the transverse distribution of velocity in the tube, but in the case of non-Newtonian velocity-profiles, the real flow-rate will be even less than the one calculated above.

In contrast to this, the lower end of the shear stress – viscosity plot can have an important meaning, by showing the presence of yield stress: the shear stress

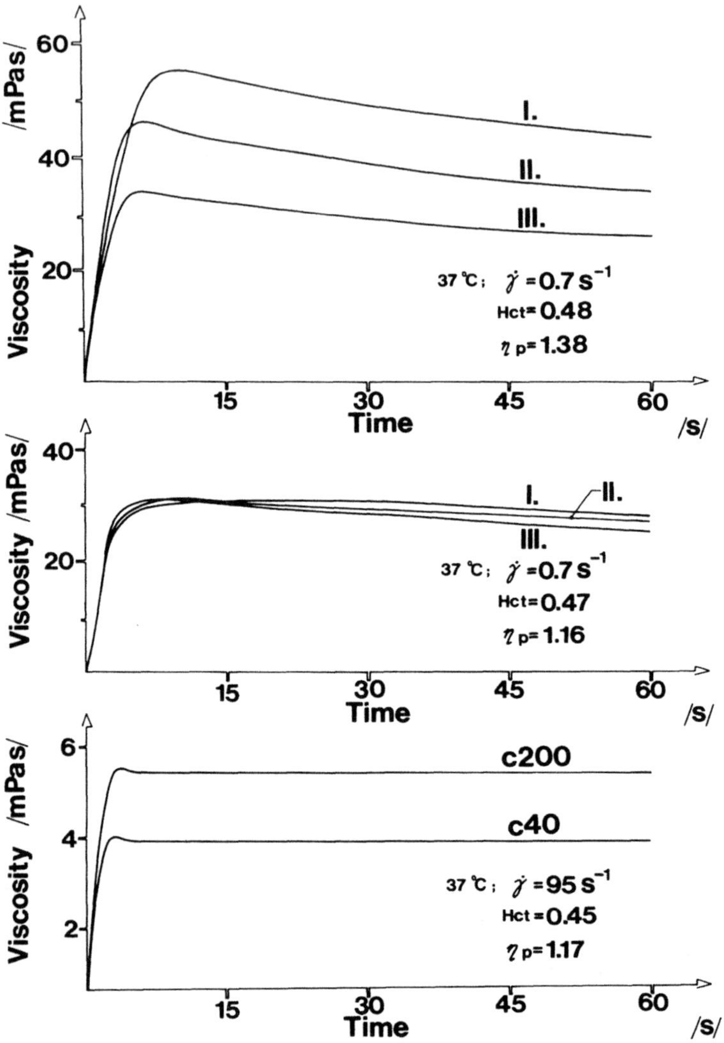

Figure 2.18. Whole blood viscosity at 37°C, plotted as function of time. Shear rate of 0.7 s^{-1} is applied in a Contraves LS-30 viscometer.
Upper plot: Heart infarction patient's blood (hematocrit = 0.48, plasma viscosity = 1.38 mPas), measured in a viscometer which was started rotating immediately after disaggregation (I), 2 min (II) and 4 min (III) later. Viscosity was high in disaggregated state, but decreased with aggregation.
Middle plot: Normal blood (hematocrit = 0.47, plasma viscosity = 1.16 mPas), curves I, II and III measured as above. Viscosity was lower and showed little change with aggregation.
Bottom plot: Washed red cells suspended in two solutions of equal viscosity (1.17 mPas): dextran 40 was added to phosphate buffer for the c40 curve, and dextran 200 added to phosphate buffer for the c200 curve. Shear rate was 95 s^{-1} and therefore no aggregation occured and viscosity did not change with time. However, suspension viscosity was higher by 38% in the presence of dextran 200, which causes aggregation at low shear.

required to initiate flow. Measurement of yield stress is only possible with controlled shear stress viscometers, and there is no routine method available for this test [48]. Moreover, the presence of a true yield stress is debatable. Nevertheless, a finite shear stress is needed to get physiologically meaningful flows.

Blood viscosity is high at low shear, where red cells aggregate, and remarkably low at high shear where red cells participate in flow by elongation, orientation and deformation [99,101]. One adaptation of red cells to flow has been also described as *tank treading*. This is the rotation of membrane around the cell interior, under high shear stress [102,103].

The contribution of red cell aggregation to low-shear blood viscosity is complex. Viscosity of a given blood sample decreases as aggregation proceeds; but blood samples with high aggregability show higher viscosity even in their aggregated state. This is demonstrated in Fig. 2.18a, where viscosity of a blood sample with high aggregability shows marked time-dependence. In contrast to this, the viscosity of normal blood with little aggregation tendency hardly changes with time (Fig. 2.18b). Fig. 2.18c demonstrates that aggregability of red cells also influences blood viscosity at high shear rates, when no cell aggregates are present. An interesting consequence of the phenomena illustrated in Fig. 2.18 is, that control of shearing history of the samples is crucially important in low shear viscosimetry [104]. Without this, aggregated samples of patients can provide viscometric readings equal to that of normal samples. This systematic error can result in faulty conclusions, e.g. when using ramp viscometry (automatic scanning of a wide shear rate range) in clinical hemorheological studies.

Several equations have been published to describe the flow curve or shear rate – viscosity curves of blood [e.g. 105,106], but they have not yet found much clinical use.

2.4.2. Plasma viscosity

The viscosity of plasma is determined by its dissolved macromolecular components and its primary component, water. The contribution of individual protein fractions is related to the mass and shape of the molecules. Fibrinogen, a large and elongated molecule, has a strong effect on plasma viscosity; smaller globular molecules, such as albumin are of less significance. Fig. 2.19 shows the relationship between concentration and viscosity of some protein solutions, in the physiologic concentration range. Albumin solution has a flat viscosity – concentration curve, whereas the viscosity of a fibrinogen solution rises steeply with increasing concentration. The effect of different protein fractions on plasma viscosity has been studied, and good correlations were found between concentrations of high molecular weight proteins and plasma viscosity [107,108]. However, human plasma is a remarkably concentrated protein solution (about 70 g/l). In this range weak protein-protein interactions, not reflected by electrophoresis tests

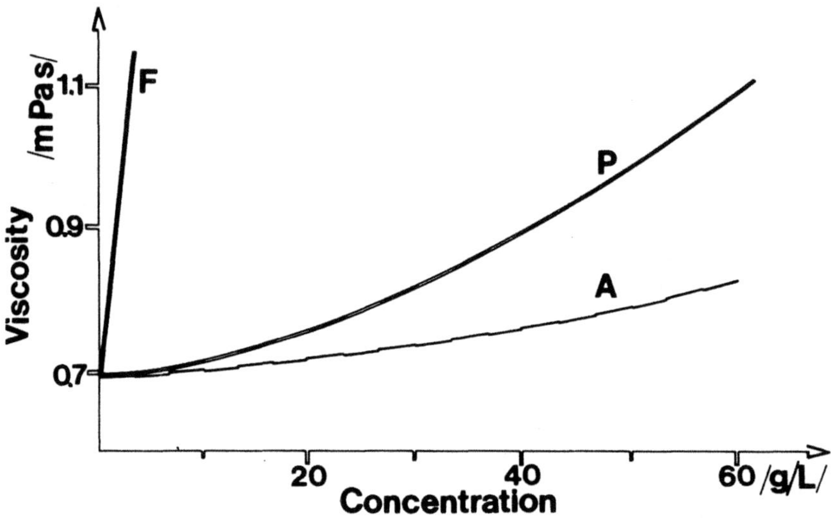

Figure 2.19. Viscosity of protein solutions plotted against concentration as measured at 37°C in a Harkness viscometer. *A*: with albumin in buffer; *P*: plasma diluted with buffer; *F*: with fibrinogen in buffer.

because of high dilution, could also have important effects, especially in pathologic samples.

The normal range of plasma viscosity is between 1.10 and 1.35 mPas at 37°C. Plasma viscosity appears to be statistically independent of age and sex, and shows only small intra-individual variation [107-111]. The value of "average normal" depends on the selection criteria for a normal or healthy group of subjects. Lower values were found in athletes than in sedentary subjects [111-112], and higher values were found in healthy subjects with positive cardiovascular risk factors [113,114]. Fig. 2.20 shows plasma viscosity distributions in 3 different groups, all measured in a Harkness viscometer at 37°C. Randomly-choosen non-hospitalized subjects (age 35–65) had a plasma viscosity range between 1.05 and 1.55 mPas (Fig. 2.20a). Young, healthy subjects (age 18–35) showed a scatter between 1.06–1.23 mPas (Fig. 2.20b). Patients with no acute disease (hospitalized for hernia or varicose vein operations, age 25–65 years) had a wider distribution, between 1.19 and 1.46 mPas (Fig. 2.20c). Individual stability of plasma viscosity is demonstrated in Fig. 2.21, summarizing several tests carried out on 2 subjects during one year.

Plasma viscosity of patients can increase up to 5–6 mPas in paraproteinemias, or to 1.5–2.0 mPas in other diseases [107]. Serum viscosity is lower than plasma viscosity, usually by 0.10–0.15 mPas, owing to the fibrinogen extraction. Fig. 2.20b shows serum and plasma viscosity-distributions in a group of healthy subjects.

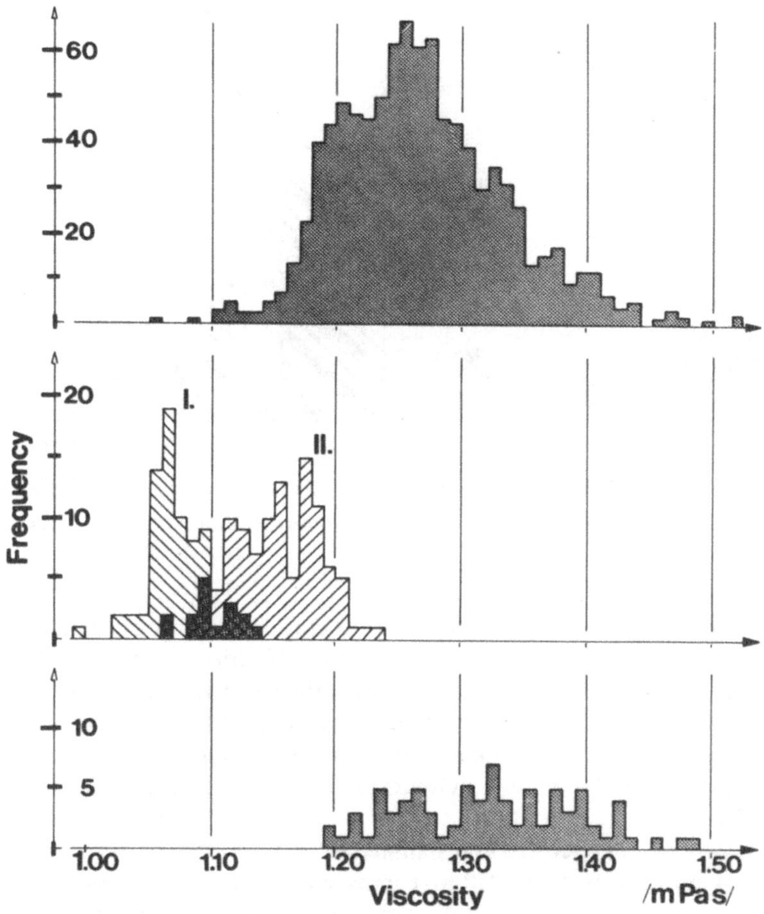

Figure 2.20. Plasma viscosity histograms.
Top: random-sampled, non-hospitalized subjects, age 35–65, N = 2000, 50% females.
Middle: healthy subjects, without any acute or chronic disease, age 16–36, n = 105, 51% females. I: serum viscosity, II: plasma viscosity.
Bottom: Hernia and varicous vein patients, with no acute disease, age 22–65, N = 82, 61% females.

2.4.3. Effect of hematocrit

The rheological properties of suspensions depend strongly on the concentration of the suspended particles present. In the case of blood, this relationship is well approximated by an exponential function: the logarithm of viscosity of red cell suspension is proportional to the hematocrit [34,36,97-99,110]:

$$\log \eta = k + k'Hct \tag{34}$$

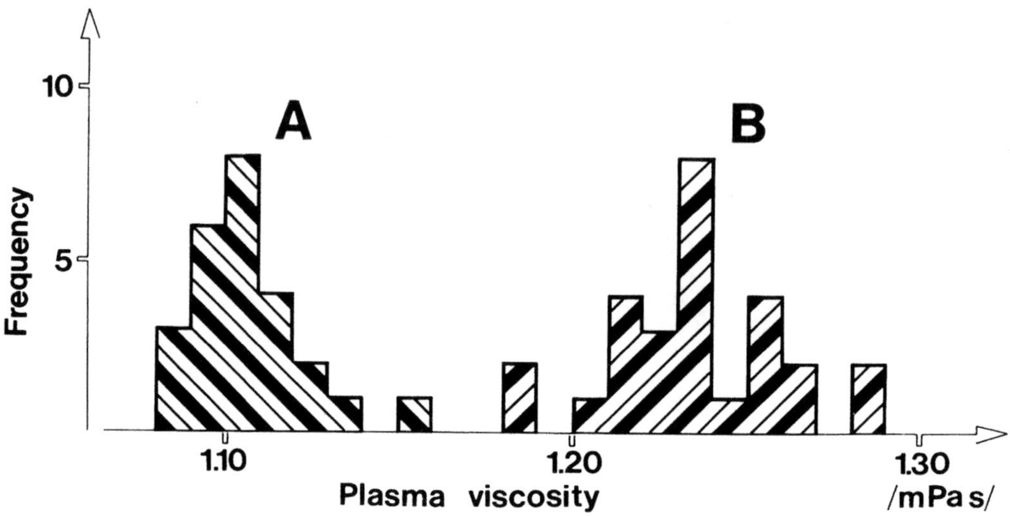

Figure 2.21. Individual stability of plasma viscosity. Subjects *A* and *B* were measured 25 and 27 times within 12 months.

where *Hct* is the suspension hematocrit, k and k' are constants for a particular blood sample. However, k and k' show considerable variation with plasma viscosity, cell aggregability, cell deformability, and with the shear imposed during the test. The first constant, k, is usually the logarithm of the plasma viscosity. The second constant, k', can be replaced by $A/f(\dot{\gamma})$; where A is a dimensionless characteristic of the sample, and $f(\dot{\gamma})$ is a defined function of the shear rate and shear-sensitivity [106].

If curves are fitted to blood-viscosity and hematocrit data of different groups of test persons, the parameters of the fitted curves can have rather different values [115]. This is merely an expression of the obvious fact that different bloods have different plasma-viscosities and different shear-sensitivities. Fig. 2.22a and 2.22b show viscosities of reconstituted normal and pathologic blood samples at various hematocrits, measured at two shear rates. The relationship between hematocrit and blood viscosity (Equation 34) makes it possible to compare intrinsic rheological properties of two blood samples of different hematocrits, by calculating blood viscosity at a standard hematocrit (see Section 2.6).

2.5. Blood sampling and handling in hemorheological tests

The mechanical properties of blood are sensitive to almost any change of blood composition, in some respects even more than in biochemical tests. Special care should be taken to prevent evaporation of water and consequent concentration of

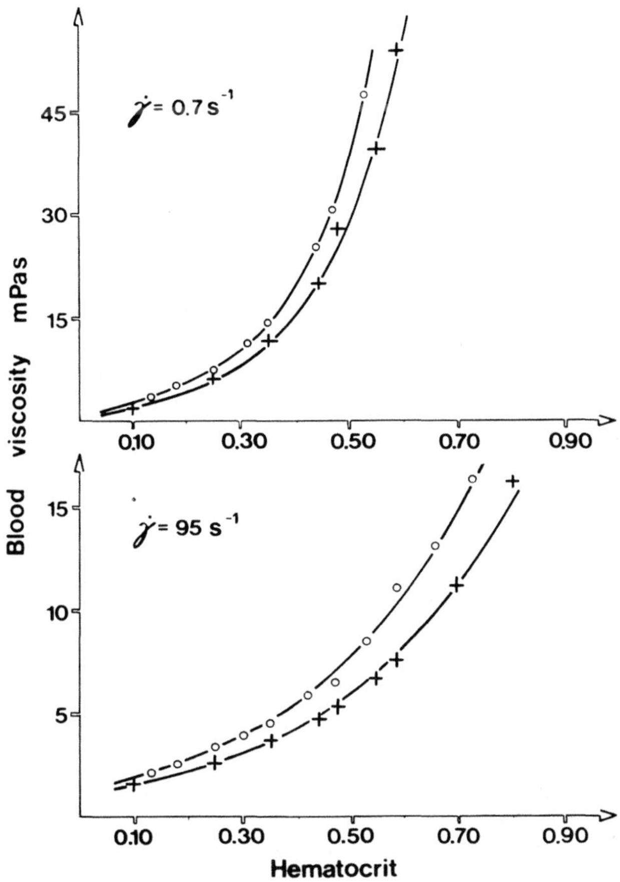

Figure 2.22. Hematocrit – viscosity relationships. + : a healthy subject, plasma viscosity 1.16 mPas; o: heart-infarction patient, plasma viscosity 1.53 mPas. Reconstituted samples measured at shear rates 0.7 s^{-1} (upper plot) and 95 s^{-1} (lower plot). Measurements were carried out in a Contraves LS-30 at 37°C. Semilogarithmic regression curves were fitted to each set of samples as shown by the curves.

the samples. In some extent, rheological properties of the blood samples depend also on the circumstances of venepuncture.

2.5.1. Postural changes

When a person moves from horizontal to vertical position, about 500 ml blood shifts into the leg veins, at the same time increasing capillary pressures, resulting in loss of fluid and small molecules into the interstitial space [116-119]. As a

Table 2.4. Effect of posture on blood composition in 10 healthy male subjects.

Blood taken from antecubital veins after 15 minutes spent	Standing	Sitting	Supine
Hematocrit	48 ±3	47 ±3	45 ±2
Plasma viscosity (mPas)	1.17±0.06	1.16±0.05	1.14±0.04
Blood viscosity at 0.7 s^{-1} (mPas)	29.2 ±5.2	26.8 ±6.1	22.7 ±4.8
Blood viscosity at 95 s^{-1} (mPas)	5.1 ±0.4	4.8 ±0.4	4.4 ±0.2

consequence, there is increased hematocrit and plasma protein concentration in the circulating blood volume and therefore increased whole blood and plasma viscosity [120]. As shown in Table 2.4, hemoconcentration occurs also in sitting. This postural source of variation can be largely eliminated, if each patient rests in a supine position for 10–15 minutes before blood collection.

2.5.2. Venous occlusion

Venepuncture can be a source of significant error if cellular or protein-bound blood components are to be determined [121-123], becuse of hemoconcentration due to prolonged occlusion. There are large individual differences in accessibility of veins and skill of venepuncturists, resulting in variable occlusion-times and pressures during blood sampling. As Table 2.5 shows, even a low occlusion pressure of 2 min duration can alter hemorheological parameters; but if the vein is freely perfused for 1 min (with siliconised cannula left in situ), the values return to baseline. Such artifacts, can be minimized by using inflatable cuffs at 40 mmHg on the upper arm, and No. 19 or 21 size siliconized cannulas to obtain blood from the antecubital veins. If longer occlusion time than 15 s, or higher occlusion pressure is necessary, the occlusion should be released for 1 min before blood withdrawal.

2.5.3. Diurnal, seasonal and climatic variations

Various circadian changes of several body functions have been described in the literature [124]. Diurnal periodicity of blood viscoity has been also observed

Table 2.5. Blood composition and venous occlusion in 10 healthy males, after 15 min lying supine.

Occlusion (40 mmHg cuff)	< 5 s	120 s	60 s relase after 120 s occlusion
Hematocrit	44 ±2	46 ±3	44 ±2
Plasma viscosity (mPas)	1.12±0.03	1.15±0.07	1.13±0.04
Blood viscosity at 0.7 s^{-1} (mPas)	23.4 ±2.2	26.5 ±4.4	24.1 ±2.7
Blood viscosity at 95 s^{-1} (mPas)	4.5 ±0.2	4.9 ±0.4	4.4 ±0.3

[35,125]. In a recent study, using small-volume specimens, no regular pattern of diurnal change was found [126]. Periodic variation of blood viscosity related to the menstrual cycle of women has been reported [127], but another study showed no such relationship [42].

Seasonal and climatic variations are probably related to plasma-volume changes [99]; but these factors have rarely been studied [128].

2.5.4. Anticoagulation and storage

Anticoagulation agents change blood viscosity if accompanied by dilution, [36,97,129,130]. The most frequently used agents are heparin (10–15 IU/ml) and EDTA (1.5 mg/ml). It is important to mix blood with anticoagulant as soon as possible to prevent microclot formation, which can easily upset viscometry. It is also advisable to carry out hemorheological tests not more than 1-2 hours after blood withdrawal. Filterability and erythrocyte aggregation tend to decrease after 2 hrs storage [60,83,131]. In the case of red cell aggregation, the mechanism of this phenomenon is not known. Filterability of heparin – anticoagulated blood deteriorates because of the effect of this anticoagulant on the leukocytes [83]. Whole blood viscosity begins to change after 4-6 hrs [132-134], but the direction of change is unpredictable. If delays between venepuncture and viscometry exceed 4-6 hours, EDTA-blood stored at 4°C yields the best results [134,135]. Plasma viscosity remains constant for several days, if blood is centrifuged and plasma kept separated at room temperature [107].

2.6. Clinical interpretation of hemorheological data

2.6.1. Plasma viscosity

Plasma viscosity can be measured with great accuracy and has remarkable individual stability [109]. Therefore, even small variations may be of pathological significance. It has long been known that plasma viscosity changes characteristically in several pathological conditions. In 1942, the substitution of a plasma viscosity test for the ubiquitous erythrocyte sedimentation rate was proposed [136].

Insofar as plasma is a Newtonian fluid, plasma viscosity does not depend on flow conditions applied or type of equipment used. However, comparison of different studies utilizing different methods is sometimes difficult. Plasma viscosity results obtained by rotational viscometers are often higher than those measured by tube viscometers, and sometimes non-Newtonian behavior is reported. Rotational viscometers are more sensitive to artifacts due to surface adsorbed proteins, resulting in spuriously high torque readings, especially at low shear. At higher shear rates instability of flow can occur, due to low viscosity, also causing higher readings. To avoid these errors, if a rotational viscometer is used, constancy of the torque/shear ratio with water or another low viscosity standard should be checked, and the highest shear within the linear range should be applied. Tube viscometers are preferable for plasma viscosity studies.

2.6.2. Blood viscosity

The rheological properties of a complex fluid, such as blood, can be described in many different ways, as indeed they are in the clinical hemorheological literature. This often makes comparison of results obtained by different researchers difficult.

Whole blood viscosity at specified shear rates
The most frequently used parameter is blood viscosity at a defined shear rate. Unfortunately, most research groups use different shear rates and viscometers: hence the direct comparison of data is not possible. Blood viscosity at high shear ($\dot{\gamma} > 50\ s^{-1}$ or $\tau > 0.25$ Pa) is mainly determined by hematocrit. The contribution of cell aggregability increases with diminishing shear, and it is the major viscosity determinant at low shear ($\dot{\gamma} < 1\ s^{-1}$ or $\tau < 0.02$ Pa). Testing at lower shear rates results in more specificity for aggregability, but also in disproportionate increase of technical difficulties and artifacts, without providing additional information.

As discussed in Chapter 4, in-vivo shear stresses are usually high in most vascular segments, suggesting that probably high-shear blood viscosity plays the major role in determining vascular resistance. However, at low shear, there are larger differences between controls and patients affected by many different diseases related to microcirculatory disfunction.

It is known that surface-adsorbed macromolecules, mainly fibrinogen, determine low-shear blood viscosity [36,97-99,137]. At the same time, probably, similar macromolecules build up the endoendothelial layer [138], determining interactions between blood cells and vessel wall. Therefore, increased low shear viscosity (and also red cell aggregability) can possibly be related to the pathological changes of the endoendothelial lining [139-141]. Such a connection could have considerable significance, because blood rheology can be studied ex vivo, whereas endothelial surface phenomena are presently not accessible to non-invasive diagnostic tools.

Whole blood viscosity at specified shear stress
A rarely-discussed consequence of measuring blood viscosity at a defined standard shear rate is that samples with higher viscosity are tested at proportionally higher shear stresses, apparently decreasing or masking part of the difference

between low and high viscosity samples and also between normal and pathological samples [143]. This measuring artifact can be avoided by measuring blood viscosity at defined shear stresses, either by using a controlled shear stress viscometer, or by interpolating the data obtained with a controlled shear rate machine. Furthermore, blood viscosity at standard shear stress is a closer reflection of the in-vivo consequences of blood rheology variations, since perfusion is due to a given pressure head in any flow system, rather than a prescribed shear rate.

Flow-curve plotting

Some sophisticated viscometers can automatically determine a portion of a flow curve. This procedure is also called ramp viscometry: the viscometer automatically scans a range of shear rates, and plots the measured shear stress or viscosity as a function of shear rate. In the case of blood, the interpretation of such curves is rather difficult, as the shearing history of the sample is different at each segment of the curve recorded. This can result in spuriously high or low readings in samples with fast sedimentation or high aggregability, respectively. In other words, results at a particular shear obtained from such a plot may not be comparable to results obtained if the sample is only exposed to that single shear rate. This effect is also related to thixotropy and is dependent on the measuring-system geometry (see Sections 2.2.5 and 2.4.1).

Apparent viscosity measured in tube viscometers

With the introduction of sophisticated rotational viscometers, tube viscometry of blood cell suspensions was largely discredited and neglected, because the shear rate profile in a tube depends on sample properties, and cannot be determined directly. One can argue however, that blood in vivo also flows in tubes, not at a constant shear rate. In addition, flow conditions (shear stress) in a tube are well defined by geometry and pressure head, and are not related to sample properties.

Tube viscometers are simpler, more accurate and cheaper than rotational machines. Therefore, they are better suited to routine clinical use, especially, if only high shear viscosity is to be measured, in which case this technique is subject to fewer artifacts. Application of tube viscometers of 0.5 mm or larger internal diameter is advisable in clinical studies, where the contribution of bulk blood rheology to vascular resistance is investigated, e.g. neonatal and adult polycythemia or paraproteinemias. In narrower tubes, the Fahreus-Lindquist effect may have some influence.

Relative viscosity

Relative viscosity is defined as the ratio of suspension viscosity to suspending-medium viscosity, and is an important parameter in rheological studies. It is an indicator of the properties of the suspended particles at fixed particle concentration. In clinical hemorheology, however, plasma viscosity and hematocrit are also variable, and these complex changes are not always correctly reflected by the relative viscosity alone. In pathological blood samples plasma viscosity and cell-aggregability increase in parallel, resulting in unchanged or even decreased relative viscosity.

Blood viscosity at standard hematocrit

Red cell concentration is the main determinant of bulk blood viscosity. Therefore, evaluation of other determinants requires elimination of hematocrit effects. This can be achieved by reconstituting and measuring blood samples at a standard hematocrit, or by calculation from the viscosity at the measured hematocrit. In the latter case application of the appropriate mathematical model is important. It has been shown that there is a linear relationship between the logarithm of blood viscosity, at a given shear rate, and the hematocrit [34,36,45,98,99]. Because the constants of this relation show significant individual variation, it is advisable to determine them individually, from the plasma viscosity and whole blood relative viscosity at the measured hematocrit. Probably the best and simplest method to achieve this is by the use of the following

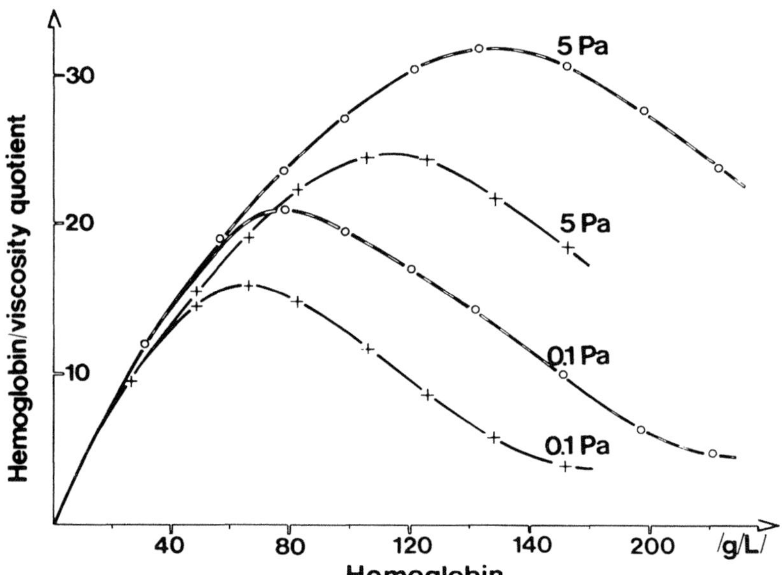

Figure 2.23. Hemoglobin/whole blood viscosity quotients. Blood viscosities were measured at 0.1 and 5 Pa shear stresses with a Carri-Med controlled shear stress rheometer. Reconstituted blood samples of a healthy control, plasma viscosity 1.18 mPas, hemoglobin 170 g/l (*o*); and of a treated myeloma patient, plasma viscosity 1.62, hemoglobin 103 g/l (+). Optimal hemoglobin concentration for oxygen transport varies with shear stress and blood properties. At low shear and deteriorated blood rheology, lower hemoglobin concentration could be beneficial.

equation:

$$\eta_{rel(45)} = [\eta_{rel(Hct)}]^{45/Hc} \tag{35}$$

wherē η_{rel} is the viscosity of blood relative to that of plasma (η/η_p). Here, 0.45 and Hct represent the standard and native hematocrits [144].

Hemoglobin / viscosity quotient
As discussed in Chapter 5, the oxygen-transport capacity of blood in the circulation is determined by its hemoglobin content and viscosity. These two variables can be combined in a clinically useful single parameter, the hemoglobin concentration/blood viscosity quotient, H/V [115,145]. Of course, the same applies to the *hematocrit/viscosity ratio*, although it is a less direct parameter, because the hemoglobin concentration of the red cells varies. Fig. 2.23 shows H/V as a function of hemoglobin concentration in control and myeloma samples. The shape and peak value of any H/V curve depends on plasma viscosity [146], red cell deformability and aggregability. It is a clinically important fact that optimal hemoglobin concentration of a given blood varies with flow conditions [99,145].

2.6.3. Blood filtration

Blood filtration is now one of the most frequently used hemorheological tests, and is sometimes regarded as a measure of red-cell deformability. However, there are many other factors also involved in most versions of this test, as explained in Section 2.3.2 above.

One can analyse this by considering the number of cells per pore in the volume filtered as an indication of possibilities of pore plugging. If only a few red cells have to negotiate each pore before the measurement is completed, the results reflect the properties of average red cells. This is the case when 0.5–1 μl of whole blood, or 10–20 μl of white-cell-depleted, diluted blood (hematocrit 0.05–0.1) is filtered through a Nuclepore filter of 13 mm diameter. If 1000 or more red cells have to travel through each pore to obtain a blood filtration result, the test is more sensitive to small, stiff subpopulations of blood cells, such as pathological red cells or leukocytes. This is the case, if 50 μl of whole blood or 500 μl of buffy-coat-depleted, diluted blood is filtered without special precautions to eliminate leukocytes. Cell-cell interactions can also influence blood filtration results, if the hematocrit is higher than 0.20–0.25 [147]. Filter-cell interactions are also of possible significance. Adherence of cells to the filter can cause plugging.

Recent data [92,95,148,149], obtained by methods eliminating filter-clogging effects, suggest that there is only a small (10% or less) difference between pore transit-times of red cells when controls and vascular or diabetic patients are compared. However, these studies apply shear stresses as high or higher than the upper limit of shear occuring in the normal circulation (5–20 Pa). To verify relative red cell rigidity as a cause of microcirculatory disturbances, requires studies applying shear stresses at least 10 times lower than those applied in presently-used filtration systems.

Nevertheless, blood filtration experiments have provided results of considerable clinical relevance. In addition, this is presently the only routine technique to study flow properties of blood under mechanical conditions with at least some similarity to the microcirculation. The changing interpretation, emphasizing leukocyte rheology rather than red cell deformability in non-hematological disorders, will probably widen the application of blood filtration in pathology and pharmacology.

2.6.4. Optical aggregometry and erythrocyte sedimentation rate

Red cell aggregation data, as measured by optical aggregometry (RCA), and sedimentation rate (ESR) are related to each other. Both tests reflect aggregation due to net attractive forces between red cells. Experimental results obtained with citrated blood (1:4 dilution) show strong correlation between the two tests, if samples are in a narrow hematocrit range (Fig. 2.24). However, correlation is

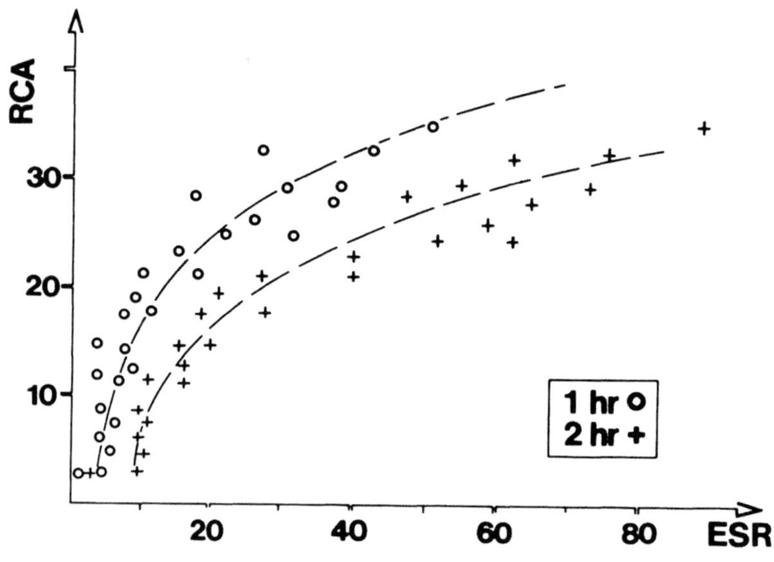

Figure 2.24. Correlation between red cell aggregation (Myrenne aggregometer) and erythrocyte sedimentation rate (Westergreen, after 1 and 2 hrs). Blood samples diluted with Na-citrate (1:4); diluted hematocrit range 0.30–0.35; diluted plasma viscosity range 0.98–1.15 mPas.

absent, if measuring blood anticoagulated with EDTA or heparin for RCA, and citrated blood for ESR [57,60]. Hematocrit variations have a large impact both on ESR and RCA: samples with low red cell concentration give spuriously high readings, whereas both tests are less sensitive to aggregation in samples with high hematocrit.

In general, ESR and plasma-viscosity tend to move in the same direction in pathological conditions; but this is an indirect relationship: the macromolecules causing increased plasma viscosity, also cause increased aggregation, and the larger aggregates sediment faster. The higher viscosity of the suspending medium itself, reduces sedimentation. Similarly, increased plasma viscosity, per se, slows-down red cell movement and decreases RCA test readings.

These tests are most valuable in studies where the viscosity of the suspending medium as well as suspension concentration are controlled and red cell aggregation is the only variable. In clinical studies, more-complex changes may be present and in some cases they can have opposite effects: e.g. patients with vascular disease have elevated hematocrit, plasma viscosity and red cell aggregability. Then RCA or ESR can be in the normal range. In contrast, therapeutic improvement of red cell aggregation, if associated with a drop of hematocrit, can result in increased RCA and ESR values.

Because of the more complex relations, transformation of measured data to a standard hematocrit is more difficult in these techniques than in blood viscometry and has not yet been developed to a point of clinical utility. Alternatively, reconstituted samples can be measured. If hematocrit and plasma viscosity are held constant, then differences in RCA or ESR can solely be interpreted as changes in red cell properties.

2.7. References

1. Fung, Y. C. 1981. Biomechanics: Mechanical Properties of Living Tissues. Springer, New York.
2. Darby, R. 1976. Viscoelastic Fluids. Marcel-Dekker, Inc. New York.
3. Flugge, W. 1967. Viscoelasticity. Blaisdell Publishing Co. Waltham, Mass.
4. Copley, A.L. and King, R.G. 1984. A survey of surface hemorheological experiments on the inhibition of fibrinogenin formation employing surface layers of fibrinogen systems with heparin and other substances. A contribution on antithrombogenic action. Thrombosis Research, 35. 237-256.
5. Blank, M. 1983. Membrane proteins in monolayers, multilayers and membranes. Ann. N. Y. Acad. Sci. 416, 128-137.
6. Matrai, A., Warburton, B. and Dormandy, J. 1984. Surface rheological observations on human plasma. Biorheology, Suppl. I; 103-105.
7. Poiseuille, J.L.M. 1840. Recherches experimentales sur le mouvement des liquides dans les tubes de tres petits diametres. Compt. Rend. 11, 961-967.
8. Merrill, E.W., Gilliland, E.R., Cokelet, G.R., Shin, H. and Wells, R.E. 1963. Rheology of human blood near and at zero flow – effects of temperature and hematocrit level. Biophys. J. 3. 199-213.
9. Whittington R.B. and Harkness J. 1968. Viscosity – temperature variations in human blood and plasma. Biorheology 5, 252.

10. Hardy, R.C. 1966. NBS viscometer calibrating liquids and capillary tube viscometers. NBS monograph 55.
11. Krieger, I.M. and Maron, S.H. 1951. Direct determination of the flow curves on non-Newtonian fluids. J. Appl. Physics 23. 147-149.
12. Cerny, L.C., Cook, F.W. and Walker, C.C. 1962. Rheology of blood. Am. J. Physiol. 202, 1188-1194.
13. Benis, A.M. 1968. A new simple low-shear capillary viscometer for blood. Biorheology 5. 263-270.
14. Walawender, W.P., Chen, T.Y. and Cala, D.F. 1975. An approximate Casson fluid model for tube flow of blood. Biorheol. 12, 111-119.
15. Matrai, A., Fendler, K. and Lissak, K. 1977. Sorozatmeresre alkalmas kapillaris mikroviszkozimeter. Kis. Orvostud. 29. 200-207.
16. Oka, S. 1960. The principles of rheometry. pp. 18-82. in Rheology Vol. III. Eirich, F.R. (ed.), Academic Press, New York.
17. Dinsdale, A. and Moore, F. 1962. Viscosity and its measurement. Chapman and Hall, London.
18. Jacobs, H.R. 1966. Meniscal Resistance in tube viscometry. Biorheol. 3. 117-140.
19. Mardles, E.W.J. 1969. The flow of liquids through fine capillaries and narrow channels: the meniscus resistance (Jamin-effect). Biorheol. 6. 1-10.
20. Harkness, J. 1963. A new instrument for the measurement of plasma viscosity. Lancet 2, 280-284.
21. Eastham, R.D. and Morgan, M. H. 1965. Plasma viscosity in clinical laboratory practice. J. Med. Lab. Tech. 22. 70-73.
22. Harris, G.J. 1972. Plasma viscometry and ESR in the elderly. Med. Lab. Technol. 29. 405-410.
23. Matrai, A., E. Ernst, P.T. Flute and J.A. Dormandy. 1984. Blood filterability in peripheral vascular disease – red cell deformability or cell sticking? Clin. Hemorheol. 4, 311-325.
24. Ernst, E., Matrai, A. Scherer, A. Schmidlechner, Ch. and Monshausen, Ch. 1985. Methodological and intra-individual variations in rheologically relevant blood tests. Clin. Hemorheol. 5, 511-514.
25. Matrai, A. and Ernst, E. 1985. Measurement of plasma viscosity – Comparison of four viscometers. Pediatric Research Societies in Europe, 2nd Joint Meeting, Munich, October 14-17.
26. Wintrobe M.M. 1981. (ed.) Clinical Hematology. Lea & Fibiger, Philadelphia.
27. Chmiel H, Anadere I, Walitza E, Witte S. 1983. The measurement of density and its significance in blood rheology. Biorheology 20, 685-696.
28. Copley, A.L. and King, R.G. 1971. Rheogoniometric study of viscosity of surface layers of fibrinogen and plasma-fibrinogen systems. Federation Proc., 30. 489-494.
29. McMillan, D.E. 1974. Surface effects of proteins in cone-plate viscometry. Biorheol. 11. 149-150.
30. King, R.G. and Copley, A.L. 1970. Modifications to the Weissenberg rheogoniometer for hemorheological and other biorheological studies. Biorheology 7. 1-4.
31. King, R.G., Chien, S., Usami, S. and Copley, A.L. 1984. Biorheological methods employing the Weissenberg rheogoniometer. Biorheology, Suppl. I; 23-34.
32. Wells, R.E., Denton, R. and Merrill, E.W. 1961. Measurement of viscosity of biological fluids by cone plate viscometer. J. Lab. Clin. Med. 57, 646-656.
33. Wells, R., Schmid-Schönbein, H. and Goldstone, J. 1971. Flow behavior of red cells in pathologic sera: existence of a yield shear stress in the absence of fibrinogen. pp. 360-365. in: Theoretical and Clinical Hemorheology, Hartert H.H. and Copley, A.L. (eds.), Springer, Berlin.
34. Dormandy, J.A. 1974. Medical and engineering problems of blood viscosity. Biomedical Engineering, 9. 284-289.
35. Ehrly, A.M. and Jung, G. 1973. Circadian rhythm of human blood viscosity. Biorheology 10, 577-583.
36. Dormandy, J.A. (Chien, S.) 1980. Blood viscosity and red cell deformability. pp. 214-266 in "Methods in Angiology", M. Verstraete (ed.), Instrumentation and Techniques in Clinical Medicine, Vol. 2. Martinus Nijhoff, Amsterdam.

37. Inglis, T.C.M., Carson, P.J. and Stuart, J. 1981. Clinical measurement of whole-blood viscosity at low shear rates. Clin. Hemorheol. 1. 167-177.
38. Ernst, E. and Matrai, A. 1982. Rotationsviskometer in der Hämorheologie. Arztl. Lab. 28. 33-38.
39. Spinelli, F.R. and Meier, Ch.D. 1974. Measurement of blood viscosity. Biorheol. 11. 301-306.
40. Gilinson, P.J., Dauwalter, C.R. and Merrill, E.W. 1963. A rotational viscometer using an A.C. torque to balance loop and air bearing. Trans. Soc. Rheol. 7. 319-331.
41. Matrai, A., Flute, P.T. and Dormandy, J.A. 1984. Improving accuracy of co-axial viscometry. Biorheology, Suppl. I; 99-101.
42. Brooks, D.E. and Easthope, P. 1981. Rheological Characteristics of blood through the menstrual cycle. Biorheology 18, 485-492.
43. Ernst, E. 1982. Zur messtechnischen Erfassung der Blutviskositaet. Labor Praxis in der Medizin, 2, 18-23.
44. Adjizian, J.C., Droulle, C., Osterman, G., Pignon, B. and Potron, G. 1984. Comparative interest of two coaxial viscometers: Ecktacytometer and Low-shear 30. Biorheology, Suppl.I; 95-97.
45. Whittington, R.B., Matrai, A. and Nicol, C.G. 1984. Characteristic parameters derived from whole-blood viscosimetry: their potential utility in diagnosis and therapy. Clin. Hemorheol. 4, 285-293.
46. Forconi, S., Guerrini, M., Pieragalli, D., Acciavatti, A. 1981. Viscosimetria ematica: approccio metodologico. La Ricerca Clin. Lab. 11. (suppl. 11). 135-144.
47. Ernst, E., Magyarosy, I., Roloff, Ch. and Drexel, H. 1984. A new simple method for measuring red cell aggregation. Biorheology, Suppl. I; 217-219.
48. Kiesewetter, H. 1981. The yield shear stress of blood in branched models of the microcirculation: Effect of hematocrit and plasma macro-molecules. Bibl.Haematol. 47. 14-20.
49. Davenport, P. and Roath, S. 1982. A variable shear stress viscometer. Clin. Hemorheol. 2. 383-387.
50. Höppler, F. 1933. Z. techn. Physik 14. 165-; cited by W. Philippoff: Viskosität der Kolloide. Theodor Steinkopff, Dresden 1942.
51. Thurston, G.B. 1972. Viscoelasticity of human blood. Biophys. J. 12, 1205-1217.
52. Anadere, I., Chmiel, H., Hess, H., Thurston, G.B. 1979. Clinical blood rheology. Biorheology 16, 171-178.
53. Born, G.V.R., Nicola, A.B. and Cusack, N.J. 1984. Functional physiology of platelets. 319-348 in Biggs, R. and Rizza, C.R. (eds.) Human Blood Coagulation, Hemostasis and Thrombosis. Blackwell, Oxford.
54. Craddock, P.R., Hammerschmidt, D., White, J.G., Dalmasso, A.P. and Jacob, HS. 1977. Complement (C5a)-induced granulocyte aggregation in vitro. A possible mechanism of complement – mediated leukostasis and leukopenia. J. Clin. Invest. 60, 260-264.
55. Brinkman, R., Zijlstra, W.G. and Jansonius, N.J. 1963. Quantitative evaluation of the rate of rouleaux formation of erythrocytes by measuring light reflection (Syllectometry). Proc. Kon. med. Akad. Wet. Ser.C66, 237-248.
56. Schmid-Schönbein, H, Volger, E. and Klose, H.J. 1972. Microrheology and light transmission of blood. The photometric quantification of red cell aggregate formation and dispersion in flow. Pflug. Arch. 333, 140-155.
57. Kiesewetter, H., Radtke, H., Schneider, R., Mussler, K., Scheffler, A. and Schmid-Schönbein, H. 1982. Das Mini-Erythrozyten-Aggregometer: Ein neues Gerät zur schnellen Quantifizierung des Ausmasses der Erythrozytenaggregation. Biomed. Technik 27, 209-213.
58. Ruhenstroth-Bauer, G., Porz, P., Boss, N., Koenig-Erich, S., Lehmacher, W. and Stamm, D. 1983. Der Erythrozyten – Aggregationswert als Mass von Hezinfarkt – Risikofaktoren und von Gefässschaeden. Münch. med. Wschr. 125(36). 771-775.
59. Nordt, F.J., Boss, N. Korndorfer, D. and Ruhenstroth-Bauer, G. 1984. Flow cytometric quantitation of erythrocyte aggregation: foundation for a diagnostic test for coronary artery disease. Clin. Hemorheol. 4, 445-454.

60. Ernst, E. 1984. Erythrozyten – Aggregation statt BKS? Labor Praxis in der Medizin 11, 451-453.
61. Stoltz, J.F., Gaillard, S., Paulus, F., Henri, O. and Dixneuf, P. 1984. Experimental approach to rouleau formation. Comparison of three methods. Biorheology, Suppl. I. 221-226.
62. Rampling, M.W., Whittingstall, P. and Linderkamp, O. 1984. The effects of fibrinogen and its plasmin degradation products on the rheology of erythrocyte suspensions. Clin. Hemorheol. 4, 533-543.
63. Jandl, J.H., Simmons, R.L. and Castle, W.B. 1961. Red cell filtration and the pathogenesis of certain haemolytic anaemias. Blood, 18. 133-148.
64. Teitel, A. and Radulescu, I. 1952. A method of determining erythrocyte plasticity. Medizina Interna, 5. 32.
65. Teitel, P. 1967. Le test de la filtrabilite erythrocytaire. Une methode simple d'etude de certaines proprietes microrheologiques des globules rouges. Nouv. Rev. franc. Hemat. 7. 195-214.
66. Teitel, P. 1977. Basic principles of the filterability test and analysis of erythrocytes' flow behaviour. Blood Cells, 3, 55-70.
67. Gregersen, M.I., Bryant, G.A., Hammerle, W., Usami, A. and Chien, S. 1967. Flow characteristics of human erythrocytes through polycarbonate sieves. Science, 157. 825-827.
68. Schmid-Schöenbein, H., Weiss, J. and Ludwig, H. 1973. A simple method for measuring red cell deformability in models of the microcirculation. Blut, 26. 369-379.
69. Ehrly, A.M. and Rossbach, P. 1973. Microrheology: studies with an 8 μm filter system. Bibl. Anat. 11. 55-62.
70. Reid, H.L., Barnes, A.J., Lock, P.J., Dormandy, J.A. and Dormandy, T.L. 1976. A simple method for measuring erythrocyte deformability. J. Clin. Pathol.29. 855-858.
71. Leblond, P.F. and Coulombe, L. 1979. The measurement of erythrocyre deformability using micropore membranes. J. Lab. Clin. Med. 94, 133-143.
72. Chien, S. 1977. Principles and techniques for assesment erythrocytes deformability. Blood Cells, 3. 71-99.
73. Dormandy, J.A. (ed.), 1983. Red Cell Deformability and Filterability. pp. 223, Martinus Nijhoff, Boston.
74. Stuart, J. 1985. Erythrocyte rheology. J. Clin. Pathol. 38, 965-977.
75. Reinhart, W.H., Usami, S., Schmalzer, E.A., Lee, M.M.L. and Chien, S. 1984. Evaluation of red blood cell filterability test: Influences of pore size, hematocrit level, and flow rate. J. Lab. Clin. Med. 104, 501-516.
76. Teitel, P. 1983. Types of filters. pp. 117-146 in: Dormandy, J.A. (ed.) Red Cell Deformability and Filterability, Martinus Nijhoff, Boston.
77. Alderman, M.J. Ridge, A., Morley, A.A., Ryall, R.G. and Walsh, J.A. 1981. Effect of total leucocyte count on whole blood filterability in patients with peripheral vascular disease. J. Clin. Pathol. 34. 163-166.
78. Dodds, A.J., Boyd, M.I., Allen, J., Bennett, E.D., Flute, P.T. and Dormandy, J.A. 1980. Changes in red cell deformability and other haemorheological variables after myocardial infarction. Br. Heart J. 44, 508-511.
79. Hanss, M. 1983. Erythrocyte filterability mesurement by the initial flow rate method. Biorheol. 20. 199-211.
80. Milligan, D.W. 1983. Red cell deformability in polycythemia vera: the influence of white cell contamination. Clin. Hemorheol. 3. 155-162.
81. Kenny, M.W., Meakin, M. and Stuart, J. 1983. Methods for removal of leucocytes and platelets prior to study of erythrocyte deformability. Clin. Hemorheol. 3. 191-200.
82. Schoerer, R. and Muth, K. 1981. Filterability of whole blood and erythrocyte suspensions under the influence of several anticoagulants. La Ricerca Clin. Lab. 11. (Suppl. 1) 109-116.
83. Lucas, G.S., Caldwell, N.M., Kenny, M.W., Meakin, M., Aillaud, M.F., Billerey, M., Juhan-Vague, I. and Stuart, J. 1983. Effect of calcium-chelating and non-chelating anticoagulants on erythrocyte and leucocyte filterability. Clin. Hemorheol. 3, 451-467.

84. Artioli, F., Gelmini, G., Pedrazzoni, M., Dall'Asta, D. and Ferretti, P.G. 1984. Erythrocyte filtration: analysis of different methods by scanning electron microscopy. Clin. Hemorheol. 4. 409-418.
85. Schmalzer, E. and Chien, S. 1984. Filterability of subpopulations of leucocytes: effect of pentoxifylline. Blood 64, 542-546.
86. Bogar, L. personal communication.
87. Chien, S., Schmalzer, E.A., Lee, M.M.L., Impelluso, T. and Skalak, R. 1983. Role of white cells in filtration of blood cell suspension. Biorheology, 20. 11-28.
88. Skalak, R., Impelluso, T., Schmalzer, E.A. and Chien, S. 1983. Theoretical modeling of filtration of blood cell suspensions Biorheology 20. 41-56.
89. Skalak, R., Hanss, M. and Chien, S. 1983. Indices of filterability of red blood cell suspensions. Biorheology, 20. 311-316.
90. Blackshear, P.L., Christianson, T.J., Majerle, R.J. and Vargas, F.F. 1979. Resistance of erythrocyte flow into pores. J. Rheology 23, 681-702.
91. Cokelet, G.R. 1981. Dynamics of erythrocyte motion in filtration tests and in vivo flow. Scand. J. Clin. Lab. Invest. 41, Suppl. 156, 77-82.
92. Matrai, A., Reid, H., Bogar, L., Flute, P.T. and Dormandy, J.A. 1985. Initial filtration rate and initial clogging in the Hemorheometre. Biorheology 22, 275-284.
93. Teitel, P. 1984. Recent progress in improving data processing in filtration measurements. Biorheology Suppl. I, 231-240.
94. Hanss, M. Koutsouris, D. 1984. Automated apparatus for the filtration initial flow rate measurement. Biorheology, Suppl. I; 275-277.
95. Matrai, A., Bogar, L., Flute, P.T. and Dormandy, J.A. 1984. Comparison of four blood filtration techniques. Clin. Hemorheol. 4, 513-523.
96. Stoltz, J.F., Duvivier, C. and Malher, E. 1984. Erythrometer: A new device for measuring erythrocyte filterability and plasma viscosity. Biorheology, Suppl. I; 255-259.
97. Merrill, E.W. 1969. Rheology of blood. Physiol. Rews. 49. 863-888.
98. Chien, S. 1972. Present state of blood rheology. pp. 1-40. in "Hemodilution, Theoretical Basis and Clinical Applications", Messmer, K. and Schmid-Schönbein, H. (eds.), Karger, Basel.
99. Chien, S. 1975. Biophysical behavior of red cells in suspensions. 1031-1131 in: The Red Blood Cell, Vol. II. Academic Press, New York.
100. Copley, A.L. and King, R.G. 1970. Rheogoniometric viscosity measurements of whole human blood at minimal shear rates down to 0.0009 sec-1. Experimentia, 26. 904-905.
101. Goldsmith, H.L. 1971. Deformation of human red cells in tube flow. Biorheology 7, 235-242.
102. Fischer, T.M., Stoehr-Liesen, M. and Schmid-Schönbein, H. 1978. The red cell as a fluid droplet; tank tread like motion of human erythrocyte membrane in shear flow. Science 202, 894-896.
103. Schmid-Schönbein, H., Rieger, H. and Fischer, T. 1980. Blood fluidity as a consequence of red cell fluidity: flow properties of blood and flow behavior of blood in vascular diseases. Angiology, 31. 301-319.
104. Meiselman, H.J., Merrill, E.W., Gilliland, E.R., Pelletier, G.A. and Salzman, E.W. 1967. Influence of total plasma osmolarity on the rheology of human blood. J. Appl. Physiol. 22. 772-781.
105. Scott-Blair, G.W. 1959. An equation for the flow of blood, plasma and serum through glass capillaries. Nature 183, 613-614.
106. Whittington, R.B., and Harkness, J. 1982. Whole-blood viscosity, as determined by plasma viscosity, hematocrit, and shear. Biorheology, 19. 175-184.
107. Harkness J. 1971. The viscosity of human blood plasma: its measurement in health and disease. Biorheology 8, 171-193.
108. Ditzel, J. and Kampmann, J. 1971. Whole blood viscosity, hematocrit and plasma proteins in normal subjects at different ages. Acta Physiol. Scand. 81. 264-268.

109. Harkness, J. 1981. Measurement of plasma viscosity. pp 79-90 in: "Clinical aspects of blood viscosity and cell deformability". G.D.O. Lowe, J.C. Barbanel and C. Forbes (eds.), Springer, Berlin.
110. Dintenfass, L. and Kammer, S. 1977. Plasma viscosity in 615 subjects, effect of fibrinogen, globulin and cholesterol in normals, peripheral vascular disease, retinopathy and melanoma. Biorheology 14, 247-251.
111. Dintenfass, L. 1976. Rheology of blood in diagnostic and preventive medicine. Butterworth, London.
112. Charm, S.E., Paz, H. and Kurland, G.S. 1979. Reduced plasma viscosity among joggers compared with non-joggers. Biorheology 16, 185-189.
113. Leonhardt, H. and Arntz, H.R. 1977. Zusammenhaenge zwischen kardiovaskulaeren Risikofaktoren und der Blutviskositaet unter besonderer Beruecksichtigung der Hyperlypoproteionaemien. Rheol. Acta 16, 368-377.
114. Ernst, E. and Matrai, A. 1985. Blutrheologie als Risikoindikator kardiovascularer Erkrankungen. Deutsch. Med. Wschrft. 110(24) 967-970.
115. Matrai, A., Bogar, L. and Fendler, K. 1979. A hematokrit es a fibrinogenszint szerepe a ver rheologiai tulajdonsagainak meghatarozasaban. Kis. Orvostud. 31. 204-212.
116. Gauer, O.H., Henry, J.P., Behn, C. 1970. The regulation of extracellular fluid volume. Ann. Rev. Physiol. 32, 547-595.
117. Tompson, W.O., Thompson, P.K. and Dailey, M.E. 1928. The effect of posture upon the composition and volume of the blood in man. J. Clin. Invest. 5, 573-604.
118. Fawcett J.K. and Wynn, V. 1960. Effects of posture on plasma volume and some blood constituents. J. Clin. Path. 13, 304-310.
119. Hagan, R.D., Diaz, F.J. and Horvath S.M. 1978. Plasma volume changes with movement to supine and standing positions. J. Appl. Physiol. 45, 414-418.
120. Ehrly, A.M. 1979. Influence of raised venous pressure on the flow properties of blood. Angiology 1, 21-26.
121. Menayr, P., Nielsen, S.L., Christiansen, C. and Axelsson C. 1979. Gross errors made by routine blood sampling from two sides using a tourniquet applied at different positions. Clin. Chim. Acta 198, 113-118.
122. Juswigg, T., Batress, R., Solomons, N.W., Pineda, O. and Milne, D.B. 1982. The effect of temporary venous occlusion on trace mineral concentrations in plasma. Am. J. Clin. Nutr. 36, 354-357.
123. Eisenberg, S. Effect of posture and position of the venous sampling site on the hematocrit and serum protein concentration. J. Lab. Clin. Med. 61, 755-760, 1963.
124. Scheving, L.E., Halberg, D.F. and Pauly J.E. (eds.), 1974. Chronobiology. Thieme, Stuttgart.
125. Seaman, G.V.F, Engel, R., Swank, R. and Hissen, W. 1965. Circadian periodicity in some physicochemical parameters of circulating blood. Nature, 207, 833-835.
126. Ernst, E., Magyarosy, I. and Matrai, A. 1985. Are there diurnal changes in hemorheological parameters? Clin. Hemorheol. 5, 269-272.
127. Dintenfass, L., Julian, D.G. and Miller, G. 1966. Viscosity of blood in healthy young women. Effect of menstrual cycle. Lancet i: 234-235.
128. Ernst, E., Matrai, A. and Magyarosy, I. 1986. Complex environmental changes alter hemorheological, hematological and biochemical variables in volunteers. Clin. Hemorheol. 6., 251-256.
129. Galuzzi, N.J., Delashmutt, R.K. and Conolly, V.J. 1964. Failure of anticoagulants to influence the viscosity of whole blood. J. Lab. Clin. Med. 64, 773-777.
130. Meiselman, H.J., Frasher, W.G. and Wayland, H. 1973. In vivo hemorheology employing outflow viscometric techniques. Biorheology 10, 361-373.
131. Reid, H. 1977. Erythrocyte deformability: Its measurement in normal man and in patients with peripheral circulatory disease. Ph. D. Thesis, University of London.
132. Barras, J.P. 1969. Blood Rheoloy. General Review. Bibl. Haemat. 33, 277-297.

133. Zingg, W., Sulew, J.C. and Morgan, C. 1973. Study of possible sources of error in clinical blood viscosity determinations with the Wells-Brookfield viscometer. Effects of fasting, food intake and sample handling. Biorheology 10, 509-515.
134. Ernst, E., Roloff, Ch., Megyarosy, I. and Drexel, H. 1984. Influence of anticoagulant, time and storing temperature on blood viscosity measurements. Clin. Hemorheol. 4, 419-422.
135. Whittington, R.B. and Harkness, J. 1984. On the capillary-tube viscometry of placental blood. Biorheology, Suppl. I; 111-114.
136. Whittington, R.B. 1942. Blood sedimentation; a study in haemo-mechanics. Proc. Roy. Soc. (B), 131, 183-190.
137. Merrill, E.W., Gilliland, E.R., Lee, T.S. and Salzman, E.W. 1966. Blood rheology. Effect of fibrinogen deduced by addition. Circ. Res. 18. 437-446.
138. Copley, A.L. (ed.), 1983. The Endoendothelial Fibrin Lining. Thrombosis Res. Suppl. V. 154 pp.
139. Dormandy, J.A. and Matrai, A. 1983. Assesment of pharmacological agents with a hemorheological action. Ann. N.Y. Acad. Sci. 416, 599-610.
140. Matrai, A., Ernst, E. and Dormandy, J.A. 1984. Die Rolle der Hämorheologie in der Medizin unter besonderer Berücksichtigung der Therapie mit Beta-Blockern. 140-148 in Heilmann, L, Kiesewetter, H. and Ernst, E. (eds.): Klinische Rheologie und Beta-1-Blockade. W. Zuckschwerdt, München.
141. Ernst, E., Weihmayr, T, Schmid, M., Bauman, M. and Matrai, A. 1985. Cardiovascular risk factors and hemorheology: physical fitness, stress and obesity. Atherosclerosis, 59, 263-269.
142. Chien, S., Usami, S., Taylor, H.M., Lundberg, J.L. and Gregersen, M.I. 1966. Effects of hematocrit and plasma proteins on human blood rheology at low shear rates. J. Appl. Physiol. 21. 81-87.
143. Matrai, A. 1980. Ph. D. thesis, Univ. Med. Sch. Pecs, Hungary, 1980.
144. Matrai, A., Whittington, R.B. and Ernst, E. 1987. A simple method to estimate whole blood viscosity at standardized hematocrit. Clin. Hemorheol. in press.
145. Dormandy, J.A. 1984. Fahreus Award Lecture: The dangereous red cell. Clin. Hemorheol. 4, 115-132.
146. Nicol, C.G. and Harkness, J. 1985. Viscosimetric monitoring of plasmapheresis. Clin. Hemorheol. 5, 45-50.
147. Schmalzer, E.A., Skalak, R., Usami, S., Vayo, M. and Chien, S. 1983. Influence of red cell concentration on filtration of blood cell suspensions. Biorheology 20. 29-40.
148. Bogar, L., Walker, T., Matrai, A. Dormandy, J.A. and Flute, P.T. 1985. Hemorheological effects of a 5-HT2 receptor antagonost (Ketanserin). Clin. Hemorheol. 5, 115-121.
149. Powell, J.E. and Stuart, J. 1984. Effect of metabolic stress and oxpentifylline on erythrocyte deformability (filterability). Clin. Hemorheol. 4, 483-491.

3
Rheology of blood cells

D.E. Brooks *+ and E.A. Evans *
*Departments of * Pathology and + Chemistry, University of British Columbia, Vancouver, B.C. Canada V6T 1W5*

3.1. Introduction

Blood rheology encompasses the flow properties of blood cell suspensions in plasma throughout the vasculature from small capillaries where cells must pass single file up to large vessels where several thousand cells occupy a cross section of the flow. The primary properties of the cellular constituents that govern whole blood rheology can be differentiated along the following lines.

In large vessels, three regimes of behavior are apparent:

1. Low shear (shear stress, $\tau < 0.01$ Pa). Here, red cell aggregation forms "polymerized cell networks" that give rise to a plastic-like response which is approximated by a yield and subsequent flow [1,2]; the important properties are cell aggregation, adhesive strengths, and cell deformability.

2. Intermediate shear ($0.01 \text{ Pa} < \tau < 0.5$ Pa). Here, cell aggregates are dispersed and individual cells are deformed by the fluid shear field [3,4,5]; the important properties are cell rigidity and conformation (e.g. discocyte-echinocyte-stomatocyte forms of red cells).

3. High shear ($\tau > 0.5$ Pa). Here, red cells are continuously deformed by the high shear field such that the outer membrane envelope circulates around the interior in a "tank tread" motion [3,4]. White cells, because of their spherical shape and dynamic rigidity, simply rotate with little cell deformation until exposed to extremely high shear stress levels ($\tau > 10$ Pa) where they begin to break up [6]. The important properties are the viscosities of the cell membrane and internal cytoplasm.

For small capillary vessels, the ratio of cell size to capillary diameter is critical. Here, cells are deformed by extension and folding on a rapid time scale when entering small vessels from larger feeding vessels. This rapid deformation is a dynamic process which occurs over a short period of time, and the relevant cell characteristic is the *dynamic cellular rigidity* that opposes entry. Thus, the important properties in cell deformation are cell geometry as well as the elastic and viscous resistances of the cell to deformation [7]. An additional factor, which is of pathological significance, is the frictional or adhesive interaction of cells with the endothelial lining.

The previous outline is cursory and by necessity somewhat subjective, but it identifies the rheological properties of the cellular constituents that are essential aspects of blood rheology: deformability of blood cells in shear flow and when entering small capillaries, cell aggregation-disaggregation and interaction with vascular endothelium. We will focus on these properties in this chapter. Other chapters will greatly expand and enrich our outline of blood flow behavior.

3.2. Dynamic deformability of blood cells

Fig. 3.1 presents a "family portrait" of the cellular constituents of blood: red cells, white cells (here a granulocyte), and platelets. Extensive research has been carried out on the mechanical properties of red cells but much less on white cells and essentially none on platelets because of their small size. We will principally discuss the deformability of red and white cells, not because this is the only area of knowledge, but because platelets easily transit small vessels without deformation and appear to act as rigid bodies in shear flow [8]. Platelet deformability has

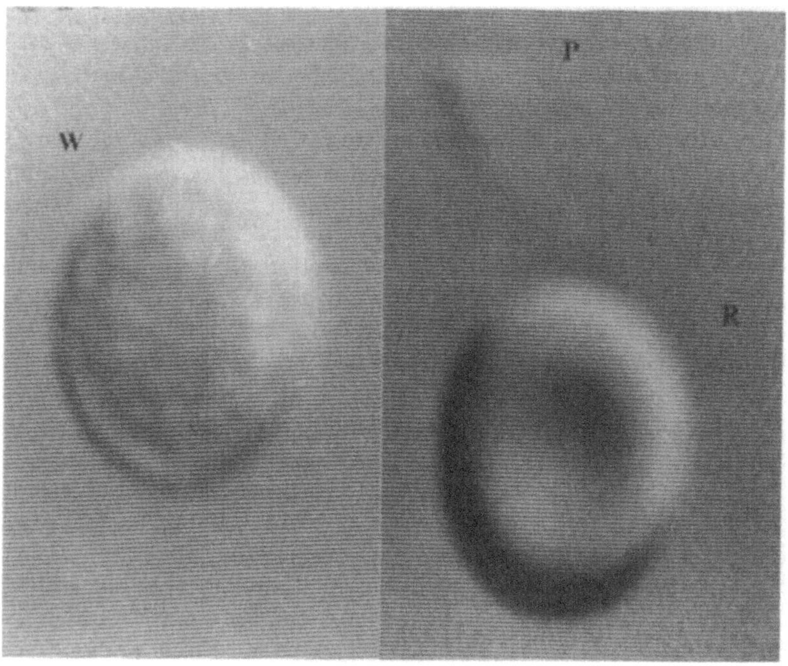

Figure 3.1 A human erythrocyte (R), a platelet (P) and a granulocyte (W), all at the same magnification. The cross sectional dimension of the erythrocyte and granulocyte are both approximately 8 μm.

been considered largely with respect to the viscoelastic properties of red and white thrombi [9] and clot contractility [10].

Rigidity and deformability are terms that describe the shape response of a body or cell to applied forces (see Chapter 2); these responses depend on several extrinsic and intrinsic factors. Extrinsic factors are gross structural features such as the surface area of the membrane in relation to enclosed volume, intracellular structure such as microfilaments, microtubules, nuclei, etc. and conformation of the cell in general. Thus, extrinsic factors are related to the size of the body, its form, and how it is assembled. On the other hand, intrinsic factors are determined by the properties of the materials which form structural elements of the cell. For example, intrinsic factors include the elastic and viscous properties of membranes, cytoplasm, nucleoplasm, and chemical factors like ionic strength and active contractile processes.

3.2.1. Blood cells deformability: "extrinsic factors"

Because of the osmotic strength of cellular contents, most deformation forces are not sufficient to alter cell volumes, as the pressures produced inside a cell are too low to drive water out of the interior. Thus, cell volumes are essentially fixed in any deformation. In addition, it has been determined experimentally (see paragraphs that follow) that cell membrane area is also a constraint, i.e. fixed. Consequently, the major extrinsic factor in blood cell deformability is the level of excess membrane surface over that of a sphere of equivalent internal volume. This is because cell deformations (for instance, extension of the cell upon entry into a small capillary) can be accomodated by changes in shape of the membrane capsule without changing internal volume or area. The most obvious effect of this extrinsic limitation is that cells are unable to enter the lumen of capillaries narrower than a critical diameter without volume reduction or area increase. Examples of this rigid, plug effect are featured in Fig. 3.2 which shows a red blood cell and a blood granulocyte aspirated by micropipettes such that the membrane surface is totally extended with a residual spherical portion of the cell left outside the pipet. The test can be used to determine surface area to volume ratio for cells. For the red cell, the normal value of surface area excess over that of a sphere is about 40%, whereas for blood granulocytes, morphometric measurements indicate that it is on the order of 80 to 90% [11], and 100 to 110% has been directly measured by micropipette aspiration, as shown in Fig. 3.2 (Evans, unpublished observation). For white cells, the membrane reservoir is in the form of a ruffled surface that encapsulates a spherical form of the cell. Another, important extrinsic factor is the morphology of the cell. For example with red cells, the disc shape of the cell can be altered into crenated or cup forms as shown in Fig. 3.3a. These shapes offer greater resistances to deformation [5] than the smooth, biconcave disc (analogous to surface "ribbing" which acts to stiffen

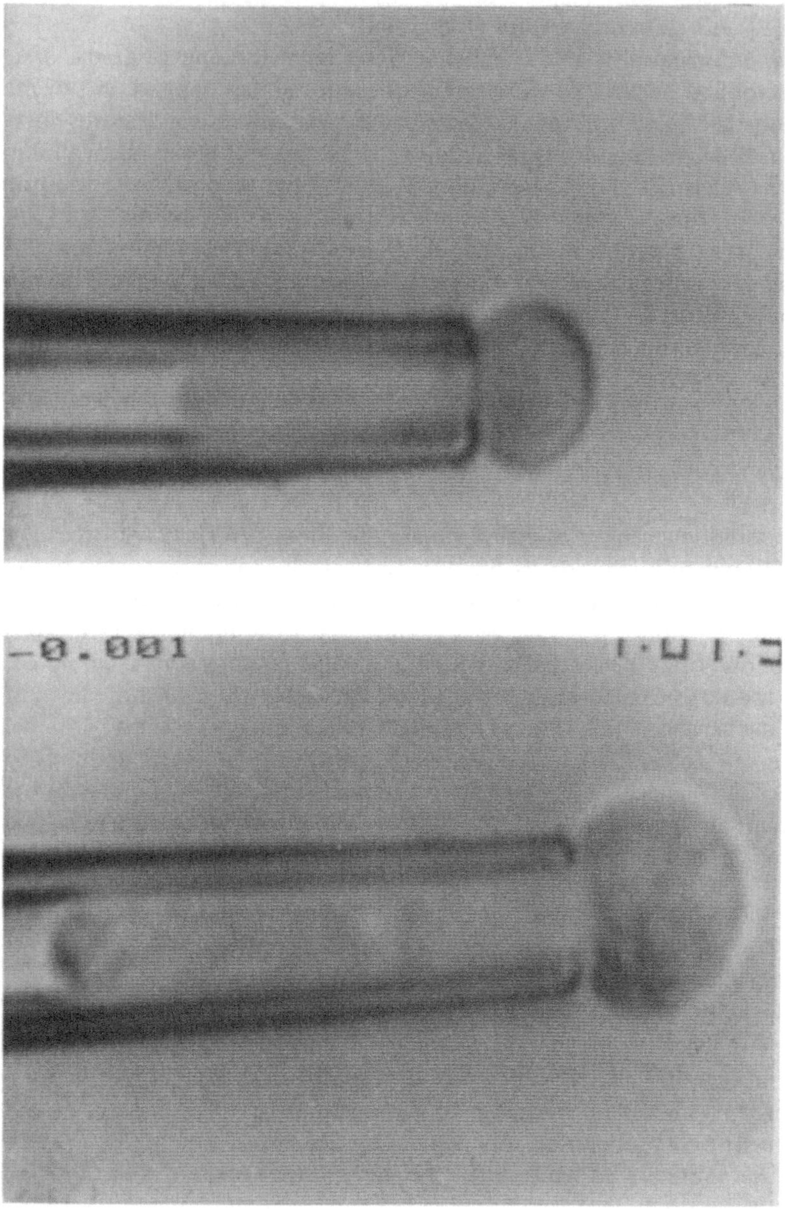

Figure 3.2 A human erythrocyte (top) and a granulocyte (bottom) aspirated to micropipettes of internal diameter 2 μm for the erythrocyte and 2.5 μm for the granulocyte.

a material against bending deformations). For white cells, there is a multiplicity of forms produced when the cell becomes active, one of which is shown in Fig. 3.3. In general, morphological alterations of red or white cells do not greatly affect cell deformability, provided that the intrinsic material properties of the cell are unchanged. Platelets also exhibit changes in geometry upon activation. They undergo rapid isovolumetric transformations from disc to spheroechinocyte forms bearing pseudopods, when stimulated by agents which render them adhesive [12].

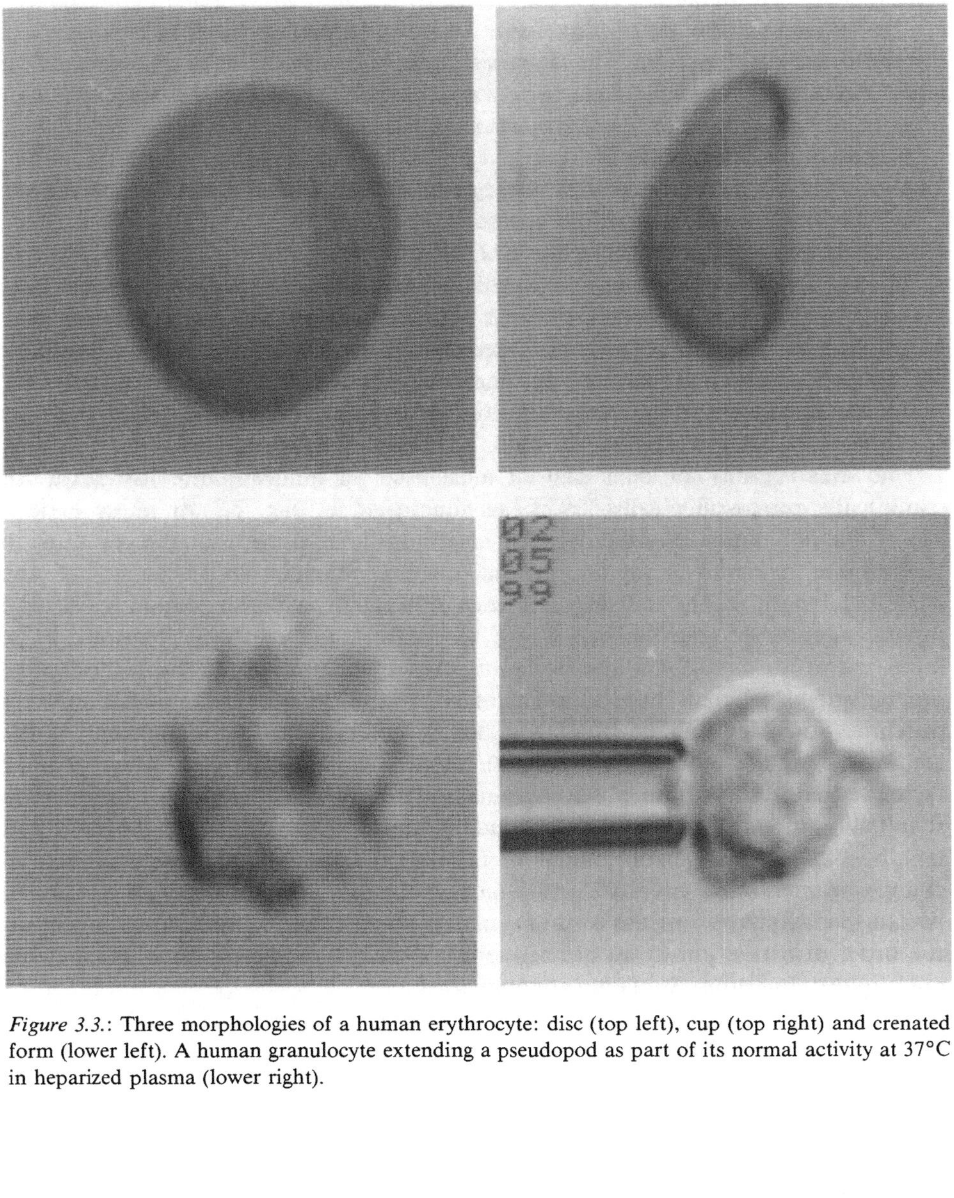

Figure 3.3.: Three morphologies of a human erythrocyte: disc (top left), cup (top right) and crenated form (lower left). A human granulocyte extending a pseudopod as part of its normal activity at 37°C in heparized plasma (lower right).

The capsular surface area increases by about 45% in this process, probably by everting some of the surface-connected canalicular network present in these cells.

3.2.2. Red blood cell deformability: "intrinsic factors"

For a simple membrane capsule like the red cell, deformability is determined by membrane elasticity and viscous properties of the membrane and cytoplasm. These properties regulate static and dynamic rigidities that resist extension and folding deformations of the red cell. The static rigidity, which reflects the rigidity of the cell when the deforming force is not limited in time, establishes the threshold for deformation. The dynamic rigidity limits the rate of deformation and reflects the time-dependent behavior of the cell. Red cell deformations can be most simply viewed as a superposition of:

a) membrane area dilation;
b) membrane extension without change in surface area (i.e. surface shear);
c) membrane bending or folding; and
d) shear and displacement of the internal cytoplasm.

The rheological approximation to red cell behavior is based on the view that the cell membrane is a viscoelastic solid which encapsulates a liquid interior [13]. In this model, membrane area compressibility, extension, and bending moduli (K, G, and B) characterize the *static rigidities* of the cell [14]; time constants for rapid elastic recovery from area dilation, extension, and bending deformations (t_a, t_e and t_f) characterize the *dynamic rigidities* of the cell [7,14].

The area rigidity of cells can be measured by micropipette aspiration of osmotically pre-swollen cells [14,15] as illustrated in Fig. 3.2. In these experiments, the cell enters the micropipette easily until the portion of the cell outside the pipette becomes a rigid spherical surface; further displacement of the aspirated length of the cell requires area dilation or volume reduction. As the pipette suction pressure is increased, the membrane isotropic tension, T, is increased proportionally. Close observation of the aspirated length in the micropipette shows a small but linear increase in this length with pipette suction pressure. Since the outside portion of the cell is spherical, displacement of the aspirated length is directly proportional to the increase in membrane area or decrease in interior volume. After correction for the small volume change (less than 0.4%), the area change is determined from the displacement of the aspirated length, L. The small displacement of the aspirated length represents fractional changes in membrane area of 2 or 3% or less; further increases in length result in lysis of the cell. Appropriate to these small area changes are suction pressures on the order of a fraction of an atmosphere. In the absence of volume change, the area rigidity modulus, K, is approximated by

$$K \sim D_0^2 \frac{dp}{dL} \tag{1}$$

where D_0 is the diameter of the spherical portion of the cell outside the pipette and dp/dL is the slope of the aspiration pressure, p, versus length, L. Results from these experiments yield values for $K \sim 0.1$–1 N/m (15). By comparison, the suction pressures needed for aspiration of cells such that the area is not required to increase are 10^3 times smaller. These lower pressures are characteristic of membrane extensional and bending rigidities.

Lipid bilayer membranes (in the liquid state) do not resist extension in the plane of the membrane unless area changes are required. In other words, the membrane modulus of extensional rigidity is zero for the lipid bilayer. On the other hand, the red cell membrane possesses a small but significant extensional rigidity such that when the red cell is extended (even though the cell area remains constant) there is an increase in static level of force in proportion to extension of the cell. The red cell membrane resistance to extension is due to the subsurface protein matrix ("cytoskeleton"). Observation of flaccid red cell aspiration (Fig. 3.4a) shows a proportional increase in aspirated length with increase in suction pressure; this stepwise increase in length versus aspiration pressure is reversible and reduction of the aspiration pressure gives a proportional reduction in length. Here, the aspiration pressures are in the range of 10–50 Pa for a suction pipette with a diameter of 1 μm. Analysis of this experiment has shown that membrane extensional rigidity, G, can be estimated from

$$G \sim R_p^2 \frac{dp}{dL} \tag{2}$$

where R_p is the pipette radius [14,16]. Experimental results have yielded values on the order of 10^{-5} N/m for the red cell membrane extensional rigidity [17,18,19].

In the measurement of membrane extensional rigidity, the bending rigidity of the membrane can be neglected provided that the surface contour of the red cell remains smooth and the extrapolated intercept of the length versus suction pressure is zero or less [20]. When the suction pressure is sufficient to produce excessively large aspiration lengths, the cell surface begins to fold (buckle) and eventually large folds occur enabling the cell to move up the pipette until limited by surface area and volume restrictions (Fig. 3.4b & c). It has been shown that the transition from smooth to "buckled" membrane contour is directly related to the ratio of membrane bending to extensional rigidities [21]. From the analysis, the bending modulus, B, is proportional to the pressure, p, at which the cell buckles or folds:

$$B \sim C R_p^3 p \tag{3}$$

where the coefficient, C, depends on the pipette inner radius, R_p, and is in the range of 0.05–0.12. Observations of normal red cells show that pressures sufficient to cause buckling are about 50 Pa for a 2μm calibre pipette [21]. From these

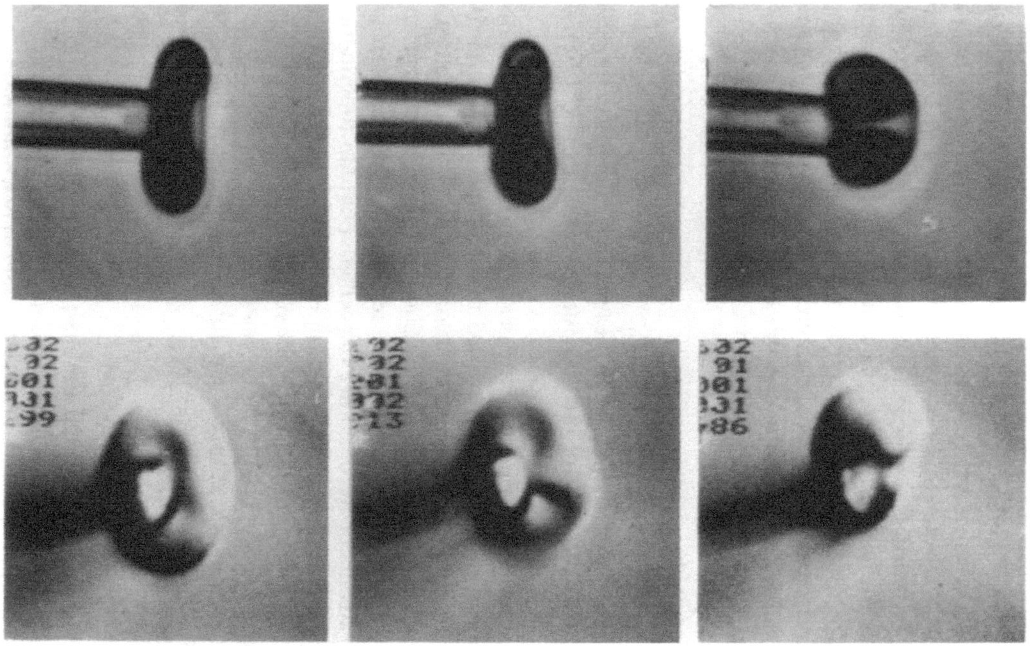

Figure 3.4 Illustrations of erythrocyte membrane extension followed by buckling. The pipette internal diameters are 1 μm. The top panel shows the aspiration sequence as viewed from the side; the bottom panel shows a similar sequence viewed from above the cell with the use of a curved pipette. The figures to the right show the onset of buckling and folding of the cell.

values, the bending modulus is determined to be on the order of 10^{-19} Nm (10^{-12} erg). Similar levels of bending modulus have been deduced for lipid bilayer membranes, where the lipid bilayer membrane is in the liquid state above the crystal transition temperature. From the measured values for extension and bending rigidities of the red cell membrane, it is clear that the bending stiffness offers significantly lower opposition to deformation than the extensional rigidity. Consequently, red cells usually fold and enter small capillaries with little stretch of their membrane surface.

The red cell membrane bending and extensional rigidities just described represent the static resistance to deformation of the cell. When cells enter small capillaries, they are deformed by extension and folding (bending) over a very small time increment which gives rise to large viscous forces that oppose the deformation. Consequently, the dynamic extension and bending rigidities of the cell become important factors in the entrance dynamics of cells. It is to be noted that the time constant for area dilation response is too fast to measure, but is estimated to be one the order of 10^{-6} second from theoretical considerations [14]. The dynamic rigidities of the cell are represented by time constants for rapid elastic recovery from extension and bending deformations [7]; these time constants are t_e and t_f respectively. The dynamic rigidities are given by dividing the product of the static rigidity and the characteristic time constant for the deformation response by the time interval over which the deformation occurs (i.e. the capillary entrance time). Based on simple rheological considerations [7,13], the characteristic time constant for membrane extensional deformation is given by the following relation

$$t_e \sim \frac{(\eta_m + \tilde{\eta}_{Hb}\delta)}{G} \tag{4}$$

where η_m is the membrane surface viscosity for extensional deformation; $\tilde{\eta}_{Hb}$ is the viscosity of the cell interior contents; δ is the characteristic thickness of the cell. By comparison, the characteristic folding time is approximated by the equation,

$$t_f \sim \frac{\tilde{\eta}_{Hb} D}{B C_m^2} \tag{5}$$

where only the cell interior viscosity appears to be significant; D is the characteristic dimension of the cell; C_m is the curvature of the fold.

The most direct approach to measurement of dynamic response times for extension and folding is to observe the time courses for rapid elastic recovery which follow the appropriate cell deformations as illustrated in Fig. 3.5. In both instances, the rate of deformation recovery is limited by viscous dissipation in both the membrane and cytoplasm. Measurement of extensional response of the

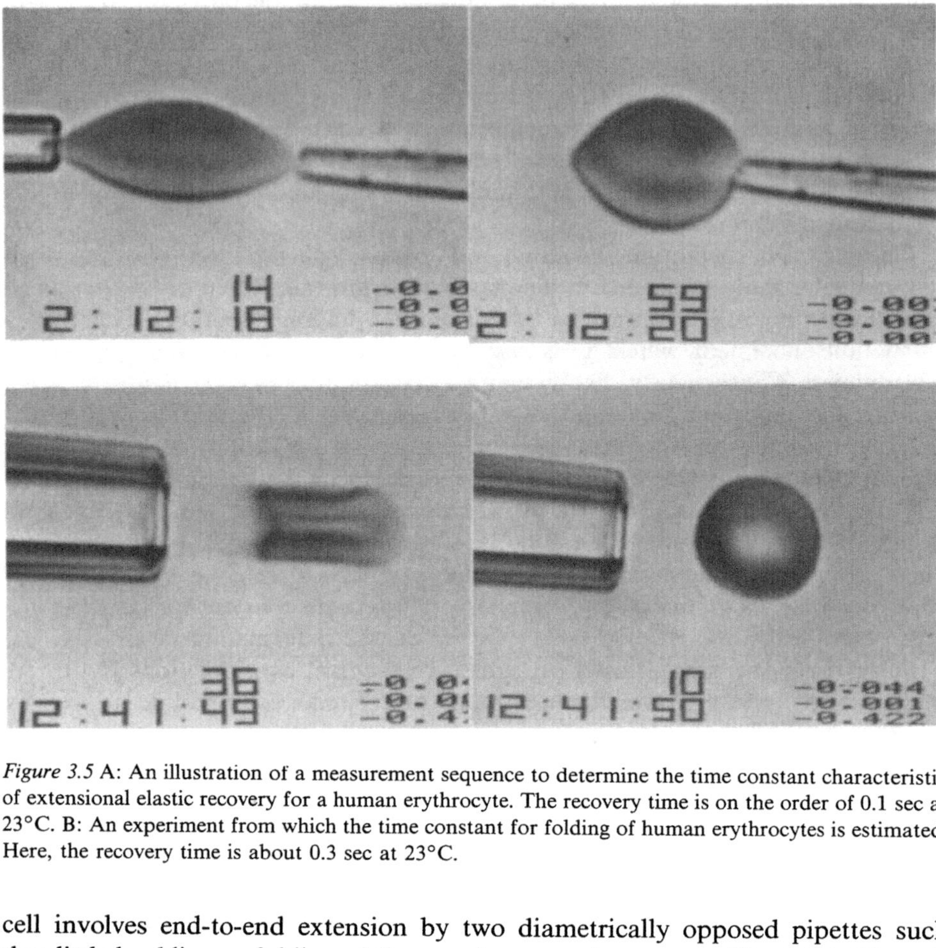

Figure 3.5 A: An illustration of a measurement sequence to determine the time constant characteristic of extensional elastic recovery for a human erythrocyte. The recovery time is on the order of 0.1 sec at 23°C. B: An experiment from which the time constant for folding of human erythrocytes is estimated. Here, the recovery time is about 0.3 sec at 23°C.

cell involves end-to-end extension by two diametrically opposed pipettes such that little buckling or folding of the membrane surface occurs (Fig. 3.5a). The cell is then quickly released and the length to width recovery time course is recorded. The time-dependent recovery of the cell shape can be analyzed using the simple visco-elastic model to give the characteristic time for extensional recovery [22]. Typically these time constants are on the order of 0.1 second for normal red cells [7,18,22]. The dynamic response of the cell to folding is tested by aspiration of red cells with large calibre pipettes such that little cell extension occurs. The cell simply folds upon entrance into the pipette (Fig. 3.5b). The cell is then rapidly expelled from the end of the pipette with a pressure pulse and the time course of the width recovery is recorded. The representative time for the cell width to recover 62% towards its final width is taken as the measure of the time constant for elastic recovery from folding. Times characteristic of the folding response are on the order of 0.3 second for normal cells [7].

3.2.3. *White blood blood cell deformability: "intrinsic factors"*

Unlike their companions, red blood cells, white blood cells are not simply membrane capsules that enclose liquid interiors. They possess a complicated cytoplasm that includes granules and a nucleus plus active, contractile elements which form a cortical layer just below the membrane [23,24]. The evidence to date indicates that the primary resistance of white cells to deformation is dynamic with a very small elastic response [25,26,27]. As with the red cell, the white cell can be easily deformed provided that the deformation does not require expansion of the surface area more than is available in the surface "ruffles". Micropipette aspiration tests have shown that passive deformations of white cells into micropipettes are essentially continuous, but exceedingly slow flow processes at low aspiration pressures [27], which become very rapid at high aspiration pressures [28]. An example of this experiment is shown in Fig. 3.6. Consequently, white cell rigidity depends very strongly on the time scale of the deformation event. For example, aspiration of a granulocyte into a pipette with lumen size half that of the cell diameter and with suction pressures on the order of 10^2 Pa causes total cell aspiration on a time scale of about 30 seconds whereas the same pipette with an aspiration pressure of 10^4 Pa causes cell aspiration within 0.1 second. For large pipettes, the rate of entry into the pipette can be roughly approximated by the relation [27,29]

$$\frac{\Delta(L/R_p)}{\Delta t} \sim CpR_p \qquad (6)$$

where the intrinsic compliance factor, C is on the order of 550–150 m/Ns. Experiments show that the white cell acts like a very viscous body with an apparent viscosity on the order of several hundred Pas for large deformations [29] and about one order of magnitude lower for very small deformations [26]. In addition to the observation that passive deformation of granulocytes is a continuous flow process only limited by the ultimate unwrinkling of the membrane envelope, there appears to be a cortical stress that establishes a threshold pressure below which a cell will not deform and that is associated with a small initial elastic response [26,27,32]. Also, granulocytes always recover their original spherical state after passive deformation, indepedent of the extent of deformation or location where the cell is aspirated. These observations indicate that the cytoplasm and granular matrix behave primarily as a highly viscous but complex liquid and that the cell membrane cortical layer (which is ruffled and folded) possesses a contractile stress responsible for the elastic recovery. Because this dynamic rigidity of the white cell is at least a thousand fold greater than that for extension of red cells, white cells can greatly impede flow in the microcirculation [30] and in vitro filtration tests [31]. It is interesting to note that the granulocyte nucleus is not rigid and can be deformed with little apparent effect on the cell

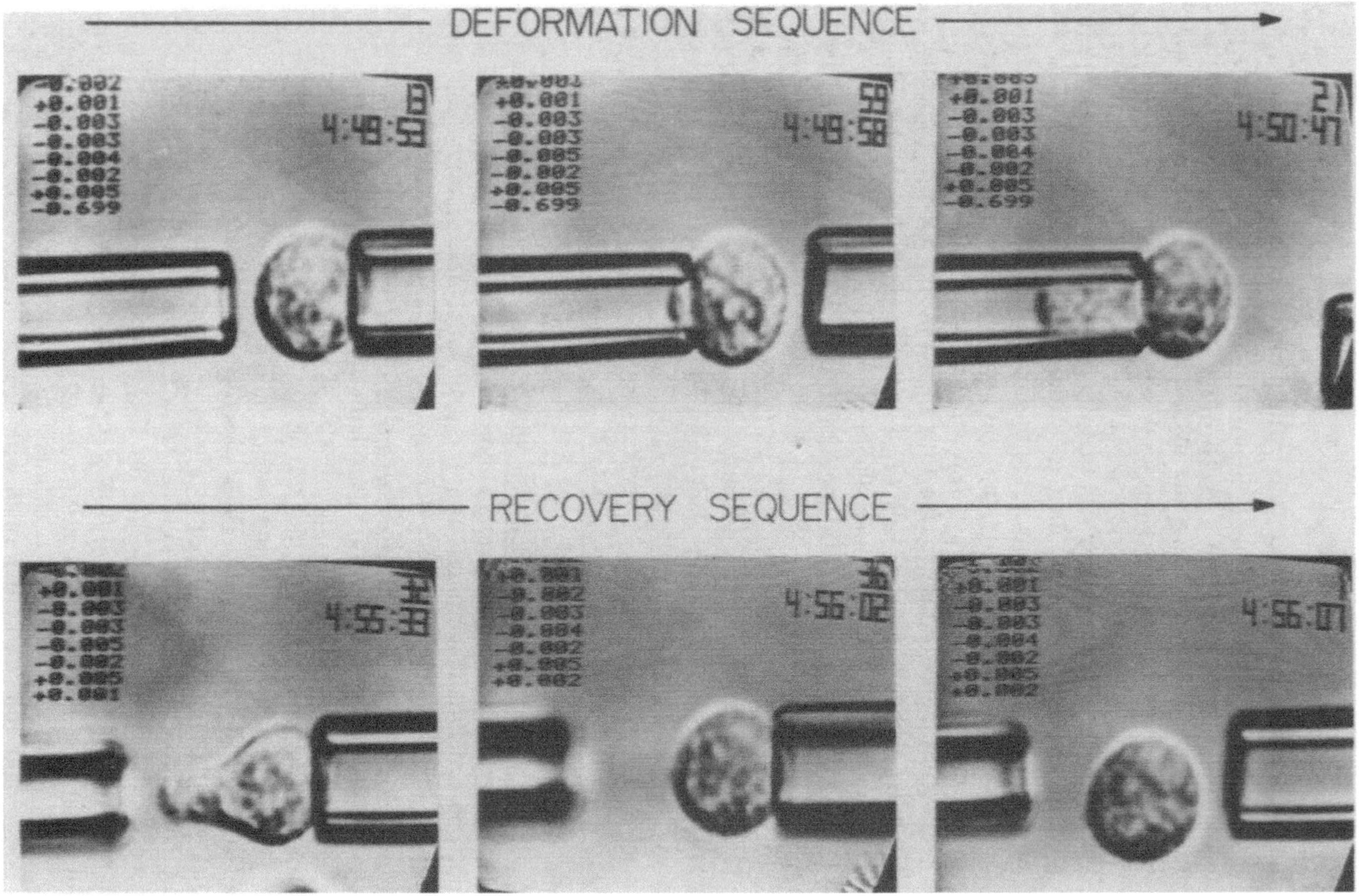

Figure 3.6 Deformation and recovery of a human granulocyte in plasma at 23° C. The top three panels show the aspiration sequence of constant pressure. After the pressure is nulled, the shape results as illustrated in the bottom three panels. The time course of each phase is given by the clock readings in the upper right hand corner of each frame.

deformability as a whole. By comparison, the nuclei of lymphocytes dominate the cell resistance to deformation in pipette aspiration experiments. Phagocytic cells like blood granulocytes are even more complicated because they have active contractile "machinery" which greatly stiffens the cell in opposition to deformation. For example, if a blood granulocyte is active, pipette aspiration pressures of one to two orders of magnitude greater than those for passive cells are required to deform the cell [32].

3.3. Rheological implications of blood cell deformabilities

In the context of the previous discussion about intrinsic deformation properties of blood cells, we will now discuss the relationship of those properties to the aspects of blood rheology which were identified in the initial paragraphs as essential, i.e. deformation of blood cells in shear flow and when entering small capillaries. For blood cells in shear flow, there are two general types of kinematic behavior: 1. tumbling or rotation of the cell as a rigid body; and 2. stable orientation of the cell with "tank tread" or convective motion of the cellular envelope around the interior contents [3]. The transition from the former, solid-like behavior to the latter, liquid drop like behavior is determined by the rigidity of the cell. For red blood cells, there is essentially a threshold level of fluid shear stress that must be applied to the cell surface in order to exceed the elastic resistance of the cell membrane to deformation. This is symbolized by the following equation,

$$\tau \sim G\epsilon/D \tag{7}$$

where ϵ is the shear strain (i.e. the fractional extension) appropriate to translocation of the cell equator up and over the toroidal rim of the cell into the dimple interior. D is the diameter of the cell. From geometry, it is possible to estimate the shear strain parameter, ϵ, and with the known values of membrane elasticity (G), the threshold shear stress is estimated to be on the order of 10^{-2} to 10^{-1} Pa. Above this threshold shear stress, the membrane will begin its tank tread motion and will convect at progressively higher rates in proportion to shear stress. When the membrane is in circulatory motion around the interior, the shear stress at the membrane is below the level deduced from the bulk shear rate; an approximate relation is given by the following equation,

$$\tau \sim \tilde{\eta}_e(\dot{\gamma} - 4D\omega/\delta) \tag{8}$$

where $\tilde{\eta}_e$ is the viscosity of the suspending medium, $\dot{\gamma}$ is the shear rate of the fluid suspension and ω is the frequency of membrane circulation around the interior; δ is the thickness of the cell. This reduced shear stress level is then opposed by membrane dynamic stresses and dissipation within the interior of the cell. An approximate relation is given by the following equations,

$$\tau \sim \frac{G\epsilon + \eta_m \epsilon \omega}{D} + \frac{4\tilde{\eta}_{Hb} D\omega}{\delta} \tag{9}$$

or

$$\tilde{\eta}_{\hat{e}}\dot{\gamma} \sim \frac{G\epsilon + \eta_m \epsilon \omega}{D} + \frac{4(\tilde{\eta}_{Hb} + \tilde{\eta}_e) D\omega}{\delta} \tag{10}$$

This relationship indicates that the rotation speed should be proportional to the fluid shear stress. This feature has been observed and quantitated in several elegant experiments [33,34]. An additional feature of red cells in shear flow is that the cell becomes progressively elongated as the shear stresses are increased which shows that the shear strain, ϵ, also increases in proportion to the shear stress. This leads to a complicated behavior that again has been well examined [34]. An excellent, approximate analysis of this fluid mechanical problem has been carried out [35] and has been used successfully to derive viscous membrane properties of red cells [36].

In contrast to the red cell, white cells simply roll in the shear field with little or no deformation unless the shear stress is very high [37]. In high shear fields they will begin to break up into fragments and eventually lyse [6]. There are two reasons for this rotational motion; one is the fact that the white cell is essentially spherical to begin with and the other is that the dynamic rigidity of the white cell is enormous (i.e. with an apparent viscosity of several hundred Pas). Approximating the white cell as a solid sphere, a fluid dynamic theory has been used to predict white cell motion and migration to vessel walls in blood flow [37]. If the cell becomes active and produces pseudopodia, the cell will exhibit rigid body rotation of a more erratic nature, again because the dynamic resistance to deformation is so large. The presence of such protrusions on white cells in blood suspensions in flow could conceivably create serious problems because of the repeated collisions between these protrusions and nearby cells.

As previously emphasized for capillary entrance dynamics, dynamic (time dependent) rigidities of blood cells are the most important parameters. Indeed, these properties will be important determinants of local flow rates and distribution within microcirculatory beds. The nominal time for entrance of a blood cell into a capillary (based on capillary flow velocity) is on the order of 0.1 second or less. Consequently, red cell resistance to deformation by extension and folding is much greater than static levels, and such rapid deformation of white cells will require pressure drops on the order of 10^4 Pa. The implications are clear, i.e. when cells enter small apertures less than their characteristic dimension, they will slow down and transit in an interruptive fashion. On the other hand, even for small apertures and low pressure differentials, cells will eventually pass through, provided that the driving forces exceed the static levels of rigidity.

3.4. Blood cell aggregation – disaggregation and interaction with vascular endothelium

3.4.1 Red blood cell aggregation: mechanisms

The previous discussion dealt with the mechanical properties of single cells and the role of cell deformability in circulatory dynamics. All of the blood cellular elements are capable of participating in aggregation/adhesion reactions in the blood stream; these multicellular products can also affect blood flow. Moreover, as is discussed elsewhere in this volume (e.g. Chapter 2), the measurement and characterization of such aggregation can provide useful clinical information.

The most common type of blood cell aggregates are *rouleaux*: the reversible, locally linear erythrocyte aggregates which form in normal blood whenever the bulk shear stress is less than about 0.05 Pa (Fig. 3.7). Rouleaux only form in the presence of certain macromolecules; washed red cells in saline undergo no

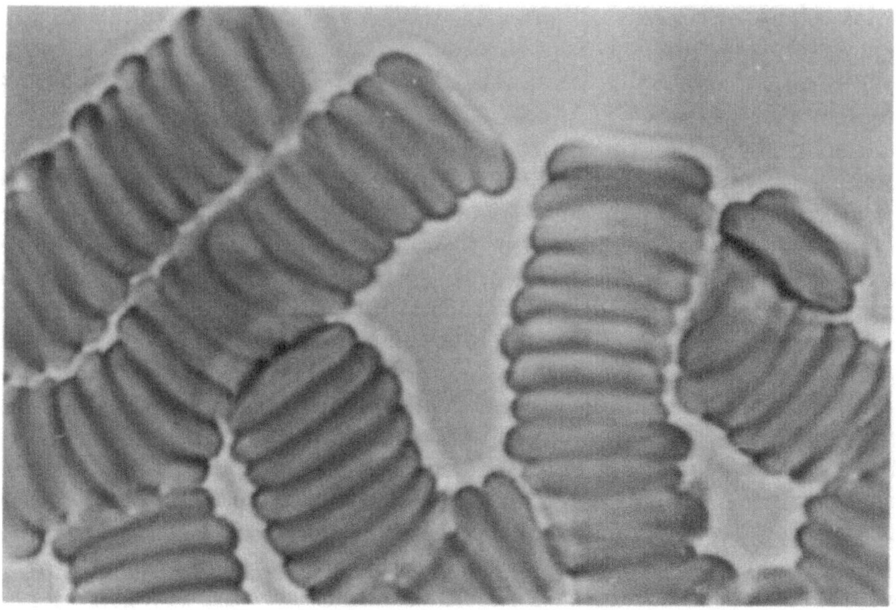

Figure 3.7 Human erythrocytes suspended in citrated autologous plasma illustrating rouleaux formation.

detectable aggregation. Normal serum also causes little if any erythrocyte aggregation. Fibrinogen is the major rouleaux-including agent in whole blood, although other high molecular weight plasma components such as alpha-2 macroglobulin and IgM contribute to the process. The addition of neutral polymers such as dextran to saline suspensions of red cells, leads to the formation of rouleaux, which are indistinguishable from those seen in anticoagulated whole blood, and this allows the aggregation to be studied in controlled solutions [38,39,40]. Such studies indicate that red cells aggregate as a result of the simultaneous adsorption of the macromolecules to adjacent cell surfaces. The molecular cross-bridges thus formed must be of sufficient strength and number to retain their patency in the face of thermal and particularly mechanical disturbances. At the biochemical level, studies of plasma protein and polymer adsorption have been carried out with erythrocytes; these have shown that the binding is weak and rapid at the relatively high solution levels associated with rouleaux formation [38,39]. Adsorption is non-specific and non-competitive (no competitive inhibitors are known) and increases linearly with concentration. Thus, the aggregate, which is formed by adsorption and molecular cross-bridging, reflects the macromolecular concentration in the suspending medium.

If the cross-bridges have a constant average surface density, the total adhesion energy will be large for large areas of intercellular contact. The maximum contact area can be attained by deformation of the cells to the limit allowed by their constant surface area and volume, but work must be done in the process to overcome the elastic energy in the membrane [41,55]. In plasma, the maximum contact area is formed at the least expense of elastic deformation energy when the cells associate face-to-face and produce the linear aggregates characteristic of rouleaux. When the adhesion energy is higher than that associated with the adsorption of physiological fibrinogen levels, more symmetric globular aggregates are produced. Here, the adhesion energy is sufficient to cause large deformations of the cells and face-to-face contact is no longer favoured. Such conditions are charcteristic of a variety of pathological situations and are responsible for the increased erythrocyte sedimentation rate observed [42]. A similar change in aggregate geometry occurs for a low density of relatively strong cross-bridges, such as those produced in antibody-induced agglutination, when the cells are sheared.

The physiological significance of normal rouleaux is not completely clear, although some circulatory phenomena appear to be affected by their formation. At low shear rates in small tubes and vessels, i.e. 30–100 μm in diameter, rouleaux formation leads to migration of red cells away from the walls of the vessel towards the region of low shear in the center, in extreme cases causing plug flow [44]. This phenomenon also results in a relative exclusion of white cells from the central region, increasing their concentration near the vessel wall [42,43]. The margination is important because these cells may then adhere to the vessel wall and migrate into the surrounding tissue as part of the inflammatory response.

White cells, therefore, need to be in frequent contact with the endothelium during normal flow if they are to respond rapidly. Finally, the formation of red cell aggregates in the post-capillary venules contributes significantly to the pressure drop in that bed, thus influencing the overall energy dissipation in the venous circulation.

Under normal conditions, the intercellular attachments in plasma are rather weak and are readily disrupted by modest shear stresses. Some pathological conditions, which increase the plasma levels of fibrinogen and other non-specifically adsorbed acute phase reactants (e.g. see Chapter 8), produce more symmetrical shear resistant aggregates that persist in regions of the circulatory bed where shear stresses are usually strong enough to disrupt rouleaux.

Types of erythrocyte aggregation other than rouleaux can occur, as was alluded to above, when more strongly bound cross-bridging macromolecules, such as antibodies, lectins, or bacterial adhesins are present. Generally, these substances interact with specific molecular structures on the cell surface; analogues to these receptor structures are effective competitive inhibitors of adsorption and aggregation. The aggregates formed in a number of these cases have been found to respond differently to moderate shear stresses. The viscosity of the cell suspension can actually increase strongly with time of shearing, rather than decrease as aggregates are broken down [45,46]. In these situations, aggregate size, symmetry, and rigidity are enhanced by shearing, with a time course that is not understood at the membrane or biochemical level. Whether or not this type of aggregation is of physiological or pathological importance remains to be seen.

3.4.2. Red blood cell aggregation: measurement

Since red cell aggregation is one of the determinants of blood flow, it is natural that viscometric measurements should be one method used to characterize the reaction. Aggregation has a large effect on whole blood viscosity at low shear rates but virtually none at high shear rates; hence, relative viscosity values at low shear rates can provide an index of the degree of aggregation present under defined conditions [47]. Such assays, along with the optical methods outlined in Chapter 2, are rapid, convenient, and can be made using relatively simple equipment. The effects of shear can be evaluated by the assay. For these reasons, they are useful clinical methods. However, since they are not amenable to detailed analysis at the single cell or membrane level, some ambiguity is associated with their interpretation. Microrheological and micromechanical measurements, on the other hand, facilitate the analysis of single cell events. Since detailed theories are available for analysis of cell adhesion, fundamental information can be obtained regarding the cross-bridging processes.

Microrheology, the measurement and interpretation of the trajectories of individual cells in defined flow fields, has been used to study blood cell aggregation [48]. Values for the force necessary to separate sphered red cells agglutinated by antibodies have been determined. In addition, information has been obtained on the aggregation behavior of both platelets [49] and white cells [50] in shear fields. One limitation of the method, however, is that the available theories apply only to spherical, rigid particles with focal or point attachments or which interact without physical contact.

Micromechanical techniques, similar to those illustrated in the section on deformability, can also be applied to the study of cell-cell interactions. In such measurements, the known mechanical (elastic) properties of cells and bilayer vesicles facilitate their use as transducers to measure the energies and/or forces which act between adherent membranes. As theoretical developments have paralleled experimental investigations of this type, considerable potential for exploitation of this approach now exists [41,51,52]. Measurements have been made to determine the *affinity* between two red cells or red cells and lipid bilayer vesicles, immersed in plasma or solutions of fibrinogen or dextran [53,54]. The affinity is the reduction in free energy per unit area of contact at equilibrium. It can be measured by recognizing, as noted above, that in order for significant areas of contact to form, work must be done in deforming the cells or membranes. At equilibrium, the affinity is equal to the rate of change of the work of deformation with respect to the change in contact area. Provided the interacting bodies are sufficiently well characterized mechanically, the work of deformation can be related to the material properties (the elastic shear and bending moduli) and the geometries of the adhering bodies at equilibrium. For instance, the shape of the end red cell "cap" on a chain of rouleaux [55] and the degree of encapsulation of a membrane vesicle by a red cell [20,56] have been used to measure affinities for red cells in plasma and dextran. Values for affinity in plasma are about 2×10^{-6} N/m; the dextran values bracket this figure depending on concentration and molecular weight [52,53]. Where it was examined (in vesicle-vesicle interactions), the formation and separation of contact in dextran appeared to be reversible, implying that in this case the work per unit area necessary to separate the two surfaces, known as the adhesion energy, was equal to the affinity [51].

While the *affinity* (the specific free energy change associated with the formation of an adhesive contact) and the *adhesion energy* (associated with the separation of the surfaces) appears to be equal in the above instance, this equality is not usually observed in the presence of more strongly bound, specific cross-bridging agents such as antibodies or lectins. In these cases, little or no spontaneous deformation of the adhering surfaces may occur, implying a low affinity value, but the work required to separate the contact can be large. In these instances, it is believed that the binding sites for the bridging molecules are sufficiently far apart that formation of an initial region of cross bridging does not "zip up" and increase the area of contact. The membrane curvature is too great at the edge of the contact area to allow further cross-bridges to form unless the surfaces are forced together externally [57,58]. It follows that the work which has to be done to separate the surfaces will depend on the size of the initial area of contact, an effect which has been observed experimentally [59].

3.4.3. Adhesion of blood cells to vessel walls

The other category of cell-cell interactions which are important in blood flow is the interaction of platelets, white cells and red cells with the vascular endothelium and, when the vessel is injured, the subendothelial lining. Since attachment of both platelets and granulocytes to the vessel wall constitutes a part of our body's natural defense mechanisms, frequent contact between these cells and the endothelium must occur under normal circumstances. If this were not the case, the accumulation of platelets at a site of vessel injury or white cells in an inflammatory locus might not occur with sufficient speed.

The frequency of wall interactions appears to be high for these cell types largely because of their interactions with erythrocytes in the flow. One mechanism, described earlier, is the exclusion and peripheral migration of leukocytes caused by aggregated erythrocytes which flow centrally through blood vessels at relatively low velocities [50]. A second mechanism has been described for white cells exiting into post-capillary venules, followed by a train of erythrocytes [50]. Here, interaction with single deformable red cells in the diverging flow field apparently forces the leukocytes to the vessel walls. This mechanism correlates well with the fact that granulocyte margination and transendothelial egress is observed in the venules of most tissues.

The frequency of platelet-wall interactions in tube flow has also been shown to depend on the presence of red cells. In this case, it was shown that the random motion induced by erythrocyte tumbling and collisions dramatically increased the diffusion of small particles across the lumen of the tube with a consequent increase in the frequency of collision with the wall [60]. Platelet adhesion is also strongly affected by the pattern of streamlines in regions where flow is disturbed and vortices exist. Evidence for greatly increased wall interactions near stagnation points, where flow around the vortex begins to reattach to the main stream, has been obtained [61]. The degree of platelet-wall adhesion was again enhanced strongly by the presence of red cells. The correlation between the sites of such disturbed flow and the appearance of platelet thrombi and atherosclerotic lesions support the relevance of these observations to the circulation in vivo.

Under normal circumstances, there is little if any adhesion of platelets to vascular endothelium. However, if the vessel wall becomes injured and subendothelial collagen fibrils are exposed to flowing blood, platelets very rapidly adhere. The molecular mechanism of adhesion is not clear, but it does not seem to require any activation of the platelet, i.e. the native platelet surface seems to have an affinity for collagen or the material which adsorbs to it when exposed to

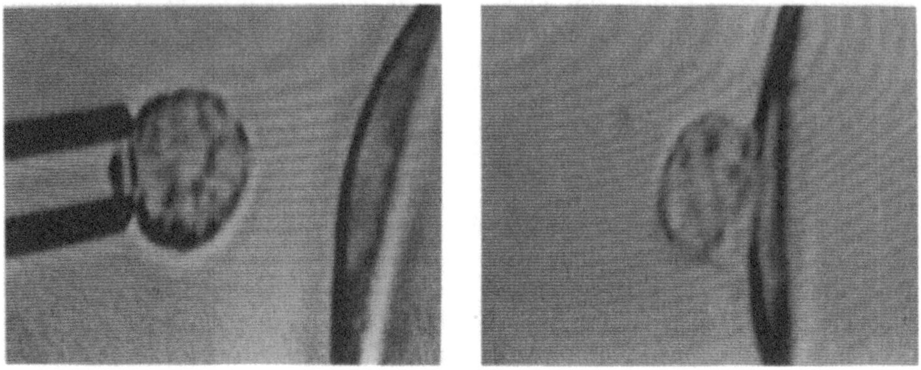

Figure 3.8 A human granulocyte, which has been maneuvered via micropipette to contact with a cultured endothelial cell, is shown adhering to the endothelial surface.

plasma. When platelets interact with collagen, however, they are then activated, resulting in the release of numerous factors; these factors activate passing platelets to cause shape changes, aggregation and adhesion and stimulate blood coagulation and fibrin formation as well [62]. The end result is a thrombus which may or may not grow and embolize, depending on the flow conditions, plug geometry and the mechanical properties of the mass.

White cell adhesion seems to be activated by soluble mediators, such as complement components, released from tissue where an inflammatory reaction is initiated [63]. Such activation enhances granulocyte adhesion to the endothelium;

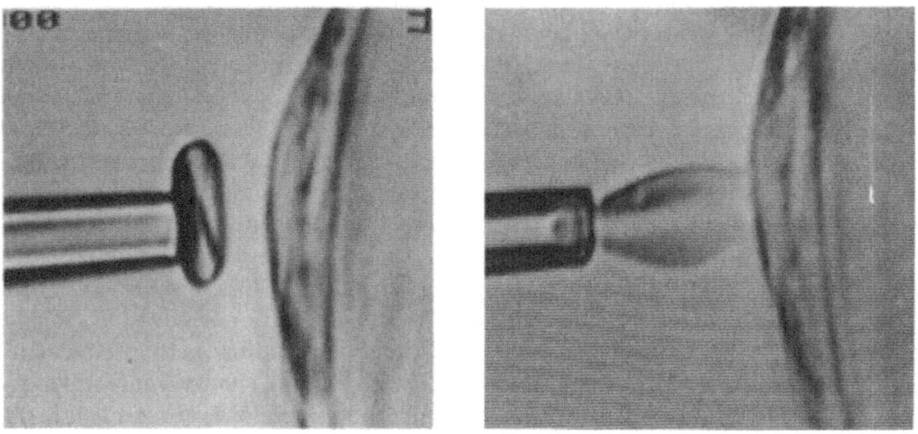

Figure 3.9 A sickle erythrocyte is shown when maneuvered for contact with a cultured endothelial cell, followed by separation from the endothelial surface. The red cell deformation demonstrates the strong adhesion.

cells cease to roll downstream along the vessel wall as adhesion becomes stronger; this is followed by migration of the cells out of the blood vessel towards the source of the inflammation. Again, the molecular mechanisms responsible for adhesion to the endothelial cells are not known. Fig. 3.8 shows a granulocyte in the process of actively adhering to an endothelial cell cultured on a sepharose bead.

Erythrocytes are considered to be the least active cells in the circulation with respect to interaction with endothelial cells. However, red cells from individuals with sickle cell disease have been found to adhere to endothelial cells in vitro at a very high frequency [64]. Moreover, measurement of the frequency and strength of adherence of sickle and normal red cells suspended in sickle or normal plasma showed that the properties of both the sickle cells and the sickle plasma were involved. It may well be that this adhesion tendency contributes to the microcirculatory disturbances present during sickle cell crisis. Fig. 3.9 shows adhesion and separation of a sickle erythrocyte to/from a cultured endothelial cell test surface.

3.5 Acknowledgements

The authors gratefully acknowledged the support in part of USPHS NIH Grant HL 26965 (EAE) and MRC of Canada Grants MT-5759 and PG24 (DEB).

3.6 References

1. Cokelet G.R., Merrill E.W., Gilliland E.R., Sh H., Britten A., Wells R.E. 1963. The rheology of human blood – measurement near and at zero shear rate. Trans. Soc. Rheology 7, 303-317.
2. Merrill E.W., Benis A.M., Gilliland E.R., Sherwood T.K., Salzman E.W. 1965. Pressure-flow relations of human blood in hollow fibers at low flow rates. J. Appl. Physiol. 20, 954-967.
3. Goldsmith H.L., Marlo J. 1972. Flow behaviour of erythrocytes. I. Rotation and deformation in dilute suspensions. Proc. Roy. Soc. Lond. B. 182, 351-384.
4. Schmid-Schöbein H., Wells R.E., Goldstone J. 1971. Fluid drop-like behaviour of erythrocytes – disturbance in pathology and its quantification. Biorheology 7, 227-234.
5. Meiselman H.J. 1978. Rheology of shape-transformed human red cells. Biorheology 15, 225-237.
6. Martin R.R., DeWitz T.S., McIntire L.V. 1979. Alterations in leukocyte structure and function due to mechanical trauma. In Hwang, Gross and Patel (eds). Quantitatve Cardiovascular Studies: Clinical and Research Applications of Engineering Principles. University Park Press, Baltimore, MD., pp. 419-454.
7. Evans E.A., Mohandas N., Leung A. 1984. Static and dynamic rigidities of normal and sickle erythrocytes: Major influence of cell hemoglobin concentration. J. Clin. Invest. 73, 477-488.
8. Bell D.N., Goldsmith H.L. 1984. Platelet aggregation in poiseuille flow II. Effect of shear rate. Microvasc. Res. 27, 316-330.
9. Hartert H. 1984. Biorheology in the practice of medicine: resonance thrombography. Biorheology 21, 19-32.

10. Jen C.J., McIntire L.V. 1982. The structural properties and contractile force of a clot. Cell Motility 2, 445-455.
11. Schmid-Schöbein G.W., Shih Y., Chien S. 1980. Morphometry of human leukocytes. Blood 56, 866-875.
12. Frojmovic M.M., Milton J.G. 1982. Human platelet size, shape, and related functions in health and disease. Physiol. Rev. 62, 185-257.
13. Evans E.A., Hochmuth R.M. 1976. Membrane viscoelastity. Biophys. J. 16, 1-11.
14. Evans E.A., Skalak R. 1980. Mechanics and Thermodynamics of Biomembranes. CRC Press, Boca Raton, FL.
15. Evans E.A., Waugh R. 1978. Osmotic correction to elastic area compressibility: measurements on red cell membrane. Biophys. J. 20, 307-313.
16. Evans E.A. 1973. New membrane concept applied to the analysis of fluid-shear and micropipette deformed red blood cells. Biophys. J. 13, 941-954.
17. Evans E.A., Lacelle P.L. 1975. Intrinsic material properties of the erythrocyte membrane indicated by mechanical analysis of the deformation. Blood 45, 29-43.
18. Chien S., Sung K.L.P., Skalak R., Usami S., Tözeren A. 1978. Theoretical and experimental studies on viscoelastic properties of red cell membranes. Biophys. J. 24, 463-488.
19. Waugh R., Evans E.A. 1979. Thermoelasticity of red blood cell membrane. Biophys. J. 26, 115-132.
20. Evans E.A. 1980. Minimum energy analysis of membrane deformation applied to pipet aspiration and surface adhesion of red blood cells. Biophys. J. 30, 265-284.
21. Evans E.A. 1982. Bending elastic modulus of red blood cell membrane derived from buckling instability in micropipet aspiration tests. Biophys. J. 43, 27-30.
22. Hochmuth R.M., Worthy P.R., Evans E.A. 1979. Red cell extensional recovery and the determination of membrane viscosity. Biophys. J. 26, 101-114.
23. Stossel T.P., Hartwig J.H., Yin H.L., Stendahl O. 1980. The motor of amoeboid leukocytes. Biochem. Soc. Symp. 45, 51-63.
24. Valerius N.H., Stendahl O., Hartwig J.H., Stossel T.P. 1981. Distribution of actin-binding protein and myosin in polymorphonuclear leukocytes during locomotion and phagocytosis. Cell 24, 195-202.
25. Bagge U., Skalak R., Attefors R. 1977. Granulocyte rheology: Experimental studies in an in vitro micro-flow system. Adv. Microcirc. 7, 19-48.
26. Schmid-Schönbein G.W., Sung K.L.P., Tözeren H., Skalak R., Chien S. 1981. Passive mechanical properties of human leukocytes. Biophys. J. 36, 243-256.
27. Evans E.A., Kukan B. 1984. Passive material behavior of granulocytes based on large deformation and recovery after deformation tests. Blood 64, 1028-1035.
28. Miller M.E., Myers K.A. 1975. Cellular deformability of the human peripheral blood polymorphonuclear leukocyte: Method of study, normal variation and effects of physical and chemical alterations. Res. J. Reticuloendothel. Soc. 18, 337-345.
29. Evans E.A., Kukan B. Viscous resistance to extension and flow of blood granulocytes: Dominated by the cell cortex. Blood (to be submitted).
30. Schmid-Schönbein G.W., Usami S., Skalak R., Chien S. 1980. The interaction of leukocytes and erythrocytes in capillary and post-capillary vessels. Microvasc. Res. 19, 45-70.
31. Chien S., Schmid-Schönbein G.W., Sung K.L.P., Schmalzer E.A., Skalak R. 1984. Viscoelastic properties of leukocytes. In White Cell Mechanics Basic Science and Clinical Aspects. H.J. Meiselman, M.A. Lichtman and P.L. LaCelle (eds.), Alan R. Liss, New York. Kroc Found. Ser. 16, pp 19-51
32. Schmid-Schönbein G.W., Skalak R., Sung K.L.P., Chien S. 1982. Human leukocytes in the active state. In White Blood Cells, Morphology and Rheology as Related to Function. U. Bagge, G.V. Born and P. Gaehtgens. (eds.) Martinus Nijhoff, The Hague, pp. 21-31.
33. Fischer T., Schmid-Schönbein H. 1977. Tank tread motion of red cell membranes in viscometric flow: Behavior of intracellular and extracellular markers. Blood Cells 3, 351.

34. Fischer T.M., Stohr M., Schmid-Schönbein H. 1978. Red blood cell (RBC) microrheology: Comparison of the behavior of single RBC and liquid droplets in shear flow. AIChE Symp. Ser. No. 182, 74, 38-45.
35. Keller S.R., Skalak R. 1982. Motion of a tank-treading ellipsoidal particle in a shear flow. J. Fluid. Mech. 120, 24-27.
36. Tran-Son-Tay R., Sutera S.P., Rao P.R. 1984. Determination of red blood cell membrane viscosity from rheoscopic observations of tank-treading motion. Biophys. J. 46, 65-72.
37. Nobis U., Fries A.R., Gaehtgens P. 1982. Rheological mechanisms contributing to WBC-margination. In Bagge U., Born G.V.R. and Gaehtgens P. (eds). White Blood Cells: Morphology and Rheology as Related to Function. Martinus Nijhoff, The Hague. pp. 57-65.
38. Brooks D.E. 1973. The effect of neutral polymers on the electrokinetic potential of cells and other charged particles. III. Experimental studies on the dextran-erythrocyte system. J. Colloid Interface Sci. 43, 700-713.
39. Jan P. K.M., Chien S. 1973. Role of surface electric charge in red blood cell interactions. J. Gen. Physiol. 61, 638-654.
40. Brooks D.E., Greig R.G., Janzen H. 1980. Mechanisms of erythrocyte aggregation. In Cokelet G.C., Meiselman H.J., Brooks D.E. (eds). Erythrocyte Mechanics and Blood Flow. Alan R. Liss, Inc. New York. pp. 119-140.
41. Evans E.A., Parsegian V.A. 1983. Energetics of membrane deformation and adhesion in cell and vesicle aggregation. In Copley A.L., Seaman G.V.F. (eds). Surface Phenomena in Hemorheology: Their Theoretical, Experimental and Clinical Aspects. Ann. N. Y. Acad. Sci. 416, 13-33.
42. Fahraeus R. 1929. The suspension stability of blood. Physiol. Rev. 9, 241-274.
43. Chien S., Usami S., Skalak R. 1984. Blood flow in small tubes. In Handbook of Physiology, Circulation. Section on Microrculation, E.M. Renk and C. Michel. (eds), Am. Physiol. Soc., Bethesda, MD. pp. 217-249.
44. Goldsmith H.L., Skalak R. 1975. Hemodynamics. Ann. Rev. Fluid. Mech. 7, 213-247.
45. Greig R.G., Brooks D.E. 1979. Shear-induced concanavalin A agglutination of human erythrocytes. Nature 282, 738-739.
46. Brooks D.E., Trust T.J. 1983. Enhancement of bacterial adhesion by shear forces: Characterization of the hemagglutination induced by Aeromonas salmonicida strain 438. J. Gen. Microbiol. 129, 3661-3669.
47. Brooks D.E. 1976. Red cell interactions in low flow states. In Grayson J., Zingg W. (eds). Microrculation I. Blood-Vessel Interactions, Systems in Special Tissues. Plenum Press, N.Y. pp. 33-52.
48. Goldsmith H.L., Gold P., Shuster J., Takamura K. 1982. Interactions between sphered human red cells in tube flow: technique for measuring the strength of antigen-antibody bonds. Microvasc. Res. 23, 231-238.
49. Karino T., Goldsmith H.L. 1979. Aggregation of human platelets in an annular vortex distal to a tubular expansion. Microvasc. Res. 17, 217-237.
50. Goldsmith H.L., Spain S. 1984. Margination of leukocytes in blood flow through small tubes. Microvasc. Res. 27, 204-222.
51. Evans E.A., Metcalfe M. 1984. Free energy potential for aggregation of mixed phosphatidylcholine/phosphatidylserine lipid vesicles in glucose polymer (dextran) solutions. Biophys. J. 45, 715-720.
52. Chien S., Sung L.A., Simchon S., Lee M.M.L., Jan, P.K.M. and Skalak R. 1984. Energy balance in red cell interactions. Ann. N.Y. Acad. Sci. 416, 190-206.
53. Buxbaum K., Evans E.A., Brooks D.E. 1982. Quantitation of surface affinities of red blood cells in dextran solutions and plasma. Biochem. 21, 3235-3239.
54. Janzen J., Evans E.A., Brooks D.E. Fibrinogen adsorption and red cell-red cell adhesion energy. (In preparation).
55. Skalak R., Zarda P.R., Jan K.M., Chien S. 1981. Mechanics of rouleaux formation. Biophys. J. 35, 771-782.

56. Evans E.A., Buxbaum K. 1981. Affinity of red blood cell membrane for particle surfaces measured by the extent of particle encapsulation. Biophys. J. 34, 1-12.
57. Evans E.A. 1985. Detailed mechanics of membrane-membrane adhesion and separation I. Continuum of molecular cross-bridges. Biophys. J. 48, 175-183.
58. Evans E.A. 1985. Detailed mechanics of membrane-membrane adhesion and separation II. Discreet, kinetically trapped molecular cross-bridges. Biophys. J. 48, 185-192.
59. Evans E.A., Leung A. 1984. Adhesivity and rigidity of red blood cell in relation to wheat germ agglutinin binding. J. Cell Biol. 98, 1201-1208.
60. Karino T., Goldsmith H.L. 1984. Role of blood cell-wall interactions in thrombogenesis and atherogenesis: A microrheological study. Biorheology 21, 587-601.
61. Karino T., Goldsmith H.L. 1979. Adhesion of human platelets to collagen on the walls distal to a tubular expansion. Microvasc. Res. 17, 238-262.
62. Mustard J.F., Packham M.A., Kinlough-Rathbone R.L. 1981. Mechanisms in thrombosis. In Blood A.L., Thomas D.P. (eds.). Hemostasis and Thrombosis. Churchill Livingstone, Edinburgh, pp. 503-526.
63. Williams T.J., Jose P.J., Forest M.J., Wedmore C.V., Clough G.F. 1984. Interactions between neutrophils and microvascular endothelial cells leading to cell emigration and plasma protein leakage. In Meiselman H.J., Lichtman M.A., Lacelle P.L. (eds). White Cell Mechanics: Basic Science and Clinical Aspects. Alan R. Liss, Inc., New York. KROC Found. Ser. 16, pp. 195-208.
64. Mohandas N., Evans E.A. 1984. Adherence of sickle erythrocytes to vascular endothelial cells: Requirement for both cell membrane changes and plasma factors. Blood 64, 282-287.

4
Structural, hemodynamic and rheological characteristics of blood flow in the circulation

P. Gaehtgens, A.R. Pries, K. Ley
Institut für Physiologie, Freie Universität Berlin, Arnimallee 22, 1000 Berlin 33, Federal Republic of Germany

4.1. Introduction

This chapter outlines some of the basic features of the circulation which appear to be of particular relevance for an understanding of hemorheological phenomena. The behavior of blood flowing through the various compartments of the cardiovascular system is determined by both its own rheological properties and the structural design and hemodynamic characteristics of the circulatory system. Thus, changes of blood rheology, which may occur in diseased states, cannot be interpreted in terms of their possible effects on blood flow in vivo, unless the hemodynamic state and possible alterations of vascular morphology are also appreciated. In fact, a multitude of pathophysiological situations or clinical disorders is characterized by an alteration, from the normal, of blood rheology and vascular hindrance; these may, in some cases, even have a common cause.

This chapter will therefore concentrate on some of the physiological aspects of the vascular system in order to define the hemodynamic conditions of blood flow in relation to vascular function. Since the circulatory system as a whole does not represent a hemodynamically uniform system, various functional compartments will have to be considered. This may then provide the background for a more detailed description of the rheological phenomena which, according to current knowledge, take place in the different vascular compartments.

4.2. Structural and hemodynamic characteristics of the vascular system

An integrative description of the structural and hemodynamic conditions of blood flow in the entire vascular system can be derived from quantitative information on vascular architecture and topology. Such a description can provide useful overall information on the distribution of blood volume, the surface area to volume ratio, and other functionally relevant features of the vascular system; application of fundamental hydrodynamic principles furthermore permits an estimation of the distribution of intravascular pressures, resistances, or flow velocities, and thus of rheologically relevant features of the vascular system. In such an approach, variations of vascular design in different vascular provinces are disregarded, although they may be quite pronounced and relevant for the specific physiological function of the various organs. In order to derive some generalized statements describing the system as a whole, a few simplifying assumptions have to be made:

a. Vessels of equal diameters are assumed to represent parallel and equivalent pathways belonging to the same cross-section of the vascular tree.
b. Temporal variation of vessel dimensions and of vessel recruitment are assumed absent.
c. Blood rheological properties are assumed to be independent of geometric and hemodynamic flow conditions.

Fig. 4.1 shows such an analysis of a composite vascular system, based on a combination of histological data [1,2] and intravital microscopic measurements [3,4], in analogy to similar estimates made by Chien [5] and Schmid-Schönbein [6]. A few important conclusions may be drawn from this analysis:

a. The arborization of the vascular tree leads to an enormous variation of the surface area to volume ratio which increases by approximately four orders of magnitude as the blood flows from the aorta into the capillary bed; this facilitates, of course, the exchange of materials between blood and tissues. The increase of surface area is brought about by an increase of the number of parallel vascular pathways which outweighs the decrease of single vessel diameter and length.

b. Since, according to the continuity principle, cardiac output must be the same as blood flows through each vascular generation, the distribution of intravascular pressure and blood flow velocity can be calculated. As shown by the variations of pressure and volume, hemodynamic parameters are not uniformly distributed within the vascular system. The greatest reduction of mean intravascular pressure is seen to occur in the arteriolar vessels, which therefore represent the site of largest vascular hindrance (*resistance vessels*). In the venous system, driving pressures are generally low.

c. As a result of pressure distribution and morphometric characteristics, wall shear stresses in the entire arterial system are in the range of 1 to 10 Pa. Under physiological conditions this leaves little room for shear-dependent changes of apparent blood viscosity to occur. A precipitous drop of wall shear stresses occurs as the blood leaves the capillaries and enters into the post-capillary venules. Under conditions of reduced cardiac output or arterial pressure, an increase of the pre- to post-capillary resistance ratio has been suggested to result from elevation of blood viscosity in the venules [5].

d. The non-uniform distribution of rheologically relevant parameters may prevent the application of Poiseuille's law to the vascular system, in view of the established non-Newtonian properties of blood. According to direct measurements [7,8], however, this conclusion is unwarranted because of the opposing effects of inhomogeneous distribution of shear stresses and intravascular hematocrit (see below) on blood viscosity.

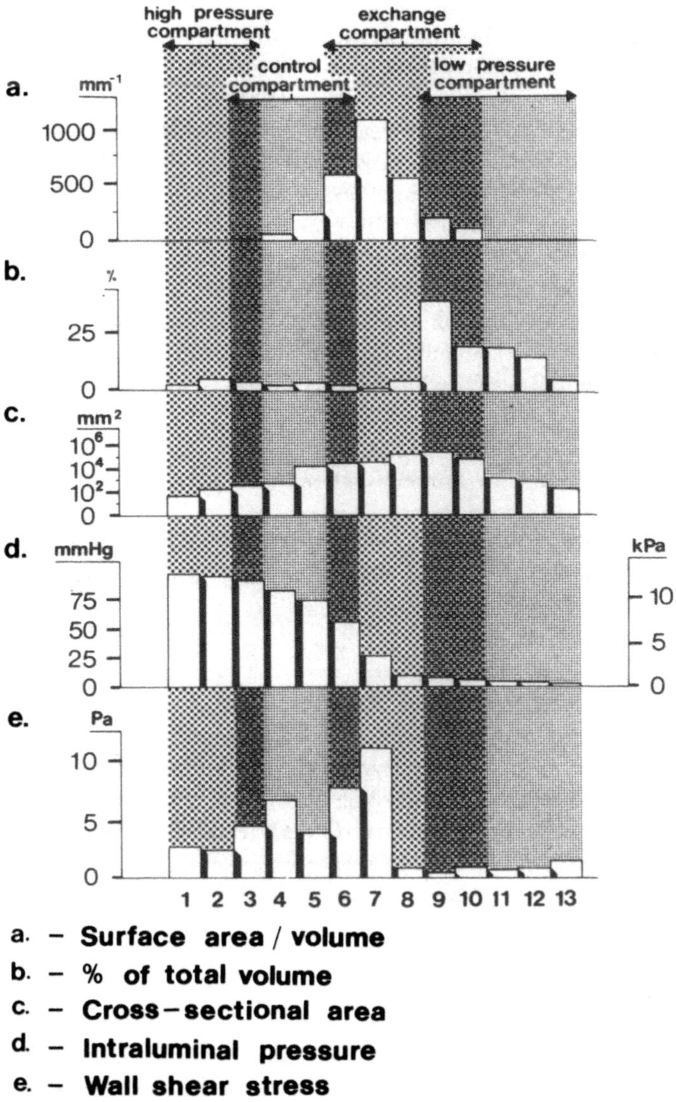

Figure 4.1. Distribution of morphological and hemodynamic parameters in the circulatory system. Data are calculated from morphometric measurements using the assumptions described in the text.

e. As can be deduced from the variation of intravascular volume, the larger part of total blood volume flows under conditions of borderline shear stresses (in terms of the shear-dependence of blood viscosity).

It must be born in mind that overall characterization of the vascular system given here is based on morphometric information and therefore represents a static description. The architectural design of the vascular system is tailored according to its basic physiological function to supply nutrients to the tissue. Changes of design (by growth of pre-existing or development of additional vascular pathways) occur under conditions of altered requirements: Large vessel stenosis may lead to the development of collateral conduit vessels, and chronically elevated functional activity or reduced supply conditions (such as hypoxia) may result in additional growth of new exchange vessels [9]. Furthermore, blood delivery to tissues is adapted to time variable metabolic activity by a variety of vascular mechanisms, as will be discussed below. Thus, the vascular system is responsive to both short-term (seconds, minutes) and long-term (days, months) imbalance between local metabolic demand and supply. Therefore, appropriate modifications of the above description, which represents an order of magnitude analysis, must be made in order to allow for a more dynamic analysis.

4.3. Functional compartments within the vascular system

From a functional point of view, the vascular system may be subdivided into at least four different "compartments" which are defined by their physiological role within the overall function of the cardiovascular system:
- the high pressure compartment of conduit vessels,
- the control compartment of resistance vessels,
- the exchange compartment of capillaries and venules,
- the low pressure compartment of capacity vessels.

No distinct demarcation line can be drawn between these compartments which overlap and vary in size depending on the physiological condition. Since variation of morphology between different vessels is related to vascular function, characteristic features can be defined which may serve as guidelines for interpretation of function.

4.3.1. The high pressure conduit vessels

The aorta and its major side branches serve as conduit pipes connecting the heart to the various organs to which blood is to be delivered. Classification of these vessels as *conduit pipes* underlines the fact that, by and large, changes in the distribution of cardiac output to the organs cannot be achieved by changes in the physiological state of these vessels. The contribution of these vessels to regional flow resistance and to total pressure drop (Fig. 4.1) is generally considered small. A more precise analysis has shown, however, that cerebral [10,11,12,13,14], myocardial [15], and skeletal muscle blood flow [16] can to some extent be affected under various physiological conditions by active constriction or dilation of the conduit arteries.

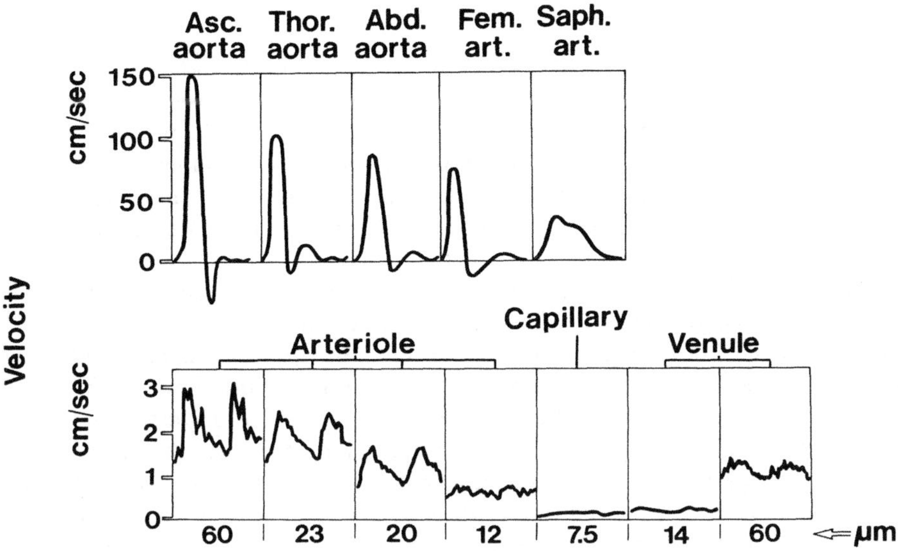

Figure 4.2. Traces of pulsatile blood flow velocity in various parts of the circulation. Although the amplitude of the pulsations decreases significantly from the ascending aorta to the capillary bed, the pulsatile nature of flow is still preserved in the most peripheral vessels.

Thus, the definition of this compartment is not so much based on the magnitude of the pressure drop occurring, but on the absolute level of intravascular pressure. By definition, intravascular and thus transmural pressure are high and mainly determined by cardiac output and total peripheral resistance. The volume of blood contained in the high pressure compartment (approx. 5–10% of total blood volume, or approx. 3–5 stroke volumes) is subjected to relatively high shear stresses, particularly during the systolic part of the cardiac cycle.

As a result of discontinuous ejection of blood from the heart, pressure as well as blood flow velocity in this vascular compartment are strongly pulsatile (Fig. 4.2). To some degree, the pulsatile nature of flow is attenuated by the elastic deformation of the vessel wall during the ejection phase (*Windkessel function*). The composition of the vessel wall is therefore adapted both to the necessity of supporting high transmural pressures and to the requirement of elastic deformation. While a large amount of elastin is present in the wall of the aorta, the more peripheral arteries exhibit an increasing proportion of smooth muscle.

Since pronounced structural changes take place in these vessels as a function of age, the dynamics of flow and pressure also vary with age: Pulse amplitude usually increases due to increasing wall stiffness, and mean intravascular pressure may also rise.

4.3.2. The control compartment

Neglecting some degree of overlap, this compartment is largely identical with the arterioles. While hemodynamic characteristics are similar to those of the conduit vessels, the major physiological function is related to local control of blood volume flow and its distribution within the tissue; this is achieved by active contraction of smooth muscle in the vessel wall. Accordingly, these vessels are characterized by a wall thickness to lumen ratio which increases towards the capillary bed.

As seen from Fig. 4.1, the major fraction of total arterio-venous pressure drop takes place in this compartment. This is the result of the decrease of single vessel diameters which is not sufficiently compensated by the increasing number of parallel pathways. However, the important physiological function of this vessel compartment is associated with the ability of these vessels to undergo significant changes of diameter: At any given level of large artery pressure, the mechanisms controlling arteriolar smooth muscle activity determine regional and local resistance to flow and thus flow rate distribution among and within tissues. Simultaneously, however, they will also affect the magnitude of "post-arteriolar" (= capillary) pressure which is one of the relevant parameters determining intra/extravascular fluid balance.

Smooth muscle activity is controlled by "endogenous" and "exogenous" mechanisms. While the former results from the intrinsic property of smooth muscle tissue to develop some degree of active myogenic tension ("basal tone"), the latter are brought about by a variety of stimuli exogenous to the muscle cell. These include

- locally produced humoral agents (metabolic regulation),
- substances circulating with the blood (hormonal regulation),
- activation of autonomic nerves (neurogenic regulation).

Under most physiological and pathophysiological conditions endogenous and exogenous control mechanisms act in concert, although their relative importance may vary [17,18,19,20,21]. As an example, neurogenically initiated release of mediator substances from cellular elements of the tissue or vascular walls may occur; likewise, locally produced substances may lead to stimulation of afferent nerve terminals, thus initiating a neurogenic reflex pathway.

Functional differences between these mechanisms may be observed with respect to the regional variations or the time scale of the observed effects: while circulating hormones result in overall adjustments of vascular conductivity without specific targets of action, neurogenic control may be regionally differential, depending on the particular nervous pathways involved. Differential sensitivity to humoral and neurogenic stimuli appears to exist within the control compartment: the more peripheral vessels exhibit higher sensitivity to humoral stimulation and lower sensitivity to neurogenic stimulation [22,23]. In general, neurogenic and myogenic mechanisms elicit faster responses compared to humoral or hormonal mechanisms, which rely on convectional or diffusional transport.

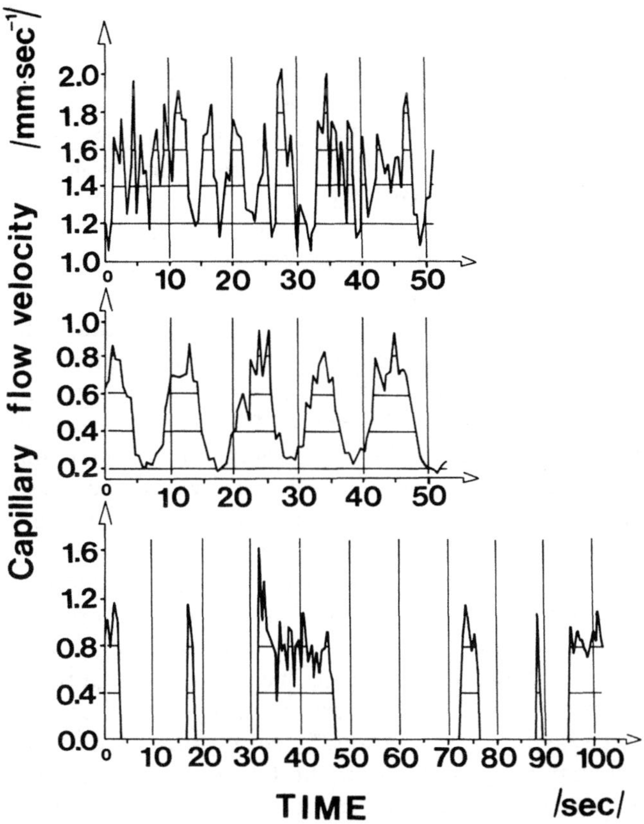

Figure 4.3. Typical traces of capillary flow velocity as a function of time.
The middle panel shows an example which could be due to arteriolar vasomotion, while the lower panel demonstrates flow intermittency due to transient white cell occlusion. Data from [28].

Due to intrinsic smooth muscle properties [24,25], arteriolar blood vessels in many organs exhibit spontaneous changes (vasomotion) of internal diameter [26,27]. Therefore blood flow through the vessels of the control compartment is not steady, but shows rhythmic variations with frequencies typically between 2 and 20 min^{-1}. The amplitude of vasomotion increases with decreasing vessel diameter, and complete closure of precapillary arterioles during the "systolic" phase of the vasomotor cycle has been observed. Since flow in capillary vessels is largely a function of phenomena occurring upstream, capillary flow will also show fluctuations (Fig. 4.3) resulting from arteriolar vasomotion [28,29,30,31]. Mechanisms regulating blood flow via arteriolar smooth muscle tone can also interfere with frequency or amplitude of vasomotion. Strong humoral or neurogenic stimulation will cause vasomotion to cease by eliciting pronounced inhibition or activation of the spontaneous contractile process in the smooth muscle cells.

In addition to the effect of vasomotion on local flow, the pulsatile nature of flow resulting from the rhythmic action of the heart is well preserved (Fig. 4.2) in the vessels of the control compartment [32,33,34]. Pulsatility may even be transmitted to the capillary level, particularly in the vasodilated state, when the pressure drop in the control compartment is reduced.

Direct measurements of pressure and flow velocity in arterioles [7,8] have confirmed the presence of relatively high wall shear stresses (5 to 15 Pa). In line with the conclusions drawn from the generalized analysis of the vascular system (Fig. 4.1), such measurements also indicate high values of average shear rates: the reduced bulk velocity ($\bar{u}$) which for a Newtonian fluid equals one eighth of the wall shear rate, was found to range between 100 and 200 sec^{-1}. Furthermore, calculations of apparent blood viscosity on the basis of such measurements demonstrated a substantial shear-dependence within the range of hemodynamic variables observed. These data appear to indicate that even within the vessel compartment discussed here the apparent blood viscosity may be an important variable contributing to the temporal and spatial variations of blood flow.

While such hemodynamic descriptions are focussed on the characteristic distribution of parameters between individual vascular segments of this compartment, one should not ignore the fact that these are part of a branching system containing divergent bifurcations. Direct measurements have shown a significant pressure drop across such bifurcations, the magnitude of which increases with decreasing daughter to parent vessel diameter ratio [35]. Both pressure and flow distribution at individual branch points may therefore be subject to local geometric conditions. In addition, the particulate nature of blood is the cause of cell/plasma separation in branched arteriolar networks; this in turn leads to non-homogeneous distribution of red cell and plasma flow to the component vessels of a network (see below). Although resistance to flow is less sensitive to alteration of hematocrit in small blood vessels, as will be discussed later, such separation effects may contribute to changes in distribution of pressures and flow in microvascular networks.

4.3.3. The exchange compartment

The major function of the vascular system is to supply metabolic nutrients to and remove waste products from the tissues. This occurs by transport through the wall of the exchange vessels. This definition is purely functional and therefore includes vessels whose hemodynamic characteristics are quite variable.

Exchange of materials between the intra- and extravascular spaces is strongly affected by the size of the exchange surface. It is therefore not surprising that vascular surface area to volume ratio reaches a maximum in this compartment. In

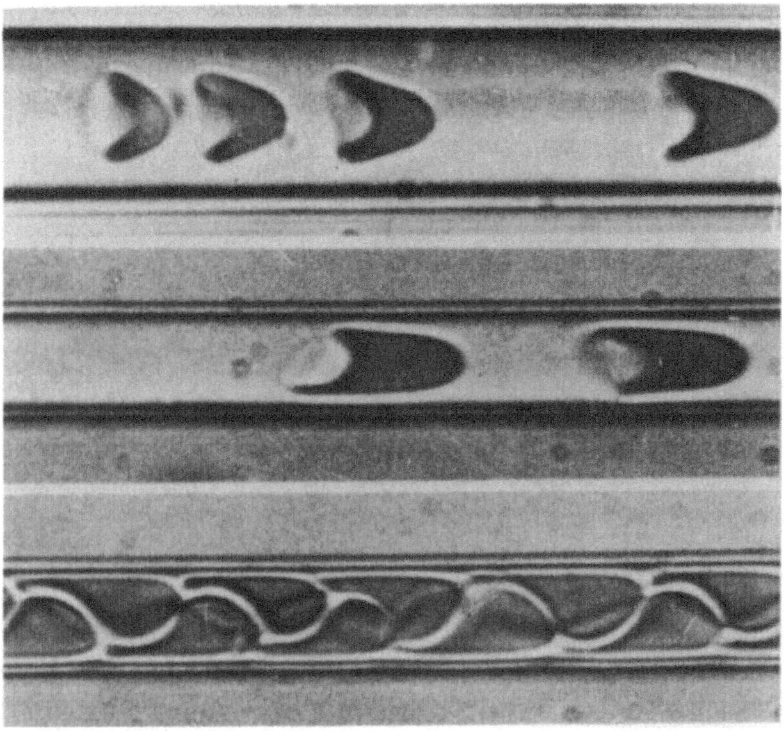

Figure 4.4. Deformation of single human red cells during flow through glass capillaries with inner diameters between 6 and 12 μm. Single file flow is seen in the two upper panels, while the bottom panel shows a multi-file arrangement in "zipper"-flow.

many tissues, e.g. skeletal muscle or myocardium, capillary diameters are smaller than resting red cell diameters, thus requiring cell deformation during passage (Fig. 4.4). However, variability of capillary diameters within any one tissue (Fig. 4.5) is substantial [36,37,38,39]. Vessel walls are characterized by a single layer of endothelial cells supported by a basement membrane. The ultrastructure of these wall elements varies greatly between different organs, depending on local function [40]. Fluid balance between the intra- and extravascular spaces is governed by hydrostatic and colloidal osmotic forces as formulated by Starling's equation.

In this context, it is worth mentioning that blood rheological properties are both a resultant and a determinant of local fluid transport. Prevalence of fluid filtration from the blood into the tissue tends to increase local hematocrit and protein concentration of the blood, while prevalence of fluid reabsorption will lead to hemodilution. On the other hand, alteration of blood rheology may lead to an alteration of pre-/post-capillary resistance ratio and thus of intracapillary pressure; this will, in turn, affect fluid balance. Because of local adjustments of

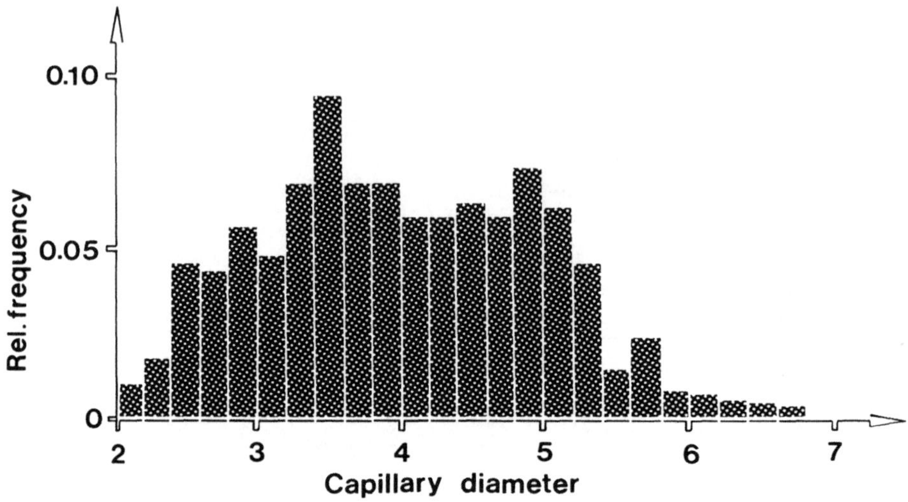

Figure 4.5. Frequency distribution of capillary diameter, as determined in the dog myocardium. Data from [38].

pressure and flow within the capillary network, this simplifying conclusion has to be modified: the apportionment of blood flow and red cell flux to the individual capillaries is determined by an interplay between smooth muscle activity in the preceding control compartment and local rheological phenomena (see below).

Blood flow through capillary vessels is often intermittent (Fig. 4.3) [28,41,42], and several mechanisms have been postulated to contribute to this phenomenon. With the exception of a few tissues, the postulated existence of "precapillary sphincters" has been questioned [36]. Whole organ studies, however, have shown that regulation of fluid exchange may be physiologically distinct from regulation of blood flow [17]. Furthermore, studies on the effect of reduced arterio-venous driving pressure on capillary perfusion have shown capillary flow to cease at positive pressures [43], thus indicating either rheological or vascular occlusion. Since the response to hypotension of precapillary resistance vessels, at least in metabolically active tissues, is relaxation and dilation rather than collapse or constriction, a rheological explanation appears to be more likely. A conclusive explanation of the observation of zero flow at positive pressures is not yet at hand. However, the yield shear stress of normal blood is too small to explain the phenomenon, and vessel occlusion by circulating white cells may be an additional cause. Intermittency of flow in single exchange vessels has been attributed to transient obstruction by circulating leukocytes [44,45], and this phenomenon has been postulated to contribute to incomplete recovery of capillary flow (*no-reflow*) following periods of ischemia [44,46,47,48].

The exchange compartment includes not only the capillaries proper but also the postcapillary venules, in which a significant part of fluid movement and most of the protein exchange between blood and tissue takes place. It is in this section of the vascular system where the exchange and low pressure compartments overlap. While the volume of blood contained in the capillaries is a very small fraction of total blood volume, it is more significant in the postcapillary venules. As shown by Fig. 4.1, the exchange compartment is also hemodynamically quite heterogeneous: While nominally high shear stresses and rates prevail in perfused capillary vessels, the values in postcapillary venules are the lowest of the entire vascular system. This is obviously the result of the substantial increase of total cross-sectional area which is found here. Since intravascular pressures are low in postcapillary venules, fluid reabsorption seems more likely to occur than filtration, if the simple Starling concept applies.

This conclusion must, however, be modified in the face of experimental observations. The equilibrium point of fluid movement, which according to the Starling hypothesis should be expected in the mid-capillary, may in fact be located in the postcapillary venules. This is due to the significantly greater permeability of these vessels not only to fluid, but also to protein; as a consequence, fluid filtration in the capillary vessels does not lead to the expected increase of colloid-osmotic pressure which is needed to reabsorb fluid into the blood downstream of the equilibrium point. Therefore, even the postcapillary venules may be considered as sites of fluid (and protein) loss from the blood, and final fluid balance is only achieved by lymph flow.

This interpretation does not allow for complete restoration of blood composition (and possibly rheological properties) during passage through the exchange compartment. In other words, the hemoconcentration resulting from outward filtration of fluid in the proximal section of the exchange compartment would not be balanced by fluid reabsorption in the distal exchange compartment, and hemoconcentration would therefore be maintained throughout the system of small postcapillary venules. As shown above, these vessels are characterized by low driving pressures, shear stresses and shear rates even under normal conditions, and an elevation of apparent blood viscosity in the presence of a net outward filtration might therefore be conceivable. If it occurs, this mechanism would certainly explain the notion that stasis of blood flow is seen predominantly in postcapillary vessels under pathophysiological circumstances. It must be stressed, however, that under physiological conditions the filtration fraction, i.e. the fraction of perfused blood which is lost into the tissue by outward filtration, is extremely small in most tissues, with the exception of the glomeruli. Therefore, the described mechanism becomes operative only when capillary blood flow is extremely reduced (with filtration maintained) and when protein permeability is elevated. The substantial protein permeability in the postcapillary venules provides a theoretical basis for a positive feedback mechanism reducing blood flow by virtue of functional coupling between exchange function and blood rheological properties.

4.3.4. The low pressure compartment

The low pressure compartment of the vascular system is defined not only by the absolute level of intravascular pressure, but also by the fact that, in contrast to the high pressure compartment, its intravascular pressure is primarily a function of blood volume and distensibility rather than cardiac output and total peripheral resistance. As seen from Fig. 4.1, more than 80% of total blood volume is contained in this compartment, which includes all large venous vessels plus, in principle, the pulmonary vessels, the atria, the right ventricle and the left ventricle in diastole. It is physiologically of great significance that blood volume can be shifted within this system, e.g. as a result of postural changes, thus affecting the filling pressure of the heart. It is also important to stress that the extent of filling, particularly in the smallest postcapillary venules, is greatly dependent on precapillary resistance: arteriolar dilatation leads to a reduction of the pressure drop across the resistance vessels, thus raising capillary and venular pressure and thereby venular blood volume. The large volume distensibility of the vessels in this compartment results from their low wall thickness to lumen ratio, but more importantly from their transition between an elliptic and a circular cross-section. While blood volume can be released from postcapillary venules as a result of venous constriction, the extent of such "mobilization" is probably small, since the small postcapillary venules are poorly equipped with smooth muscle cells and seem to respond poorly to neurogenic or metabolic stimuli (in contrast to the larger venules and veins). Hence physiological blood volume shifts in this compartment are mainly considered passive events.

In the context of rheological considerations, the vessels of this compartment may be of considerable interest because of the hemodynamic characteristics of flow. It is well known that flow in these vessels may easily be sluggish and, even under physiological circumstances, almost stagnant at times. Since wall shear stresses are low (1 Pa and less), the blood in these vessels may be exposed to changes of the chemical environment for a considerable length of time. This enables mediators released from blood cells (e.g. platelets or leukocytes) to react with the vessel walls, and, conversely, mediators released from vessel wall elements to react with blood cells or other blood constituents. Coagulation phenomena are consequently much more commonly seen in the low pressure compartment than in the arterial system. Also, the low shear regime present in venous vessels is more likely to allow the apparent viscosity of the blood to be elevated, particularly under conditions where significant fluid filtration from the blood to the tissues occurs, such as in the dependent limbs or in venous occlusion. As discussed above, this is one of the reasons why in low flow states of various etiologies stasis occurs predominantly in the peripheral sections of the low pressure system.

4.4. Blood cell rheology in the circulation

Since only limited data are available on the effective rheological behavior of the blood in the circulation, the following summary includes extrapolation from data obtained in vitro, i.e. in artificially perfused tubes. For the physical phenomena described here, the in vitro findings are probably relevant to the situation in vivo.

Blood is a heterogeneous suspension containing different cells of different dimensions in different concentrations. Cell diameters vary by one order of magnitude from the platelets (approx. 1–2 μm) to granulocytes and monocytes (approx. 8–12 μm). Blood cell concentrations vary by approximately three orders of magnitude between white cells ($5 \times 10^3/\mu$l) and red cells ($5 \times 10^6/\mu$l). In addition, these particles exhibit different mechanical and rheological properties.

The rheological behavior of the blood flowing through the vascular system (in which vessel diameters vary by more than three orders of magnitude) is determined by interactions of these cells with the vessel walls. The relative importance of these two phenomena in determining the effective resistance to blood flow will be a function of the diameter ratio between blood cell and blood vessel. It is obvious that this diameter ratio is an important parameter to classify rheological phenomena observed in blood flow in vivo and in vitro. In the following an absolute scale of vessel diameters is used to differentiate between flow regimes in larger and smaller vessels. The relative importance of cell to cell interaction decreases from category I to III, while the importance of cell to vessel wall interactions increases:

I. Bulk flow regime; Vessel diameter > 300 μm.
Blood cell diameters are negligibly small compared to vessel diameter.

II. Transition zone;
a: Vessel diameter between approximately 300 and 30 μm. Blood cell diameters are small compared to vessel diameter, but a cell concentration profile across the vessel is present.
b: Vessel diameter between approximately 30 and 8 μm. Several cells can be accomodated in one vessel cross section.

III. Single file flow regime; Vessel diameter < 8 μm. Only one cell can be accommodated in a vessel cross section.

It should be stressed that the vessel diameter range used here for the purpose of classification is only an approximation and may vary with circulatory conditions and the effective rheological properties of the blood. In the case of strong aggregation of the red cells, for instance, a flow regime corresponding to the "transition zone" may already be present in much larger vessels, since the effective particle diameter is increased by the process of aggregation.

4.4.1. Bulk flow regime I

In the flow regime of category I, which is present in all vessels of the high pressure compartment and in the larger vessels of the control compartment, the rheological behavior of the flowing blood can be deduced from its bulk properties which are mainly determined by cell-to-cell interactions. Thus, measurements of the apparent viscosity of blood as obtained in macro-viscometers can be applied to the situation in the living macrocirculation (the conduit vessels).

As already described in Chapter 2, the apparent viscosity of whole blood depends on hematocrit, plasma viscosity, deformability and aggregability of red cells. Since many of these determinants are affected by the flow conditions, knowledge of shear stresses and shear rates in these vessels will allow predictions of rheological behavior. The contribution of white cells and platelets, which normally occupy less than 1% of the blood volume, can be neglected; this is obviously different under conditions of pathological alteration of blood cell concentrations [49].

4.4.2. Transition zone IIa

It was experimentally shown in tube flow that red blood cells in extremely dilute suspensions exhibit a tendency to migrate towards the tube axis [50,51]. This is consistent with theoretical considerations which predict a centripetal movement of deformable fluid drops [52]. The rate of this movement increases with increasing flow rate and is most prominent in the high shear region close to the tube wall.

With increasing particle concentration, however, the interactions and collisions between the cells lead to diffusional forces which counteract inward movement of particles and tend to displace them from the central flow regions [51,53]. Under steady state conditions a profile of cell concentration or hematocrit is established which reflects the dynamic equilibrium between centripetal and centrifugal forces at each point across the tube. Although a precise measurement of the hematocrit profile has not yet been feasible, there is experimental evidence for the existence of a relatively cell depleted marginal region of less than 5 μm width [54,55,56]. The hematocrit profile in the central part of the tube cross section depends on bulk flow rate and hematocrit, but in general shows an increased cell concentration towards the axis of the tube [53].

In tubes perfused with Newtonian fluids a parabolic velocity profile is established (Chapter 2). Since the apparent viscosity of blood increases with decreasing shear, the velocity profile of blood flowing through a tube or vessel is blunted [53,57,58]. The extent of blunting is further enhanced by the non-uniform distribution of red cells across the vessel and varies with flow rate and hematocrit.

4.4.2.1. Fahraeus effect

Blood flow in tubes is characterized by the existence of cross sectional profiles of hematocrit and velocity. Both profiles show high values in the central flow regions and minimal values close to the tube wall. From these considerations Fahraeus concluded in 1928 [59] that the hematocrit of blood contained in a given section of a tube or vessel (tube hematocrit, H_T) should be lower than the hematocrit of the blood collected from the outflow (discharge hematocrit, H_D). This can be deduced as follows.

Since the red cell concentration in regions of high flow velocity is greater than in the regions of low flow velocity, the red cells will, on average, travel faster than the blood. Therefore, the ratio of cell velocity (v_c) divided by blood velocity (v_b) will be larger than unity. Consider a cross sectional plane of the tube, e.g. the tube outlet. The area of such a plane will be occupied by red cells and plasma in proportion to their share of the volume contained in the tube which is given by the tube hematocrit (H_T). Since the red cells travel through that plane at a velocity (v_c) higher than the bulk velocity (v_b), the red cells will make up a share of the volume transmitted through that plane (discharge hematocrit H_D) higher than H_T. The ratio between H_T and H_D is therefore given by the velocity quotient v_b/v_c:

$$H_T/H_D = v_b/v_c.$$

This Fahraeus effect is quantitatively significant only in vessels with diameters below about 300 μm. Fig. 4.6 shows the ratio of H_T and H_D due to the Fahraeus effect as a function of vessel diameter, as determined in vitro by various authors. Three salient aspects of the experimental data are substantiated by theoretical considerations.

First, the hematocrit ratio asymptotically approaches unity, if the vessel diameters exceed about 300 μm. This is due to the fact that in large vessels the marginal region of reduced local hematocrit is very small compared to the vessel diameter. At the lower end of the diameter range shown in Fig. 4.6 (single file flow regime), the hematocrit ratio again approaches unity. As the vessel diameter approaches the theoretical minimum of 2.7 μm which can be passed by a red cell, the cells will occupy the entire cross section of the vessel, with the exception of a very thin plasma layer at the wall. In this case, red cell velocity will be practically equal to blood velocity, and therefore H_T/H_D equal to unity. It was demonstrated experimentally that in a glass tube of 3.3 μm diameter the ratio H_T/H_D was 0.93, which corresponds to a plasma layer thickness of approx. 0.1 μm [60].

In an intermediate range of vessel diameters (10 to 20 μm), which corresponds to transition zone IIb, the Fahraeus effect is maximal at normal hematocrits. The lowest values of H_T/H_D observed approach the theoretical lower limit which is 0.5 under the conditions of near zero hematocrit and infinitesimally small red cell diameter. This limit results from the fact that the maximum velocity (v_{max}) in a parabolic velocity profile is twice the average velocity. In practice, however, this low value of H_T/H_D cannot be reached, since red cells have finite dimensions and determination of Fahraeus effect is normally performed at hematocrits considerably higher than zero. For this case a more realistic minimum of H_T/H_D can be calculated with the assumption that all red cells travel in a central flow

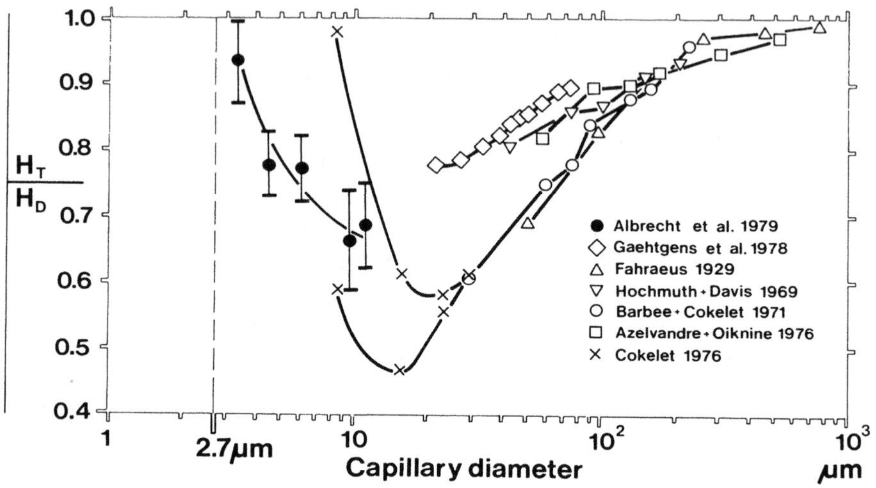

Figure 4.6. Variation of the Fahraeus effect as a function of vessel diameter according to in vitro determinations by various investigators [59,60,63,72,109,110,111]. From [92].

region (core) with a hematocrit of unity. Fig. 4.7 shows the effect of two possible velocity profile shapes in the tube on the relationship between discharge hematocrit and the hematocrit ratio. The more probable assumption of a blunted profile yields, for a H_D of 0.4, a minimal H_T/H_D ratio of 0.63.

4.4.2.2. Fahraeus-Lindqvist effect

Since the apparent viscosity of blood strongly depends on hematocrit, the dynamic hematocrit reduction should also lead to a reduction of apparent viscosity. This is called the *Fahraeus-Lindqvist effect* [61,62]. Fig. 4.8 shows the changes of apparent blood viscosity as a function of vessel diameter, as obtained by various investigators in vitro. In the diameter range between 300 and 30 μm the effective blood viscosity can be predicted using the hematocrit reduction resulting from the Fahraeus effect and the apparent blood viscosity determined in macro-viscometers [63].

4.4.3. Transition zone IIb

In the distal sections of the control and low pressure compartments where vessel diameters (10–30 μm) are in the range of 2- to 5-times the effective red cell diameter, interactions between red cells and other blood cells (especially white cells), and between blood cells and vessel wall become increasingly important.

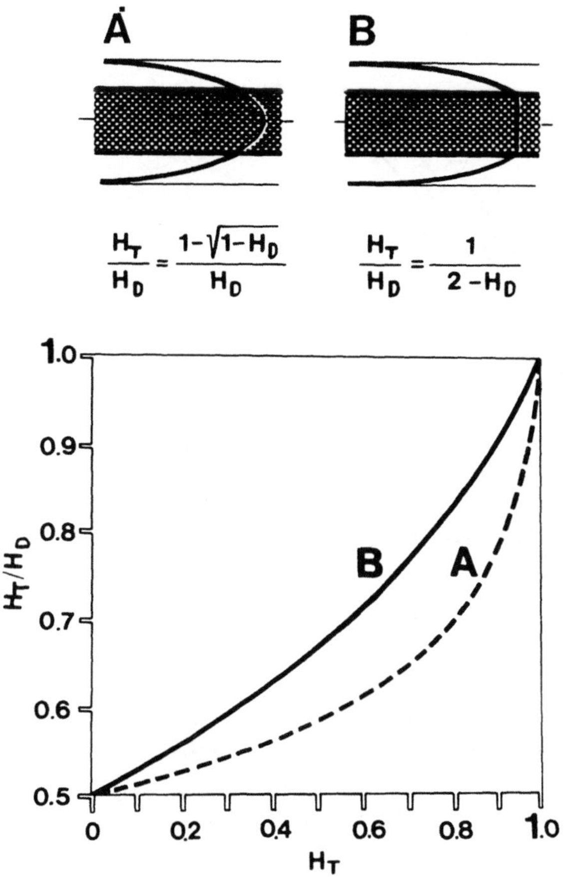

Figure 4.7. Estimation of the hematocrit dependence of the Fahraeus effect in small vessel flow, assuming two different shapes of the velocity profile in the central core, as shown in the drawings above. A: parabolic profile. B: blunted profile.

Since, in principle, the hematocrit of the flowing blood is a determining factor of apparent blood viscosity, it is important to state that the dynamic reduction of hematocrit within a single unbranched vessel (Fahraeus effect) is maximal in this range of vessel diameters. In addition, single vessel hematocrit in this diameter range is also affected by inhomogeneous distribution of cells and plasma within a microvessel network. Such a distribution may result from phase (cell/plasma) separation phenomena occurring at individual vessel bifurcations. In the presence of uneven flow rate distribution at the bifurcation, the daughter branches may receive blood with hematocrits differing from the hematocrit in the parent vessel

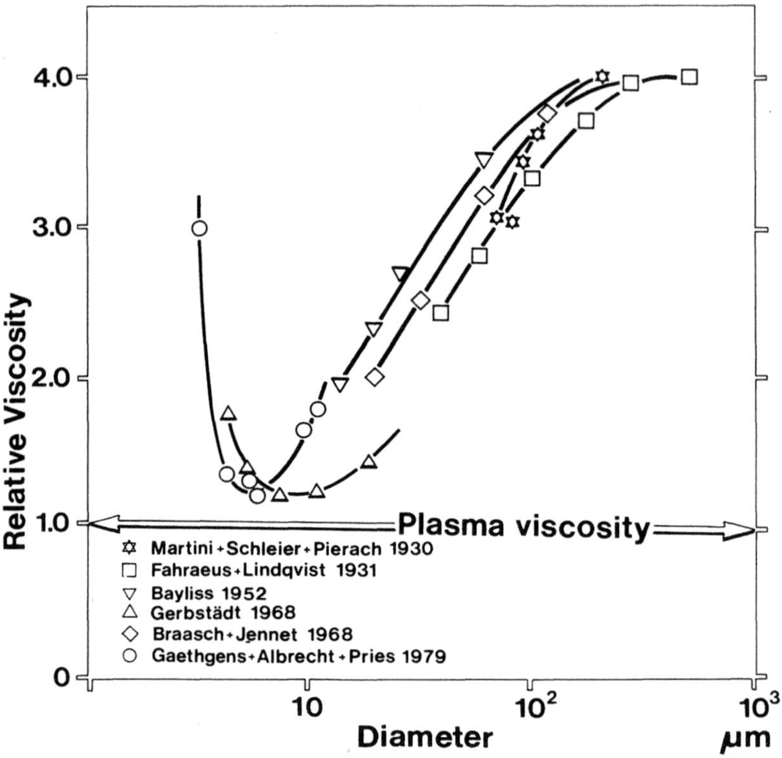

Figure 4.8. Variation in apparent blood viscosity (expressed relative to plasma viscosity) with vessel diameter, as determined by various investigators in vitro [50,61,62,92,112,113].

[64]. The branch which receives the higher flow fraction also receives a higher hematocrit than its counterpart (Fig. 4.9).

The phenomenon of phase separation has been extensively described in studies in vitro [56,65,66], in which the physical variables governing this process were defined. In essence, plasma skimming and red cell screening effects have been differentiated. Plasma skimming [67] results from phase separation within the feeding vessel due to axial migration of the red cells. Therefore, a daughter branch at a bifurcation may be primarily fed from the relatively cell depleted region close to the wall of the feeding vessel. Plasma skimming has been observed in vivo by several authors [68,69,70,71]. Red cell screening [72] is defined as a separation phenomenon which occurs immediately at the branch point due to the balance of forces acting on the individual red cell in the direction of one or the other branch [56]. It is therefore independent of the radial red cell distribution in the feeding vessel and plays a role only in the diameter range below approx. 12 µm.

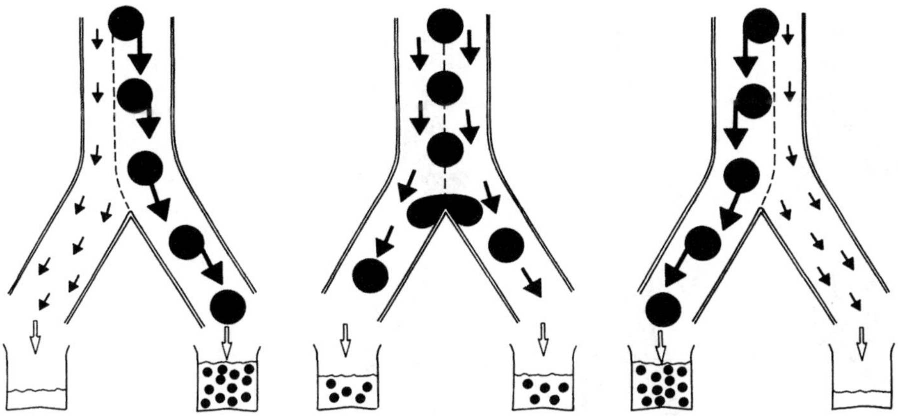

Figure 4.9. Schematic drawing of the red cell distribution at a microvessel bifurcation. As symbolized by the reservoirs below, the vessel branch receiving the higher volume flow will also receive the higher discharge hematocrit.

In a microvascular network, these phenomena lead to a large number of vessels with reduced hematocrit and lower flow rate compensated by a few vessels exhibiting higher hematocrit values. Although there is only limited in-vivo evidence for the precise relationship between fractional volume flow and fractional red cell flux at bifurcations in the diameter range discussed here, intravital microscopic studies yield indirect evidence for the relevance of this phenomenon [73].

Phase separation and Fahraeus effect result in a hematocrit reduction in microvessels with diameters of approximately 10 to 20 μm to about 40 to 50% of large vessel hematocrit [74,75,76,77]. On the basis of these observations one would expect a substantial decrease of apparent blood viscosity in these vessels. Calculations of blood viscosity from direct measurements of pressure and flow velocity in vivo [7,8] have indeed shown a small decrease of viscosity in the microvessels. A quantitative comparison between these in-vivo data and the above predictions is, however, not possible, since hematocrit measurements could not be performed. Nevertheless, the range of viscosity values obtained in these in vivo studies appears to be surprisingly high. This may be indicative of the presence of additional rheological phenomena which lead to increased resistance to flow.

In microvessels of the transition zone, interactions between red and white cells become increasingly important. Since the white cells occupy a comparatively large fraction of the vessel cross section, they travel at a speed which is still higher than the mean bulk flow velocity, but lower than the mean red cell velocity. Therefore, the red cells pile up behind the white cell to form a "red cell train", i.e. a region behind the white cell with significantly elevated hematocrit [78,79]. This phenomenon, which occurs with or without red cells overtaking the

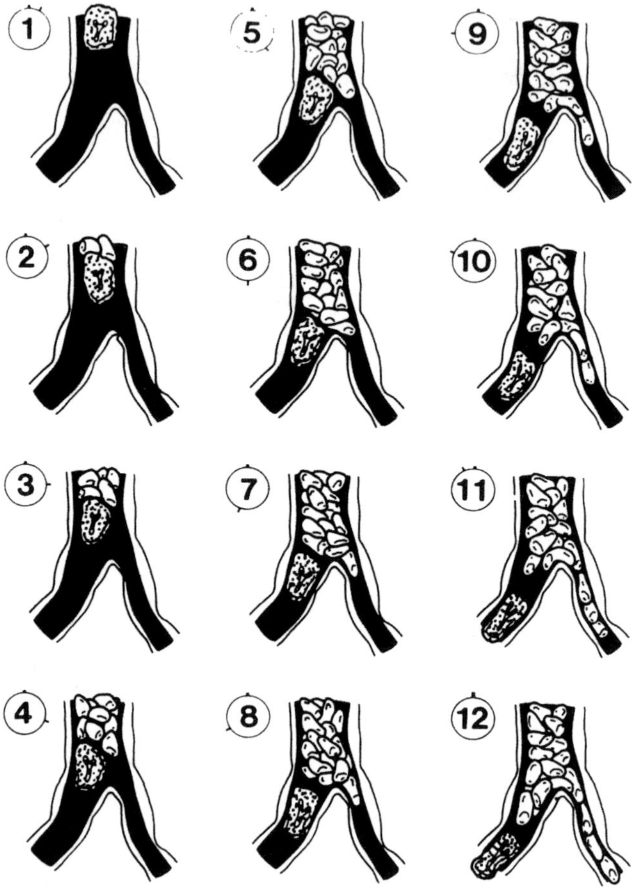

Figure 4.10. A single leukocyte followed by a red cell train entering a microvessel bifurcation. While the white cell enters the left branch, most of the following red cells are seen to enter the opposite branch.

white cell, is also observed in the microcirculation [42]. The significance of train formation for overall resistance in vivo is not known. In vitro studies suggest that resistance to flow is significantly elevated if red cell trains are formed [78]. Train formation due to the presence of white cells is likely to also play a significant part in the distribution of volume flow and red cell flux at microvascular branch points (Fig. 4.10).

The above described discrepancy between apparent blood viscosity obtained in living vessels of the category discussed here and the predictions from Fahraeus and Fahraeus-Lindqvist effects may also be the result of the interaction between the white cells and the vascular endothelium: White cells adhering to the endothelium will reduce the available flow cross-section resulting in elevated flow resistance [75,80]. Margination is a prerequisite for this phenomenon to occur. Studies both in vivo [81] and in vitro [82,83,84,85,86] have identified the rheological mechanisms of margination which depend on red cell-white cell interactions during flow. This phenomenon occurs largely in the small venules, preferentially under inflammatory conditions [87,88].

Although the contribution of white cells to bulk viscosity of whole blood is small due to their low concentration, they play a significant part in vessels below 30 μm diameter. This influence on resistance must be a function of their local concentration. There are indications that white cells may distribute non-uniformly within the microcirculation.

The contribution of platelets to the microrheological behaviour of blood cannot be evaluated at the present time. Due to their interaction with the larger blood constituents, platelets travel in a more marginal position and at a lower speed within the microvessel [89,90]. Typically, these cells are not aligned with their major axis parallel to the flow direction [91].

4.4.4. Single file flow regime III

Diameters of the smallest vessels in the microcirculation are similar to the resting red cell diameter; in true capillaries of some organs, vessel diameter may even be less than red cell diameter. Under such geometric conditions the rheology of flow is governed not by the bulk properties of blood, but by the mechanical properties of the single cells and their interactions with the vessel wall. Although the term "apparent viscosity" is used here and in the preceding discussion, it may not be appropriate under such flow conditions, since it implies the concept of a continuum.

The red cells occupy a considerable portion of the flow cross section available in vessels of this diameter range (< 8 μm). Therefore, the magnitude of the Fahraeus effect decreases strongly with diameter but is largely independent of hematocrit [60]. However, as shown by Fig. 4.8, the apparent viscosity may continue to be low in this flow regime, as long as vessel diameter is clearly above the critical value of 2.7 μm. This is thought to result from the unique flow behavior of single red cells in capillary flow, which is characterized by non-axisymmetric deformation, stable orientation, and a tanktreading motion of the membrane around the cell contents [6,92,93,94,95,96]. While the latter phenomenon may be of limited effect on flow resistance at normal capillary hematocrits, it is probably very important under conditions of elevated local cell concentration, such as in "zipper flow" [83] or within red cell trains. It can also be seen from Fig. 4.8 that even small variations of capillary dimensions in the range discussed here may lead to pronounced changes in apparent viscosity. This prediction from measurements in vitro lends qualitative support to observations made in living capillaries [8] which show apparent viscosity to vary by a factor of approximately 5 as the red cell diameter increases from 70 to 90% of capillary diameter [8,80].

Separation effects described above lead to a strongly positive correlation between fractional volume flow and hematocrit at capillary branch points. The phenomenon is more pronounced here than in larger vessels, since cellular distribution to the daughter vessels of a bifurcation shows an "all-or-none" behavior which is also strongly influenced by an off-center position of the red cells arriving at the branch point [70].

It has been speculated [64,70,97] that the relationship between the distribution of flow and hematocrit at capillary bifurcations results in an "autoregulation" of red cell flux in single capillaries, since flow resistance might be expected to increase as flow rate increases. However, the magnitude of the resistance changes which are caused by an alteration of red cell volume fraction is significantly dependent on capillary diameter. Thus, the quantitative estimation of the resistance distribution within a complex capillary network is limited by the large variability of diameters encountered in such a network. It must also be expected that this effect will be strongly affected by the passage of white cells which lead to larger changes of local resistance than the individual red cells. Therefore, "apparent blood viscosity" in small capillaries will also be subjected to time-dependent changes.

Both the resistance to flow in an unbranched vessel and the distribution of flow at branch points may be significantly affected by pathological alteration of red cell deformability. This was, for instance, shown for human sickle cells [98,99] as well as for artificially altered red cells [100,101,102].

In part, the rheological effects of leukocyte passage through small vessels has already been described above. In view of the dimensions [103] and microrheological properties of these cells [44,46,104,105], it may not be surprizing that capillary flow can be completely interrupted during leukocyte entry ("plugging"). As stated above, this is one of the mechanisms responsible for flow intermittency in these vessels even at physiological conditions. Leukocyte deformation in small vessels is a slow phenomenon, particularly at low driving pressures [44], and observations in vivo [45] have shown that duration of capillary occlusion due to white cells increases significantly, if arterial blood pressure is reduced. In low-flow states, capillary plugging as well as leukocyte adhesion in post-capillary venules may therefore lead to transient or even permanent occlusion of considerable parts of the microvascular network, thus leading to heterogeneous flow distribution, sustained increase of precapillary resistance, and impairment of tissue function [47,48,106,107,108].

4.5. Summary and conclusions

The vascular system can be considered to consist of several compartments, which are defined on the basis of the morphological design and the physiological function of the constituting blood vessels. Hemodynamic blood flow conditions in these compartments vary considerably. The flow behavior of the blood in the circulation is therefore a function not only of its intrinsic rheological properties, but also of the hemodynamic characteristics of these compartments.

While blood flow in the circulation is affected by various rheological phenomena resulting from the properties of the composite suspension and those of the individual cellular elements, the hemodynamic relevance of these properties varies, depending on the vessel diameter considered. In the macrocirculation, the rheological behavior of blood is dominated by its bulk properties. In the microcirculation, single cell properties, microrheological differences between different blood cell species, and interaction between cells and vascular wall become increasingly relevant.

The circulatory consequences of characteristic alterations of blood rheological properties observed in certain diseases may therefore be quite variable. As an example, a reduction of red cell deformability leads to impairment of blood flow predominantly in the small blood vessels, particularly in the control and exchange compartments. Increased apparent viscosity of blood due to enhanced red cell aggregability will result in an increased resistance to flow mainly in the larger vessels. Since such elevation of viscosity will be most pronounced at low shear rates, major effects are to be expected in the low pressure compartment.

By affecting the delivery of blood to and the distribution of blood flow within tissues, alterations of blood rheology under pathological conditions will also compromise the exchange of materials between the intra- and extravascular space; thereby, tissue function can be impaired. Predictions of such effects in the individual case must also consider the adaptive long-term changes in vascular morphology and architecture.

4.6. References

1. Mall, F. 1888: Die Blut- und Lymphwege im Dünndarm des Hundes. Ber. Sächs. Ges. Akad. Wiss. 14: 151.
2. Schleier, J. 1918: Der Engergieverbrauch in der Blutbahn. Pflügers Arch. 173: 172-204.
3. Wiedeman, M.P. 1962: Lengths and diameters of peripheral arterial vessels in the living animal. Circulat. Res. 10: 686-690.
4. Wiedeman, M.P. 1963: Dimensions of blood vessels from distributing artery to collecting vein. Circulat. Res. 12: 375-381.
5. Chien, S. 1969: Blood rheology and its relation to flow resistance and transcapillary exchange, with special reference to shock. Adv. Microcirc. 2: 89-103.
6. Schmid-Schönbein, H. 1977: Microrheology of erythrocytes and thrombocytes, blood viscosity and the distribution of blood flow in the microcirculation. In: Handbuch der allg. Pathologie, III/7: Mikrozirkulation (H. Meesen, Ed.), Berlin, Heidelberg, New York: Springer-Verlag, pp. 289-384.
7. Lipowsky, H.H., Kovalcheck, S., Zweifach, B.W. 1978: The distribution of blood rheological parameters in the microvasculature of cat mesentery. Circulat. Res. 43: 738-749.

8. Lipowsky, H.H., Zweifach, B.W. 1977: Methods for simultaneous measurement of pressure differentials and flow in single unbranched vessels of the microcirculation for rheological studies. Microvasc. Res. 14: 345-361.
9. Miller, A.T., Hale, D.M. 1970: Increased vascularity of brain, heart, and skeletal muscle of polycythemic rats. Amer. J. Physiol. 219: 702-704.
10. Dieckhoff, D., Kanzow, E. 1969: über die Lokalisation des Strömungswiderstandes im Hirnkreislauf. Pflügers Arch. ges. Physiol. 310: 75-85.
11. Kanzow, E., Dieckhoff, D., Holzgraefe, H., Langhorst, P. 1969: über den Einfluss von Durchblutungs- und Druckänderungen auf den Druckabfall in den Arterien des Hirnkreislaufs. Pflügers Arch. ges. Physiol. 312: R32 (Abstr.).
12. Shapiro, H.M., Stromberg, D., Lee, D.R., Wiederhielm, C.A. 1971: Dynamic pressure in the pial arterial microcirculation. Amer. J. Physiol. 221: 279-283.
13. Stromberg, D.D., Fox, J.R. 1972: Pressures in the pial arterial microcirculation of the cat during changes in systemic arterial blood pressure. Circulat. Res. 31: 229-239.
14. Mshedlisvili, G.I., Ormotsadze, L.G., Nikolashvili, L.S., Baramidze, D.G. 1967: Reaction of different parts of the cerebral vascular system in asphyxia. Exp. Neurol. 18: 239-252.
15. Bassenge, E., Holtz, J., Kolin, A., Graser, G. 1981: Observations on coronary conductance artery vasomotion by induction angiometry and ultrasonic dimension technique. Basic. Res. Cardiol. 76: 524.
16. Gerová, M., Gero, J. 1969: Range of sympathetic control of the dog femoral artery. Circulat. Res. 24: 349-360.
17. Mellander, S., Johansson, B. 1968: Control of resistance, exchange and capacitance functions in the peripheral circulation. Pharmacol. Rev. 20: 117-196.
18. Duling, B.R. 1984: Oxygen, metabolism, and microcirculatory control. In: Microcirculation, (G. Kaley and B.M. Altura, Eds.), Baltimore: University Park Press, Vol. II, pp. 401-4029.
19. Rosell, S. 1978: Nervous control of the microcirculation. In: Microcirculation, (G. Kaley, B.M. Altura, Eds.), Baltimore: University Park Press, Vol. II, pp. 371-400.
20. Rosell, S. 1980: Neuronal control of microvessels. Ann. Rev. Physiol. 42: 359-371.
21. Burnstock, G., Griffith, S.G. 1983: Innervation of microvascular smooth muscle. Progr. Appl. Microcirc. 3: 19-39.
22. Zweifach, B.W. 1961: Functional behaviour of the microcirculation. Springfield, Ill.: C. Thomas Publ.
23. Vanhoutte, P.M. 1978: Heterogeneity in vascular smooth muscle. In: Microcirculation, (G. Kaley and B.M. Altura, Eds.), Baltimore: University Park Press, Vol. II, pp. 181-309.
24. Johansson, B., Bohr, D.F. 1966: Rhythmic activity in smooth muscle from small subcutaneous arteries. Amer. J. Physiol. 210: 801-806.
25. Siegel, G. 1983: Principles of vascular rhythmogenesis. Prog. Appl. Microcirc. 3: 40-62.
26. Funk, W., Endrich, B., Messmer, K., Intaglietta, M. 1983: Spontaneous arteriolar vasomotion as a determinant of peripheral vascular resistance. Int. J. Microcirc. Clin. Exp. 2: 11-25.
27. Funk, W., Intaglietta, M. 1983: Spontaneous arteriolar vasomotion. Prog. Appl. Microcirc. 3: 66-82.
28. Johnson, P.C., Wayland, H. 1967: Regulation of blood flow in single capillaries. Amer. J. Physiol. 212: 1405-1415.
29. Arfors, K.E., Bergqvist, D., Intaglietta, M., Westergren, B. 1975: Measurement of blood flow velocity in the microcirculation. Uppsala J. Med. Sci. 80: 27-33.
30. Tuma, R.F., Lindbom, L., Arfors, K.E. 1977: The effect of tissue oxygen tension on reactive hyperemia in skeletal muscle. Bibl. Anat. 15: 425-428.
31. Lindbom, L. 1983: Microvascular blood flow distribution in skeletal muscle. An intravital microscopic study in the rabbit. Acta Physiol. Scand. Suppl. 525.
32. Gaehtgens, P. 1970: Pulsatile pressure and flow in the mesenteric vascular bed of the cat. Pflügers Arch. ges. Physiol. 316: 140-151.

33. Intaglietta, M., Richardson, D.R., Tompkins, W.R. 1971: Blood pressure, flow, and elastic properties in microvessels of cat omentum. Amer. J. Phsiol. 221: 922-928.
34. Gross, J.F., Intaglietta, M., Zweifach, B.W. 1974: Network model of pulsatile hemodynamics in the microcirculation of the rabbit omentum. Amer. J. Physiol. 226: 1117-1123.
35. Zweifach, B.W. 1974: Quantitative studies of microvascular structure and function. I. Analysis of pressure distribution in the terminal vascular bed in cat mesentery. Circulat. Res. 34: 843-857.
36. Eriksson, E., Myrrhage, R. 1972: Microvascular dimensions and blood flow in skeletal muscle. Acta Physiol. Scand. 86: 211-222.
37. Potter, R.F., Groom, A.C. 1983: Capillary diameter and geometry in cardiac and skeletal muscle studied by means of corrosion casts. Microvasc. Res. 25: 68-84.
38. Bassingthwaighte, J.B., Ypintsoi, T., Harvey, R.B. 1974: Microvasculature of the dog left ventricular myocardium. Microvasc. Res. 7: 229-249.
39. Plyley, M.J., Sutherland, G.J., Groom, A.C. 1976: Geometry of the capillary network in skeletal muscle. Microvasc. Res. 11: 161-173.
40. Hammersen, F. 1977: Bau und Funktion der Blutkapillaren. In: Handbuch der allg. Pathologie, III/7: Mikrozirkulation, (H. Meessen, Ed.), Berlin, Heidelberg, New York: Springer-Verlag, pp. 134-229.
41. Palmer, A.A. 1959: A study of blood flow in minute vessels of the pancreatic region of the rat with reference to intermittent corpuscular flow in individual capillaries. Quart. J. Exp. Physiol. 44: 149-159.
42. Branemark, P.I., Lindström, J. 1963: Studies in the function of nutritive capillaries in the connective tissue in rabbit's ear chamber. J. Anat. (Lond.) 97: 323-332.
43. Reneman, R.S., Slaaf, D.W., Lindbom, L., Tangelder, G.J., Arfors, K.E. 1980: Muscle blood flow disturbances produced by simultaneously elevated venous and total muscle tissue pressure. Microvasc. Res. 20: 307-318.
44. Bagge, U. 1976: Granulocyte rheology. Blood Cells 2: 481-490.
45. Gaehtgens, P., Ley, K., Pries, A.R., Müller, R. 1985: Mutual interaction between leukocytes and microvascular blood flow. Prog. Appl. Microcirc. 7: 15-28.
46. Bagge, U., Johansson, B.R., Olofsson, J. 1977: Deformation of white blood cells in capillaries. A combined intravital and electron microcopic study in the mesentery of rabbits. Adv. Microcirc. 7: 18-28.
47. Amundson, B. 1979: Skeletal muscle microcirculation and metabolism in hemorrhagic shock. Thesis, Dept. of Anatomy, Univ. of Göteborg, Sweden.
48. Engler, R.L., Schmid-Schönbein, G.W., Pavelec, R.S. 1983: Leukocyte capillary plugging in myocardial ischemia and reperfusion in the dog. Amer. J. Pathol. 111: 98-111.
49. Lichtman, M.A., Gregory, A., Kearney, E. 1973: Rheology of leukocytes, leukocyte suspensions, and blood in leukemia. J. Clin. Invest. 52: 350-358.
50. Bayliss, L.E. 1965: The flow of suspensions of red blood cells in capillary tubes: Changes in the "cell free" marginal sheath with changes in the shearing stress. J. Physiol. 179: 1-25.
51. Goldsmith, H.L. 1971: Red cell motions and wall interactions in tube flow. Federation Proc. 30: 1578-1587.
52. Schmid-Schönbein, G.W., Zweifach, B.W., Kovalcheck, S. 1977: The application of stereological principles to morphometry of the microcirculation in different tissues. Microvasc. Res. 14: 303-317.
53. Goldsmith, H.L., Marlow, J.C. 1979: Flow behaviour of erythrocytes. II. Particle motion in concentrated suspensions of ghost cells. J. Colloid Interface Sci. 71: 383-407.
54. Bayliss, L.E. 1959: The axial drift of the red cells when blood flows in a narrow tube. J. Physiol. 149: 593-613.
55. Bugliarello, G., Sevilla, J. 1970: Velocity distribution and other characteristics of steady and pulsatile blood flow in fine glass tubes. Biorheology 7: 85-107.
56. Pries, A.R., Albrecht, K.H., Gaehtgens, P. 1981: Model studies on phase separation at a capillary orifice. Biorheology 18: 355-367.

57. Gaehtgens, P., Meiselman, H.J., Wayland, H. 1970: Velocity profiles of human blood at normal and reduced hematocrit in glass tubes up to 130 μm diameter. Microvasc. Res. 2: 13-23.
58. Schmid-Schönbein, G.W., Zweifach, B.W. 1975: RBC velocity profiles in arterioles and venules of the rabbit omentum. Microvasc. Res. 10: 153-164.
59. Fahraeus, R. 1928: Die Strömungsverhältnisse und die Verteilung der Blutzellen im Gefässsystem. Klin. Wschr. 7: 100-106.
60. Albrecht, K.H., Gaehtgens, P., Pries, A., Heuser, M. 1979: The Fahraeus effect in narrow capillaries (i.d. 3.3 to 11.0 μm). Microvasc. Res. 18: 33-47.
61. Martini, P., Pierach, A., Schreyer, E. 1930: Die Strömung des Blutes in engen Gefässen. Dtsch. Arch. Klin. Med. 169: 212-222.
62. Fahraeus, R., Lindqvist, T. 1931: The viscosity of blood in narrow capillary tubes. Amer. J. Physiol. 96: 562-568.
63. Barbee, J.H., Cokelet, G.R. 1971: Prediction of blood flow in tubes with diameters as small as 29 μm. Microvasc. Res. 3: 17-21.
64. Yen, R.T., Fung, Y.C. 1978: Effect of velocity distribution on red cell distribution in capillary blood vessels. Amer. J. Physiol. 235: H251-H257.
65. Dellimore, J.W., Dunlop, M.J., Canham, P.B. 1983: Ratio of cells and plasma in blood flowing past branches in small plastic channels. Amer. J. Physiol. 244: H635-H643.
66. Fenton, B.M., Carr, R.T., Cokelet, G.R. 1985: Non-uniform red cell distribution in 20 to 100 μm bifurcations. Microvasc. Res. 29: 103-126.
67. Krogh, A. 1921: Studies on the physiology of capillaries. II. The reactions to local stimuli of the blood vessels in the skin and web of the frog. J. Physiol. 55: 412-422.
68. Jodal, M., Lundgren, O. 1970: Plasma skimming in the intestinal tract. Acta Physiol. Scand. 80: 50-60.
69. Johnson, P.C. 1971: Red cell separation in the mesenteric capillary network. Amer. J. Physiol. 221: 99-104.
70. Schmid-Schönbein, G.W., Skalak, R., Usami, S., Chien, S. 1980: Cell distribution in capillary networks. Microvasc. Res. 19: 18-44.
71. Svanes, K., Zweifach, B.W. 1968: Variations in small blood vessel hematocrit produced in hypothermic rats by micro-occlusion. Microvasc. Res. 1: 210-220.
72. Cokelet, G.R. 1976: Macroscopic rheology and tube flow of human blood. In: Microcirculation, (J. Grayson, W. Zingg, Eds.), New York: Plenum Publ. Corp., Vol. 1, pp. 9-31.
73. Klitzman, B., Johnson, P.C. 1982: Capillary network geometry and red cell distribution in hamster cremaster muscle. Amer. J. Physiol. 242: H211-H219.
74. Johnson, P.C., Blaschke, J., Burton, K.S., Dial, J.H. 1971: Influence of flow variations on capillary hematocrit in mesentery. Amer. J. Physiol. 221: 105-112.
75. Lipowsky, H.H., Usami, S., Chien,S. 1980: In vivo measurements of "apparent viscosity" and microvessel hematocrit in the mesentery of the cat. Microvasc. Res. 19: 297-319.
76. Sarelius, I.H., Duling, B.R. 1982: Direct measurement of microvessel hematocrit, red cell flux, velocity, and transit time. Amer. J. Physiol. 243: H1018-H1026.
77. Kanzow, G., Pries, A.R., Gaehtgens, P. 1982: Analysis of the hematocrit distribution in the mesenteric microcirculation. Int. J. Micr. Clin. Exp. 1: 67-79.
78. Gaehtgens, P., Pries, A.R., Nobis, U. 1984: Flow behaviour of white cells in capillaries. In: White Cell Mechanics, (H.J. Meiselman, M.A. Lichtman, P.L. LaCelle, Eds.), New York: A.R. Liss Publ., pp. 147-157.
79. Secomb, T.W., Pries, A.R., Gaehtgens, P. 1985: Estimation of Fahraeus effect through analysis of red blood cell trains in microvessels. Microvasc. Res. 29: 249 (Abstr.).
80. Chien, S. 1985: Role of blood cells in microcirculatory regulation. Microvasc. Res. 29: 129-151.
81. Schmid-Schönbein, G.W., Usami, S., Skalak, R., Chien, S. 1980: The interaction of leukocytes and erythrocytes in capillary and post-capillary vessels. Microvasc. Res. 19: 45-70.
82. Vejlens, G. 1938: The distribution of leukocytes in the vascular system. Acta Path. Microbiol. Scand., Suppl. 33: 11-239.

83. Nobis, U., Pries, A.R., Gaehtgens, P. 1982: Rheological mechanisms contributing to WBC-margination. In: White Blood Cells, Morphology and Rheology as Related to Function, (Bagge, U., Born, G.V.R., Gaehtgens, P., Eds.), The Hague, Boston, London: M. Nijhoff Publ., pp. 57-65.
84. Bagge, U., Blixt, A., Strid, K.G. 1983: The initiation of post-capillary margination of leukocytes: Studies in vitro on the influence of erythrocyte concentration and flow velocity. Int. J. Micr. Clin. Exp. 2: 215-227.
85. Goldsmith, H.L., Spain, S. 1984: Margination of leukocytes in blood flow through small tubes. Microvasc. Res. 27: 204-222.
86. Nobis, U., Pries, A.R., Cokelet, G.R., Gaehtgens, P. 1985: Radial distribution of white cells during blood flow in small tubes. Microvasc. Res. 29: 295-304.
87. Dahlén, S.E., Björk, J., Hedqvist, P., Arfors, K.E., Hammarström, S., Lindgren, J.A., Samuelsson, B. 1981: Leukotrienes promote plasma leakage and leukocyte adhesion in post-capillary venules: In vivo effects with relevance to the acute inflammatory response. Proc. Natl. Acad. Sci. USA. 78: 3887-3891.
88. Tuma, R. 1985: White cell adherence in microvessels. Prog. Appl. Microcirc. 7: 31-42.
89. Beck, M.R., Eckstein, E.C. 1980: Preliminary report on platelet concentration in capillary tube flows of whole blood. Biorheology 17: 455-464.
90. Tangelder, G.J. 1982: Distribution and orientation of blood platelets flowing in small arterioles. Thesis, Dept. of Biophysics and Physiology, Rijksuniversiteit Limburg, Maastricht, The Netherlands.
91. Teirlinck, H.C., Tangelder, G.J., Slaaf, D.W., Muijtjens, A.M.M., Arts, T., Reneman, R.S. 1984: Orientation and diameter distribution of rabbit blood platelets flowing in small arterioles. Biorheology 21: 317-331.
92. Gaehtgens, P. 1980: Flow of blood through narrow capillaries: Rheological mechanisms determining capillary hematocrit and apparent viscosity. Biorheology 17: 183-189.
93. Gaehtgens, P., Dührssen, C., Albrecht, K.H. 1980: Motion, deformation, and interaction of blood cells and plasma during flow through narrow capillary tubes. Blood Cells 6: 799-812.
94. Gaehtgens, P., Schmid-Schönbein, H. 1982: Mechanisms of dynamic flow adaptation of mammalian erythrocytes. Naturwiss. 96: 294-296.
95. Secomb, T.W., Gross, J.F. 1983: Flow of red blood cells in narrow capillaries: role of membrane tension. Int. J. Micr. Clin. Exp. 2: 229-240.
96. Schmid-Schönbein, H., Gaehtgens, P., Fischer, T., Stöhr-Liesen, M. 1984: Biology of red cells: non-nucleated erythrocytes as fluid drop-like cell fragments. Int. J. Micr. Clin. Exp. 3: 161-196.
97. Gaehtgens, P., Pries, A., Albrecht, K.H. 1979: Model experiments on the effect of bifurcations on capillary blood flow and oxygen transport. Pflügers Arch. ges. Physiol. 380: 115-120.
98. Chien, S. 1981: Hemorheology in disease, pathophysiological significance and therapeutic implications. Clin. Hemorheol. 1: 419-442.
99. Lipowsky, H.H., Usami, S., Chien, S. 1982: Human SS red cell rheological behaviour in the microcirculation of cremaster muscle. Blood Cells 8: 113-126.
100. Driessen, G.K., Haest, C.W.M., Heidtmann, H., Kamp, D., Schmid-Schönbein, H. 1980: Effect of reduced red cell "deformability" on flow velocity in capillaries of rat mesentery. Pflügers Arch. ges. Physiol. 388: 75-78.
101. Driessen, G.K., Scheidt-Bleichert, H., Sobota, A., Inhoffen, W., Heidtmann, H., Haest, C.W.M., Kamp, D. 1982: Capillary resistance to flow of hardened (diamide treated) red blood cells (RBC). Pflügers Arch. ges. Physiol. 392: 261-267.
102. Driessen, G.K., Fischer, T.M., Haest, C.W.M., Inhoffen, W., Schmid-Schönbein, H. 1978: Flow behaviour of rigid blood cells in the microcirculation. Int. J. Micr. Clin. Exp. 3: 197-210.
103. Schmid-Schönbein, G.W., Shih, Y.Y., Chien, S. 1980: Morphometry of human leukocytes. Blood 56: 866-875.
104. Schmid-Schönbein, G.W., Sung, K.L.P., Tözeren, H., Skalak, R., Chien, S. 1981: Passive mechanical properties of human leukocytes. Biophys. J. 36: 243-256.

105. Chien, S., Schmid-Schönbein, G.W., Sung, K.L.P., Schmalzer, E.A., Skalak, R. 1984: Viscoelastic properties of leukocytes. In: White Cell Mechanics, (Meiselman, H.J., Lichtman, M.A., LaCelle, P.L., Eds.), New York: A.R. Liss Publ., Krock Found. Sci. 16, pp. 19-51.
106. Bagge, U., Amundson, B., Lauritzen, C. 1980: White blood cell deformability and plugging of skeletal muscle capillaries in hemorrhagic shock. Acta Physiol. Scand. 108: 159-163.
107. Braide, M., Amundson, B., Chien, S., Bagge, U. 1984: Quantitative studies on the influence of leukocytes on vascular resistance in a skeletal muscle preparation. Microvasc. Res. 27: 331-352.
108. Bagge, U., Braide, M. 1985: Microcirculatory effects of white blood cells in shock. Prog. Appl. Microcirc. 7: 43-50.
109. Gaehtgens, P., Albrecht, K.H., Kreutz, F. 1978: Fahraeus effect and red cell screening during tube flow of human blood. I. Effect of variation of flow rate. Biorheology 15: 155-161.
110. Hochmuth, R.M., Davis, D.O. 1969: Changes in hematocrit for blood flowing in narrow tubes. Bibl. Anat. 10: 59-65.
111. Azelvandre, F., Oiknine, C. 1977: Effet Fahraeus et effet Fahraeus-Lindqvist: Résultats expérimentaux et modèles théorétiques. Biorheology 13: 315-335. C.R. Acad. Sci. Paris 284, pp. 577-580.
112. Gerbstaedt, H., Vogtmann, C., Rüth, P., Schöntube, E. 1966: Die Scheinviskosität von Blut in Glaskapillaren kleinster Durchmesser. Naturwiss. 53: 526.
113. Braasch, D., Jennet, W. 1968: Erythrozytenflexibilität, Hämokonzentration und Reibungswiderstand in Glaskapillaren mit Durchmessern zwischen 6 bis 50 μm. Pfügers Arch. ges. Physiol. 302: 245-254.

5
Physiological and pathophysiological significance of hemorheology

Shu Chien
Division of Circulatory Physiology and Biophysics, Department of Physiology, College of Physicians and Surgeons, Columbia University, New York, NY 10032, United States of America

The biophysical principles and the rheological properties of blood cells presented in Chapters 2 (Matrai et al) and 3 (Brooks and Evans) form the basis for the discussion on flow behavior of blood in the circulation in vivo in Chapter 4 (Gaehtgens et al). In this Chapter, we shall further apply the above information to analyze the role of blood rheology in affecting circulatory dynamics, nutrient transport, and transcapillary exchange under physiological and pathophysiological conditions. The aim is to provide a common background for the specific discussions on blood rheology in various clinical disorders in the subsequent chapters.

5.1. The role of hemorheology in circulatory physiology

5.1.1. Vascular hindrance and blood viscosity as determinants of resistance

The primary function of the circulatory system is to transport nutrients, metabolites, hormones and other materials to and from tissues. The cardiac output from the left ventricle together with the total peripheral resistance in the systemic circulation set the level of the arterial pressure, which provides the perfusion pressure head for blood flow through various organs and tissues. The resistance (R) to flow is defined as the ratio of the pressure drop from arteries to veins $(p_A - p_V)$ to the rate of blood flow (Q).

$$R = \frac{p_A - p_V}{Q} \qquad (1)$$

Thus the blood flow to a given region varies directly with the pressure drop and inversely with the flow resistance in the region.

$$Q = \frac{p_A - p_V}{R} \tag{2}$$

In streamline or laminar flow, when there is no turbulence, the resistance results from viscous dissipation of energy between adjacent fluid laminae, and it is equal to the product of blood viscosity (η_B) and vascular hindrance (Z).

$$R = \eta_B Z \tag{3}$$

The vascular hindrance represents the contribution of the vascular geometry per se (at a constant viscosity) to the resistance in streamline flow [1,2]. When both the resistance and blood viscosity are measured, vascular hindrance can be calculated as

$$Z = \frac{R}{\eta_B} = \frac{p_A - p_V}{Q\eta_B} \qquad (4), (4a)$$

According to the Poiseuille-Hagen law (see Chapter 2), which applies quantitatively to a fluid with a Newtonian viscosity η flowing in a rigid tube with radius r and length L, the relationship between the pressure drop Δp and the flow q through this tube is expressed as

$$\frac{\Delta p}{q} = \frac{8\eta L}{\pi r^4} \tag{5}$$

For N parallel tubes with a total flow of Q, Equation 5 becomes

$$\frac{\Delta p}{Q} = \frac{8\eta L}{\pi r^4 N} = \frac{128\eta L}{\pi D^4 N} \qquad (6), (6a)$$

where D is the tube diameter. The right hand sides of equations [5] and [6] represent the resistance in a single tube and N parallel tubes, respectively. The hindrance through N parallel tubes is thus equal to $8L/\pi r^4 N$.

Because of the existence in the circulatory system of complex geometries, flow pulsatility, vessel distensibility, and non-Newtonian blood viscosity, the Poiseuille-Hagen law cannot be quantitatively applied to blood flow in vivo. Nevertheless, the vascular hindrance is goverened by the same parameters L, r and N as in tube flow.

$$Z = f\left(\frac{L}{r^x N}\right) \tag{7}$$

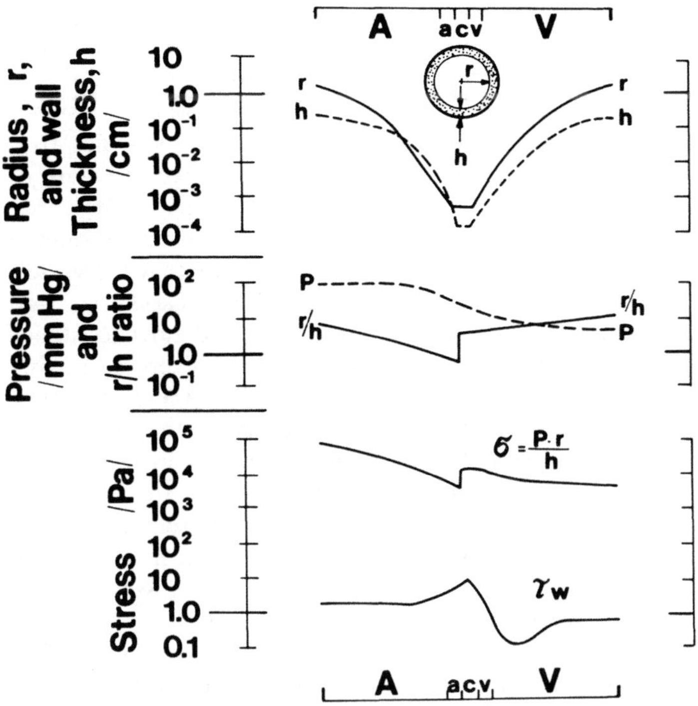

Figure 5.1. Variations in number of parallel vessels (N), diameter (D), wall shear rate ($\dot{\gamma}_w$), wall shear stress (τ_w), Reynolds number (Re), mean velocity (v), segmental hindrance (Z_{seg}/L) and resistance per unit length (R_{seg}/L), relative to the corresponding values in the aorta) in different segments of the systemic circulation. Geometric data are based on ref. (4,5,6). Blood viscosity is assumed to be equal to 4 mPas in all vessel segments. The values shown in this figure are approximate estimates and do not reflect the variations in different organs and fluctuations during the cardiac cycle.

The notation $f(\ )$, which refers to "a function of", is used to indicate the lack of a quantitative description of the mathematical relationship for vascular hindrance in the circulatory system. Equation 7 shows that vascular hindrance in vivo varies directly with vessel length and inversely with the vessel radius and the number of parallel vessels. The vessel radius has a strong influence on vascular hindrance, as indicated by its exponent x, which has been found to be approximately 4 in the small vessels which are the major contributors to resistance [3]. Thus a reduction in vessel radius to one-half causes marked increases in vascular hindrance and flow resistance by approximately 16 fold. The vessel length does not change significantly, while the number of parallel vessels (especially capillaries) can alter as a result of variations in vasomotor activities in response to changes in local metabolic demands; the predominant factor in determining vascular hindrance is the vessel radius (Equation 7). The segmental hindrance of each generation of vessels can be estimated as L/r^4N. The segmental hindrance per unit length ($Z_{seg}/L = 1/r^4N$) for each vessel generation relative to that in the aorta is plotted in Fig. 5.1. The segmental resistance per unit length ($R_{seg}/L = \eta_B/r^4/N$) is proportional to the segmental hindrance per unit length, if blood viscosity is assumed to be constant throughout the various segments of the vascular tree. Although blood viscosity is known to vary in the circulatory system, because of differences in intravascular hematocrit and flow conditions, the changes are relatively small and, as a first approximation, blood viscosity can be considered to be invariant in the circulation for this purpose. Fig. 5.1 shows that the vessels with small diameters, i.e. the very small arteries, arterioles, capillaries and venules, contribute most significantly to vascular hindrance and flow resistance under physiological conditions. It is to be noted, however, that severe narrowing of large vessels may lead to significant increases in vascular hindrance and flow resistance in vascular disease. The arterioles possess a significant amount of smooth muscle, which can induce marked changes in their radius in response to neurohumoral factors; hence they play the most important role in controlling resistance and are usually referred to as the major resistance vessels. In view of the dominant role of radius in controlling vascular hindrance, an increase in Z usually indicates a narrowing of the lumen of the resistance vessels, and a decrease in Z usually indicates a widening.

The above discussions on flow resistance are based primarily on laminar flow and viscous dissipation. With increasing flow, there may be the onset of turbulence, and the resistance will be that due to inertial dissipation in addition to viscous dissipation. The likelihood of the occurrence of turbulence can be estimated from the Reynolds number (Re), which is a dimensionless parameter.

$$Re = \frac{2r\rho v}{\eta} = \frac{2Q\rho}{\pi r \eta} \qquad (8), (8a)$$

where r is the vessel radius (m), σ is fluid density (kg/m^3), v is mean linear velocity (m/s), and η is fluid viscosity (Pas). In a straight tube with a uniform radius, the critical Reynolds number (Re_c) is approximately 2,000 (Fig. 5.2). The value of Re_c becomes lower in tubes with complicated geometry, especially in a dilated lumen downstream to a narrow constriction; under these conditions turbulence can set in at Re as low as 10–100 [7]. Under physiological conditions of blood flow, significant turbulence occurs only in large vessels where Re values are high; the Re values in the microcirculation, where the resistance vessels are located, are so low (Fig. 5.2.) that it is extremely unlikely to have turbulence [8]. Therefore, in most conditions, especially in high viscosity and low flow states, one needs to consider only the viscous resistance. The contribution of turbulence to resistance may become significant in conditions with low blood viscosity, e.g. anemias, when the low η_B and the ensuing high v can raise Re to above Re_c.

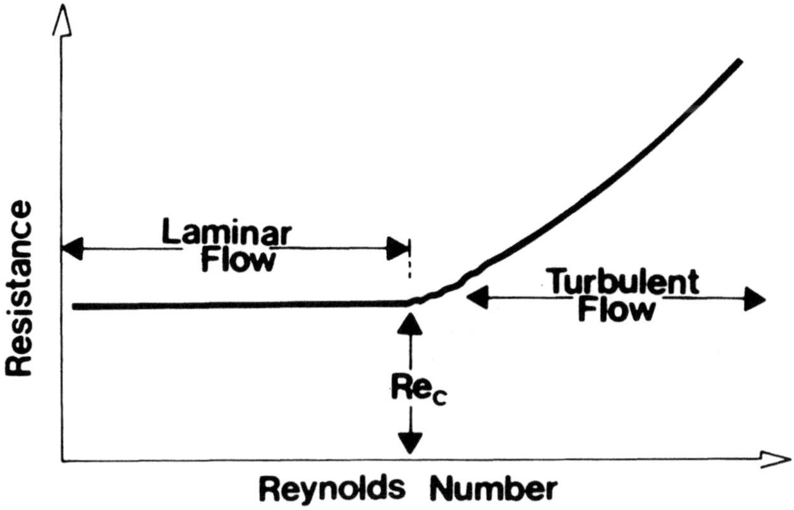

Figure 5.2. Effects of Reynolds number on flow resistance. Note the increase in resistance when the flow pattern undergoes transition from laminar to turbulent at the critical Reynolds number (Re_c). As discussed in the text, Re_c is a function of the geometry of the flow system.

5.1.2. Fundamental determinants of blood viscosity

The viscosity of blood, as that of other liquids, varies inversely with temperature. At a given temperature η_B is primarily a function of cell concentration, plasma viscosity, cell aggregation and cell deformation [2]. Because the red blood cells (RBCs) occupy the largest volume fraction of blood cells, RBC concentration (or hematocrit, Hct) is a major determinant of η_B. White blood cells (WBCs) and platelets are much lower in their volume concentrations (sum $< 1\%$), and they normally have no significant influence on the flow behavior of blood in large vessels. In very narrow vessels, however, WBCs may cause microvascular plugging due to their rigidity and larger volume [9-12], thus becoming a significant rheological factor in some pathological conditions, as already discussed in Chapters 3 and 4.

The viscosity of normal human plasma at 37°C is approximately 1.2 mPas [13,14]. Plasma viscosity (η_P) is a function of the concentration and molecular size of plasma proteins, especially those with molecular asymmetry, i.e. fibrinogen and some globulin fractions. The ratio η_B/η_P is referred to as the relative viscosity (η_r). η_r of a blood sample with Hct adjusted to a constant level, e.g. 0.45, serves to normalize variations in Hct and η_P among samples, and η_r value at low shear rates may be used to estimate variations in RBC aggregation.

Red cells aggregate to form rouleaux as a result of bridging of cell surfaces by fibrinogen and some globulin fractions. This aggregation occurs under low flow

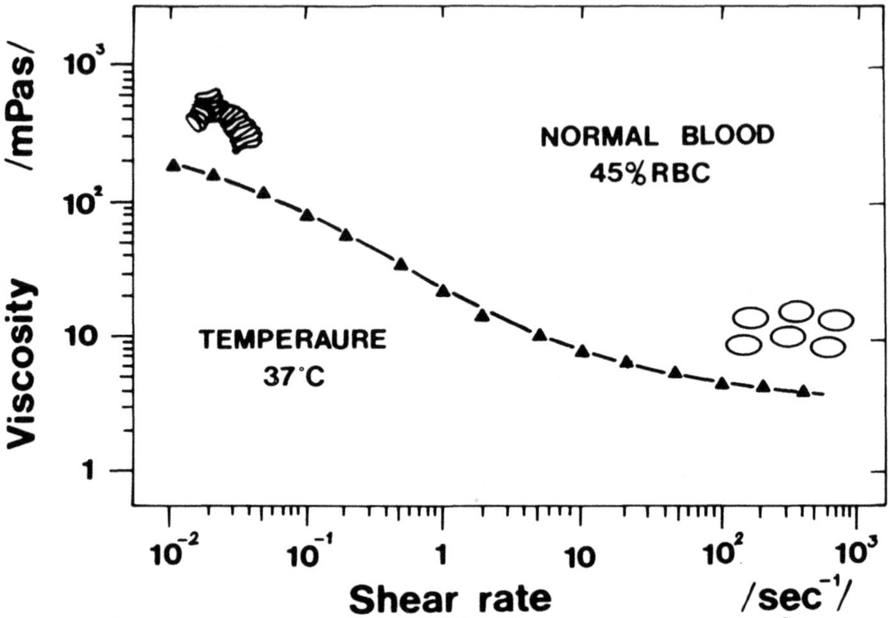

Figure 5.3. Logarithmic plot showing the relationship between the viscosity of normal human blood and shear rate. The insert sketches show the aggregation of red blood cells at low shear rates and their disaggregation and deformation at high shear rates. From (87).

conditions when the shear stress is insufficient to disperse the rouleaux. An increase in shear stress causes a progressive disaggregation of rouleaux and a decrease in η_B (Fig. 5.3).

Normal human RBCs are remarkably deformable, and the degree of RBC deformation depends on the level of shear stress acting on the cell surface. With an increase in either the shear rate or the fluid viscosity surrounding the cells, especially the latter, the deforming stress causes elongation of RBCs with their long axis aligned with flow [15,16]. As a result the viscous resistance resulting from the presence of RBCs decreases, and η_B becomes lower at high shear. Therefore the shear thinning property of blood is the result of the shear dependent variations in RBC aggregation and deformation. The mechanisms of RBC aggregation and deformation are discussed in Chapter 3.

5.1.3. Blood rheology in relation to circulation in vivo

Due to the complexity of vascular geometry and the non-Newtonian behavior of blood, it is difficult to determine the shear rate ($\dot{\gamma}$) and shear stress τ in the circulation in vivo. A rough estimate of the wall shear rate in a blood vessel can be obtained as $4v/r$, which is derived for a Newtonian fluid in Poiseuille flow with a parabolic velocity profile (Chapter 2). The wall shear stress is equal to $\Delta pr/2L$, where Δp is the pressure drop along a vessel length L, and it is also equal to the product of wall shear rate and viscosity. The approximate values for shear rate and shear stress in various parts of the circulation are given in Fig. 5.1.

Because blood is a non-Newtonian fluid, the velocity profile is blunted in the center and steepened at the wall [2,17], thus increasing the wall shear rate above that predicted for a Newtonian fluid. The actual wall shear rate in the circulatory system is further complicated by the pulsatile nature of the flow, the distensibility of the wall and the geometric features of the vascular tree. At a branch point, the fluid enters with a relatively flat velocity profile, and it takes a traverse distance of several vessel diameters before the velocity profile can be fully developed [8]. Because of the frequent occurrence of vascular branching in the circulatory system, the velocity profile is usually not fully developed [18]; the shear rate distribution across the vessel cross section becomes non-axisymmetric and is usually steepened near the wall (Fig. 5.4). Based upon the above considerations, the wall shear rate values given in Fig. 5.1 should be considered only as an order of magnitude estimate. The radial distribution of shear rate across the vessel is accompanied by a radial distribution of cell concentration [19]. Since blood viscosity is a function of shear rate (and shear stress) as well as cell concentration, it is also non-uniform across the vessel section; the high shear rate and the low cell concentration near the wall tend to lower the viscosity there. Thus, the non-Newtonian behavior of blood results in an increase of shear rate and a lowering of viscosity at the wall, but it has relatively little effect on the wall shear stress, which is a product of these two parameters being affected in opposite directions. Therefore the values of wall shear stress shown in Fig. 5.1 are probably more reliable than those of wall shear rate. For non-Newtonian fluids, in contrast to the nonlinear profile of shear rate across the tube, the shear stress still varies linearly from the a maximum at the wall to zero in the tube center.

Under physiological flow conditions, the shear stress in the arteries is sufficiently high to cause RBC deformation and disaggregation, resulting in a low η_B. The highest shear stress is normally found in the capillaries; this serves to insure the stress deformation of RBCs where it is needed. Furthermore, as pointed out in Chapter 4, the hematocrit in tubes with diameter smaller than approximately 300 μm is lower than that in the feed reservoir or the discharge [20,21]. Measurements in the microcirculation in vivo have also shown that the microvessel Hct (H_μ) in small vessels with diameters below 100 μ is lower than that found in the large systemic vessels (H_{sys}) [22-24]; this further contributes to a reduction in η_B in small vessels. Therefore, the high vascular hindrance in a narrow capillary due to the small vessel radius (Equation 7) is compensated by a lower η_B, thus preventing a markedly elevated resistance (Equation 3). It is only in capillaries with diameters smaller than 4–5 μm that the η_B would rise because of

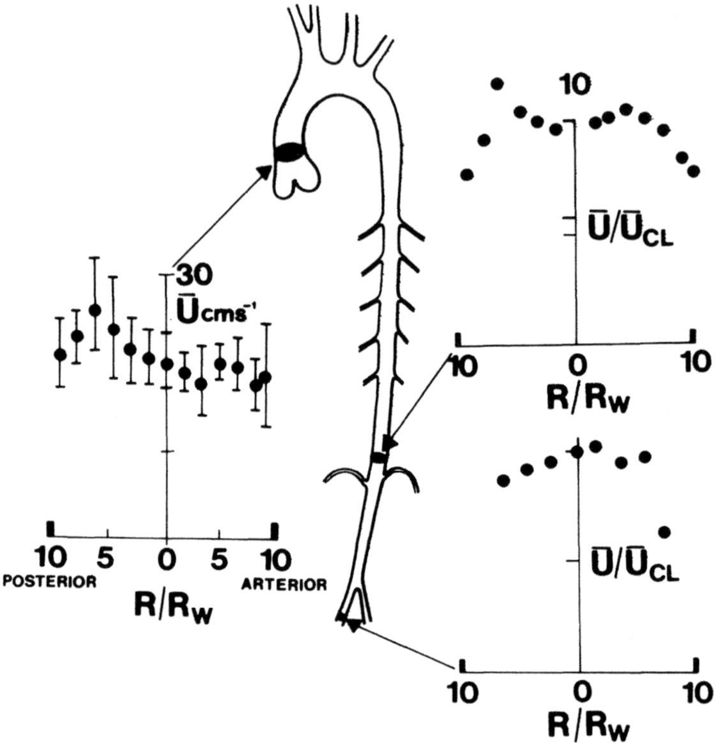

Figure 5.4. Velocity distribution in the ascending aorta, lower thoracic aorta and femoral artery of man. U: mean velocity; U_{CL}, center-line velocity; R/R_w, radial position normalized to the wall radius. From (18).

the need of marked RBC deformation in passing through these narrow vessels [19,25]. The increase of η_B in small capillaries becomes more pronounced when RBC deformability has been reduced, e.g. in sickle cell disease [26], or when there is an elevation of the concentration of WBCs, which are more rigid than RBCs [9, 27-30], e.g., in leukemia [31].

The postcapillary venules and small veins have the lowest shear stress in the circulations (Fig. 5.1), and they represent the most likely sites of RBC aggregation. The existence of lower shear rates in the postcapillary than the precapillary segments may also affect transcapillary fluid exchange in low flow states [32]. In the normal circulation the shear stress is high in both the pre- and post-capillary segments, and the difference in shear may not be associated with a significant difference in η_B. With a reduction in shear stress down to the shear-dependent portion of the $\eta_B - \tau$ curve, the lower shear in postcapillary segment would lead to a high η_B (Fig. 5.5). Such a preferential elevation of postcapillary η_B would

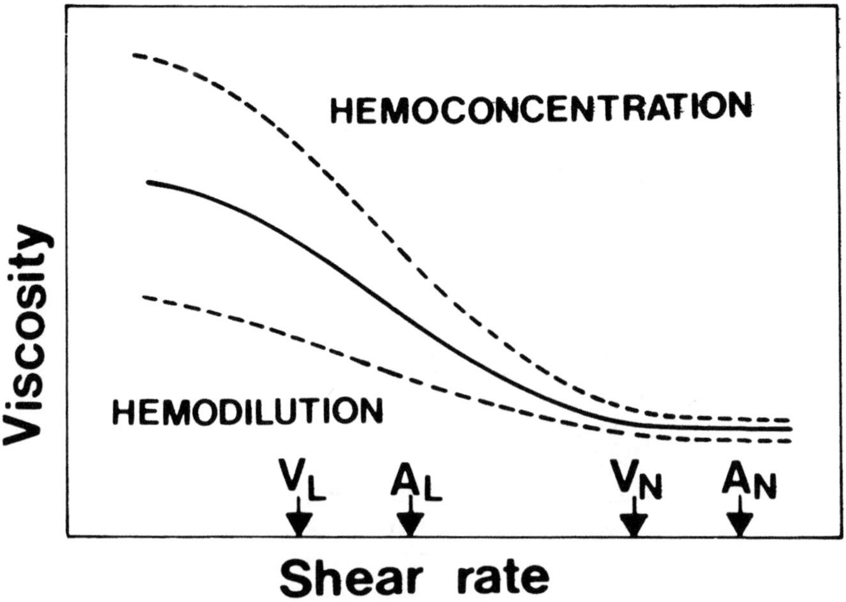

Figure 5.5. Viscosity - shear rate plot showing the disproportionate influence of flow alteration on viscosity of postcapillary (V) and precapillary (A) segments. Solid line indicates the relation for normal blood. The normal shear rate in the postcapillary segment (V_N) is lower than that in the precapillary segment (A_N). In low flow states, the shear rates in these segments are reduced to V_L and A_L, respectively. The broken lines above and below the solid curve indicate the relations obtained when the shear dependence of blood viscosity is altered by hemoconcentration and hemodilution, respectively. From (32).

cause an increase in the post-/precapillary resistance ratio and raise the capillary pressure. Experimental evidence in support of this prediction has been recently reported in studies on muscle microcirculation [33]. The effect of shear-dependent blood viscosity on transcapillary fluid exchange would be more pronounced if the $\eta_B - \dot{\gamma}$ curve becomes steeper as a result of hemoconcentration (Fig. 5.5). Such a vicious cycle involving rheologically induced fluid loss through capillaries may play a significant role in some forms of low flow state (see Section 5.2. below).

As discussed above, the microvessel hematocrit is lower than the systemic hematocrit in the large vessels. The H_μ/H_{sys} ratios in the larger arterioles and venules (diameter > 70 μm) are close to 1, but the value decreases in smaller vessels to a minimum of about 1/4 at the capillary level (Fig. 5.6, bottom panel). By measuring the pressure drop (Δp) across the vessel over a known length with the use of the servo-nulling micropipette technique [34,35], the vessel diameter by image shearing [36], and the volumetric flow rate calculated from the red cell velocity (V_{rbc}) determined by the dual-slit technique [37] using photodiodes and

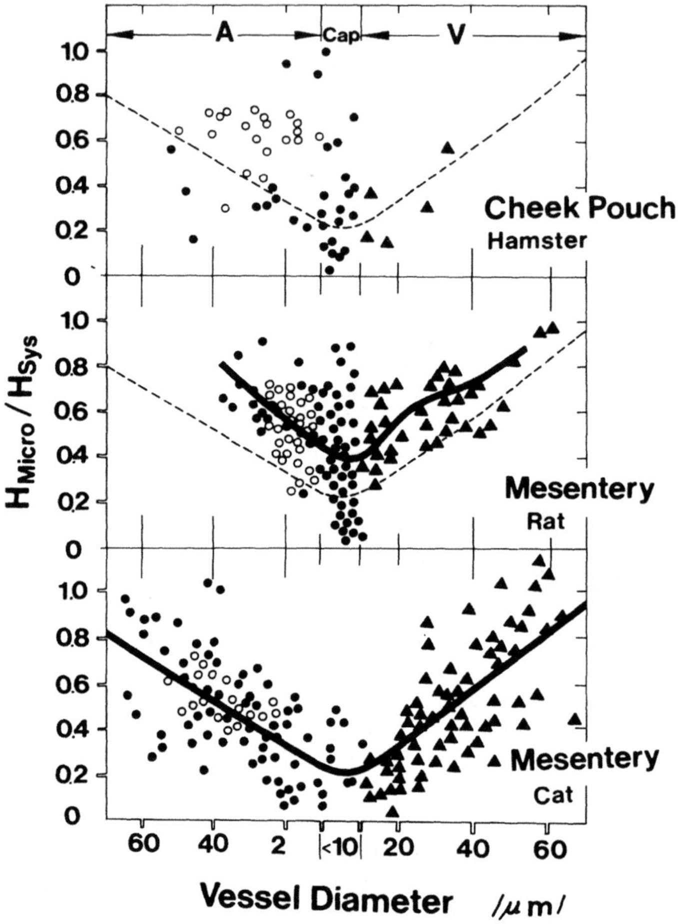

Figure 5.6. Arteriovenous distribution of microvessel hematocrit (H_{micro}) plotted as a ratio to the corresponding systemic hematocrit (H_{sys}). The data were obtained in hamster check pouch by Sarelius and Duling (24), rat mesentery by Kanzow et al (Intern. J. Microcirc. 1: 67, 1982), and cat mesentery by Lipowsky et al (22). Circles are data from arterioles; dots, capillaries; triangles, venules. The solid curves in the middle and lower panels represent cubic spline statistical fit of the data. The minimum H_{micro} appears to lie within the narrowest vessels ($D < 10$ μm). For the purpose of comparison, the solid line in the bottom panel is drawn as dashed lines in the top and middle panels. From (58).

on-line cross-correlation [38], one can determine all the parameters required to compute the apparent blood viscosity (η_a) in a single microvessel by using the Poiseuille-Hagen law.

$$\eta_a = \frac{\pi}{128} \frac{D^4}{Q} \frac{\Delta p}{L} \tag{9}$$

where

$$Q = \frac{\pi D^2}{4} \frac{V_{rbc}}{1.6} \tag{10}$$

The empirical factor of 1.6 is used to convert V_{rbc} to the bulk velocity of blood [39]. The computed apparent viscosity shows a significant correlation with the hematocrit simultaneously determined in the same microvessels, and the $\eta_a - H_\mu$ regression line agrees with the viscosity – hematocrit relationship obtained from in vitro bulk viscosity measurement (Fig. 5.7). These results indicate that the in vitro viscosity – hematocrit relationship can be applied to the in vivo microcirculation, provided that the microvessel hematocrit is known.

When an isolated part of the body is perfused by blood with varying Hct the flow resistance changes in the same direction as the blood viscosity [40-43]. The relative resistance of the perfused organ (resistance ratio of blood perfusion to perfusion with the suspending medium), however, is lower than the η_r determined in a viscometer. This discrepancy is often explained on the basis of the Fåhraeus-Lindqvist effect [44], i.e. a lowering of η_B in narrow vessels which is related to the lowering of Hct therein [20,45]. It is to be noted, however, that while inertial resistance is negligible for the flow of blood in vivo, it may become

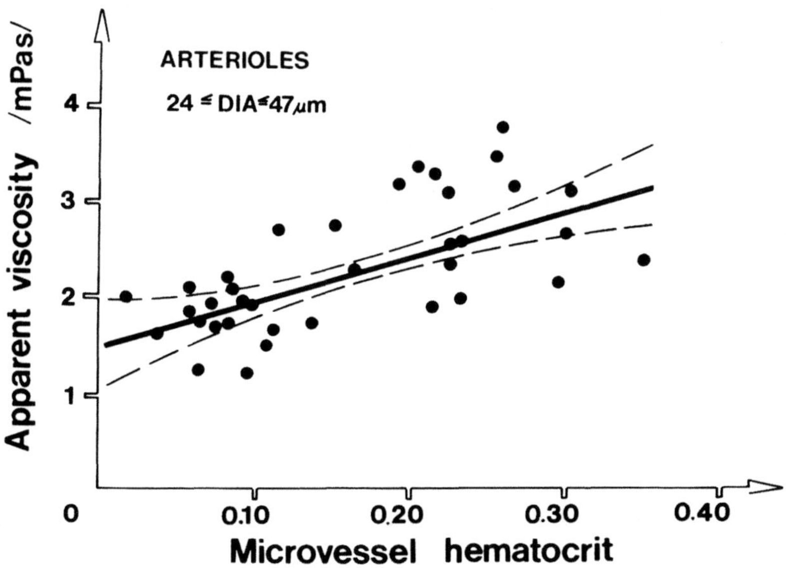

Figure 5.7. "Apparent blood viscosity" vs. hematocrit as determined in vivo for six arterioles in the cat mesentery. The solid line represents a linear regression of the in vivo data, bracketed by ± 95 % confidence limits (dashed lines). The solid line agree with the in vitro viscometry data for cat blood at a shear rate of 2000 s^{-1}. Modified from (22).

significant for the cell-free suspending medium because of the low fluid viscosity in conjunction with the complex vascular geometry in vivo; this may cause an elevation of the resistance value for the suspending medium and hence a lowering of the relative resistance value (blood/suspending medium) in vivo [8,42].

Although blood viscosity is one of the two major determinants of flow resistance (Equation 3), hemodynamic investigations on cardiovascular diseases usually are centered on changes in vascular hindrance, mainly because of the strong 4th power influence of vessel radius, which can change rapidly and markedly in a variety of physiological and pathophysiological conditions. It is to be noted, however, that the influences of vascular hindrance and blood viscosity on resistance are not additive, but rather multiplicative. Therefore, changes in either one of the two determinants of resistance can superimpose on the other, and the effects can thus be amplified. As will be discussed in Section 5.2. of this Chapter, the coexistence of rheological and vascular abnormalities may play a significant part in the pathogenesis of many clinical disorders and that hemorheological manipulations may have therapeutic values in improving blood flow and metabolic transport in vascular disorders.

It should also be noted that blood viscosity and vascular hindrance are not independent entities. A change in vascular hindrance, by altering blood flow and shearing conditions, can affect the blood viscosity, which is shear-dependent (Fig. 5.3). An alteration in blood viscosity, by changing the local hemodynamic and metabolic conditions through its effects on blood flow, can initiate autoregulatory variations in vascular hindrance [46,47].

5.1.4. Influence of blood rheology on oxygen transport

The rate of oxygen delivery (JO_2) to tissues is equal to the product of blood flow and the arterial blood oxygen content (AO_2).

$$JO_2 = QAO_2 \tag{11}$$

From Equation (4a) blood flow can be expressed as

$$Q = \frac{p_A - p_V}{\eta_B Z} \tag{12}$$

The arterial blood oxygen content is mainly that carried with the hemoglobin (Hb), and this is

$$AO_2 = kSO_2(MCHC)Hct \tag{13}$$

where k is a constant ($= 1.34$ ml O_2/g Hb), SO_2 is the percent HbO_2 saturation in the arterial blood, and MCHC is the mean corpuscular hemoglobin concentration (in g/dl). Combination of Equations [11], [12] and [13] yields:

$$JO_2 = k\frac{SO_2(MCHC)Hct(p_A - p_v)}{\eta_B Z} \quad (14)$$

Increases in values of the terms in the numerator in this equation facililate O_2 delivery by increasing arterial O_2 content or blood flow, whereas increases in values of the denominator decrease O_2 delivery by reducing blood flow. If $p_A - p_v$, SO_2 and MCHC are normal, the rate of O_2 delivery can be expressed as:

$$JO_2 = k'\frac{Hct}{\eta_B Z} \quad (15)$$

where k' is a constant. If Z is also unchanged, then the rate of oxygen delivery varies with the ratio of hematocrit to blood viscosity (Hct/η_B). As a consequence of the relationship between $1/\eta_B$ and Hct (Fig. 5.8), the parameter Hct/η_B, which is a reflection of JO_2 under conditions of normal cardiovascular and respiratory functions, exhibits a maximum value when plotted against Hct (Fig. 5.8b). At low levels of Hct (<30 %), the decrease in O_2 carrying capacity of the blood causes a drop of oxygen delivery despite the low η_B and high Q. At high levels of Hct (>50 %), the steep rise in η_B and the ensuing sharp decrease in blood flow overwhelm the linear increase in O_2 carrying capacity, and oxygen delivery again drops. Thus, an optimum range of Hct for maximum oxygen delivery by normal blood at the physiologically high shear conditions is between 0.30 and 0.50. The effect of variations of hematocrit on oxygen delivery has been studied in the mesenteric microcirculation of the cat [48]. The rate of oxygen delivery was estimated from RBC flux in the microvessel, which was calculated as the product of the blood flow and the discharge hematocrit [21] from the vessel. The microvessel RBC flux follows a bell-shape curve, having a maximum at the resting hematocrit value (Fig. 5.9, right panel). Such a relationship between oxygen delivery and hematocrit found in the microvasculature is similar to what has been obtained at the macrocirculatory level (49,50) (Fig. 5.9, left panel). In both cases oxygen transport is maximized at the resting hematocrit.

A change in the η_B vs. Hct relationship (Fig. 5.10) would cause alterations of the JO_2 – Hct curve and the optimum Hct level. Such shifts of the optimum Hct occur when η_B becomes elevated at a given Hct level in various hematological and cardiovascular disorders (Section 5.2.).

Equation (15) indicates that an increased Z has the same effect as an elevated η_B on oxygen delivery as estimated by Hct/$\eta_B Z$. Therefore, in conditions with high vascular hindrance, e.g. intense vasoconstriction, the JO_2 curve is suppressed and the optimum Hct is shifted to lower levels. Under conditions of vasodilation,

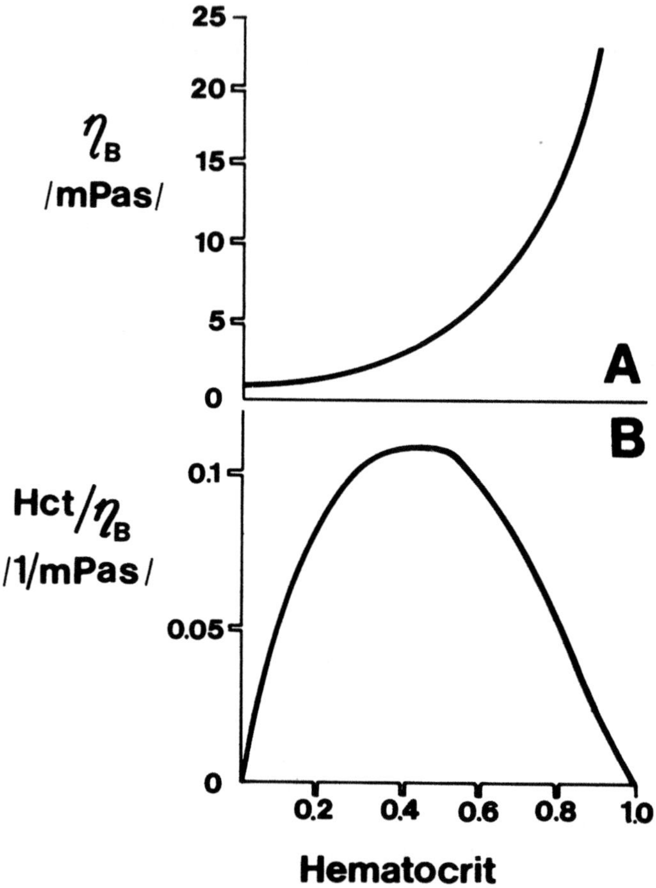

Figure 5.8. Effects of hematocrit (Hct) variations on blood viscosity (η_B) at shear rate of 500 s^{-1} (upper panel) and the ratio Hct/η_B (lower panel), which reflects the rate of oxygen transport for given cardiopulmonary function. Note the range of optimum Hct for maximum oxygen transport.

e.g. in muscular exercise, the decrease in vascular hindrance would shift the optimum Hct to higher levels [51].

The above considerations are based upon the rate of oxygen delivery; a more important parameter is the rate of oxygen utilization or comsumption (MO_2), which is equal to the product of blood flow and the arterial-venous difference in O_2 content.

$$MO_2 = Q(AO_2 - VO_2) \tag{16}$$

$$MO_2 = JO_2 EO_2 \tag{17}$$

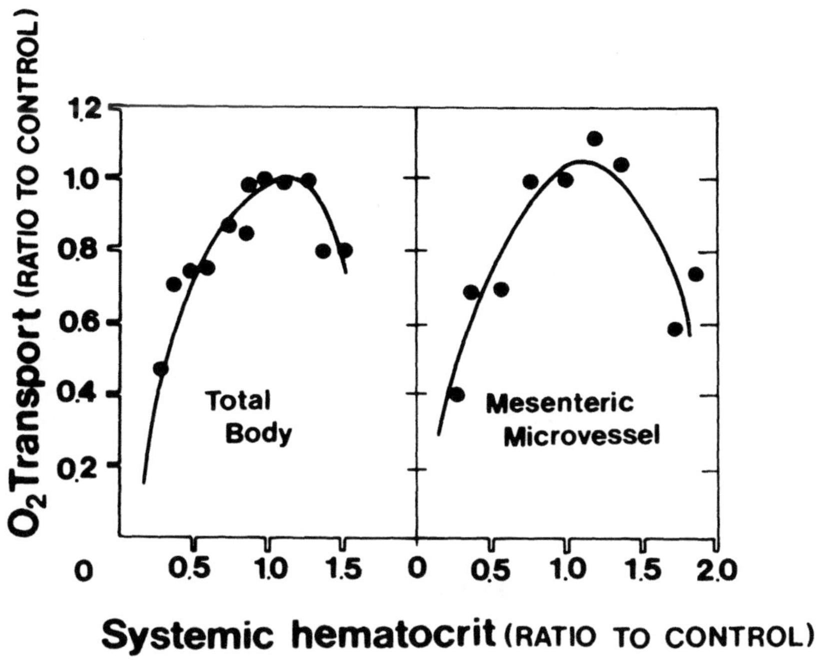

Figure 5.9. Effects of variations in systemic hematocrit on oxygen transport as estimated from red cell flux (= flow x discharge hematocrit) in a cat mesenteric arteriole (right) and the total systemic circulation of dogs (left). All data are shown as ratio to control values. From (58).

where EO_2 is the oxygen extraction ratio and equals $(AO_2 - VO_2)/AO_2$. The rate of oxygen consumption by tissues is affected by the processes influencing oxygen unloading from Hb and oxygen diffusion to tissue cells. The unloading process depends on the local pH [52], red cell content of organic phosphates [53] and possibly also red cell deformability [54,55]. In the coronary circulation, where the myocardial O_2 extraction is already near maximum under normal conditions, oxygen consumption (Fig. 5.11a) varies almost directly with oxygen delivery (Fig. 5.11b), as EO_2 remains essentially constant [49,50] (Fig. 5.11c). In the other parts of the systemic circulation, however, a decrease in oxygen delivery is usually compensated by an increase in EO_2, and hence the range of optimum Hct for MO_2 is broader than that for JO_2 (Fig. 5.11).

Despite the various simplifications and assumptions used in the theoretical derivations of the optimum Hct concept as shown in Fig. 5.8, the results agree well with the optimum hematocrit for O_2 delivery and utilization found in experimental studies in vivo [49,50,56,57]. It appears that the physiological mechanisms for the control of red cell volume and plasma volume are coordinated such that the hematocrit level is regulated to be in the optimum range.

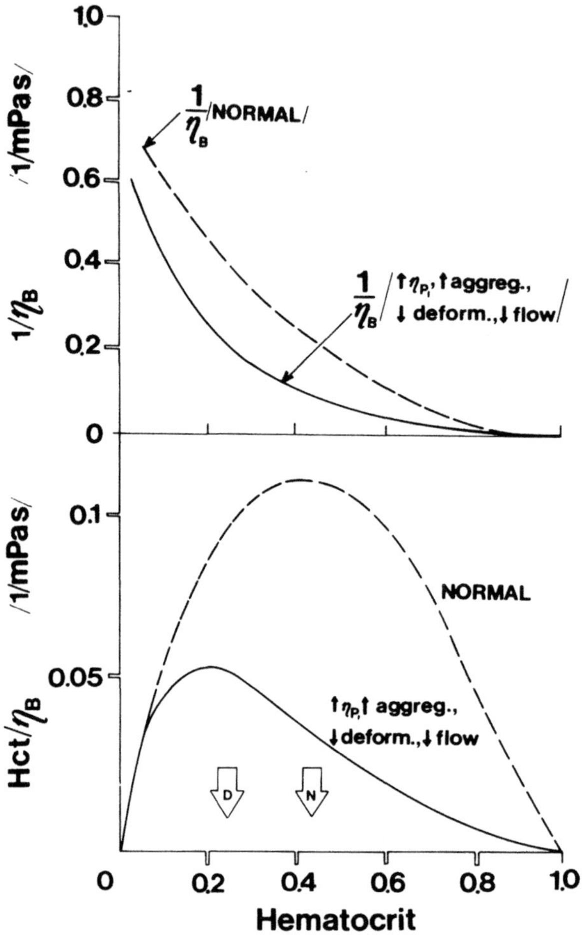

Figure 5.10. Effects of variations in hematocrit (Hct) on O_2 transport as reflected by the calculated parameter Hct/η_B (bottom panel). Top panel shows the variations in Hct and $1/\eta_B$ with Hct. Dashed lines: Results obtained when Hct is the only variable, with other hemorheological parameters remaining normal. Solid lines: Results obtained when there are increases in plasma viscosity (η_P), red cell aggregation or red cell rigidity, or a decrease in flow rate. Arrow marked *N* shows normal Hct level, and that marked *D* shows Hct level found in patients with sickle cell disease or multiple myeloma. From (87).

When the optimum Hct is shifted in various physiological conditions, the control mechanisms operate to provide again the optimum Hct under the circumstance. A good example is the compensatory increase of Hct at high altitudes, where the reduction in pO_2 of the inspired air leads to a decrease in arterial O_2 content at a given Hct. In this case, it may be more advantageous to increase Hct despite the

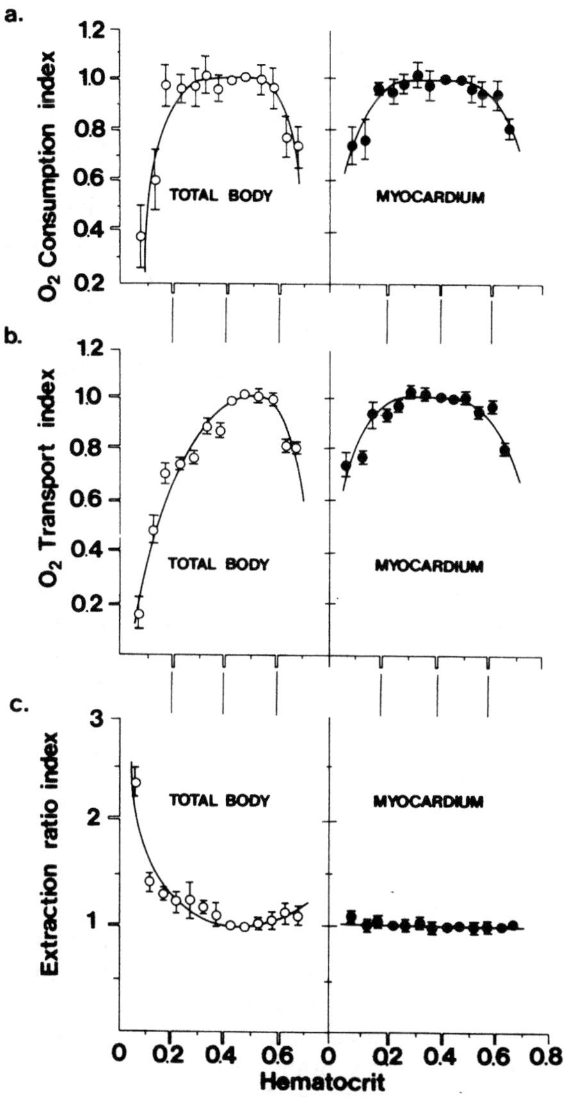

Figure 5.11. Effects of hematocrit variations in the dog on oxygen consumption (A), oxygen transport (B) and oxygen extraction (C) in the total body (left sides) and myocardium (right sides). The index value for each parameter is calculated by dividing the experimental value by the corresponding control value obtained at hematocrit of 0.45. Vertical bars denote S.E.M. Modified from (49).

accompanying increase in blood viscosity. As will be discussed in Section 5.2. of this Chapter, the volume control mechanisms also provide the appropriate Hct in a variety of clinical conditions when the optimum levels has been shifted due to rheological or cardiovascular abnormalities. The control mechanisms are mediated by regulating the plasma volume through transcapillary fluid shifts and/or the cell volume through the balance between erythropoiesis and red cell destruction, but the precise nature of the feedback control which provides the coordination between these two mechanisms and the ensuing optimum Hct has not been established.

The discussion thus far has centered primarily on the whole body. Each organ and tissues may have different levels of optimum Hct because of the regional variations in vascular hindrance [47]. In various physiological and pathophysiological conditions, the neurohumoral influences on regional vascular hindrances would further enhance the heterogeneity of regional optimum Hct. For immediate survival, it is more important to consider the heart and the brain, but for long-term physiological functioning it is also necessary to include other organs.

5.1.5. Influence of leukocytes on blood flow in the microcirculation

The effects of WBCs on blood flow in the microcirculation have already been discussed in Chapters 3 and 4. Because of their larger volume and lower deformability, WBCs can exert significant influences on blood flow through narrow vessels [58]. The presence of WBCs in the fluid used to perfuse the rat hindquarter causes a significant rise in flow resistance [11]. The entry of a WBC into a narrow capillary leads to a slowing of the local flow rate [59]. Because only plasma can overtake the WBC through the narrow clearance between the WBC and the capillary wall, there is usually a plasma column in front of the WBC, and behind the WBC there would be a train of RBCs travelling at the same reduced velocity as the leading WBC [59,60]. This leads to a non-homogeneity of the distribution of cells and plasma along the length of a capillary.

The rheological behavior of WBCs in narrow vessels has a significant influence on the distribution of blood cells at branch points. In a divergent bifurcation composed of narrow vessels (e.g. $< 10\ \mu m$ in diameter), the RBCs tend to travel in a single file near the center line of the parent vessel; therefore a slight discrepancy in the partition of flow between the two branches would cause nearly all of the BRCs to enter from the parent vessel into the branch with the higher flow. The entrance of a WBC into one branch (A in Fig. 5.12) of such a bifurcation would reduce the flow in that branch and increase the flow in other branch (B in Fig. 5.12). The partition of the flow lines in the parent vessel would be such that all RBCs near the center line are swept into branch B (Fig. 5.12). The preferential distribution of RBCs into branch B would continue until the increase in resistance due to multiple RBCs in that branch would match that due to the WBC in branch A, or until the WBC leaves branch A into the next generation of vessels.

The above discussions indicate that, in a microvascular bifurcation, fractional RBC flux into a daughter branch is often not equal to the fractional flow into that branch. If these two parameters are equal to each other, then one would obtain the diagonal line in Fig. 5.13. In narrow capillaries ($D < 10$ μm), where the blood cells travel near the center line, the experimental data show that the partition of RBC flux is very sensitive to changes in flow partitioning, as indicated by the S-shaped curve in Fig. 5.13. A 60/40 percent distribution of blood flow may lead to the passage of all RBCs arriving at the bifurcation into the higher flow branch. These results obtained on capillary bifurcations in the rabbit ear chamber in vivo [59] agree with the results obtained in an in vitro system [61] and from theoretical considerations [62].

At bifurcations of larger microvessels, i.e. arterioles and venules from 20 to 90 μm in diameter [58], the radial distribution of RBCs in the parent vessels is more uniform, and the partitioning of RBC flux is essentially proportional to the flow partitioning (Fig. 5.13b), instead of being S-shaped. These results are similar to those reported by Klitzman and Johnson [23]. Therefore, the relationship between the partitioning of RBC flux and that of blood flow at a branch point is dependent on the vessel diameter and blood cell concentration profile in the parent vessels.

WBCs may become adhered to the venular endothelium, especially in low flow

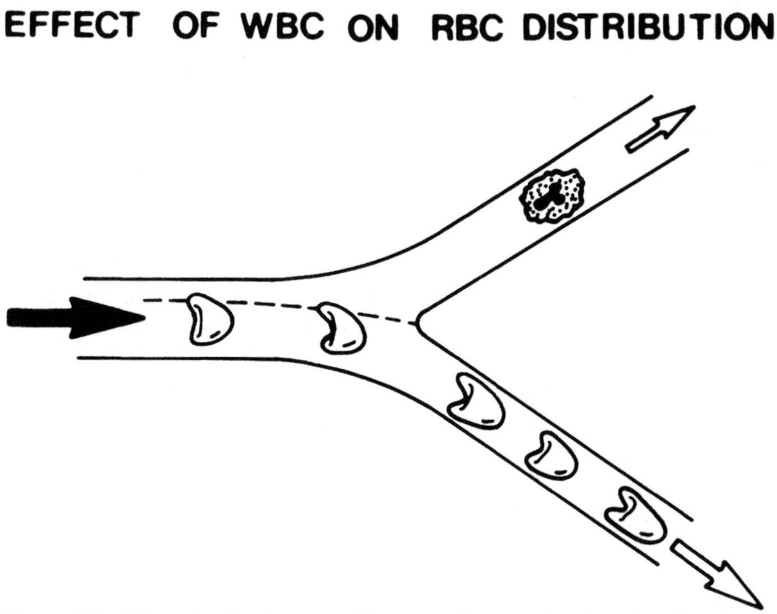

Figure 5.12. Schematic drawing of a divergent microvascular branch point showing the influence of WBC on RBC distribution. The entrance of a WBC into one branch (A) causes the subsequently arriving RBCs to enter the other branch (B). From (58).

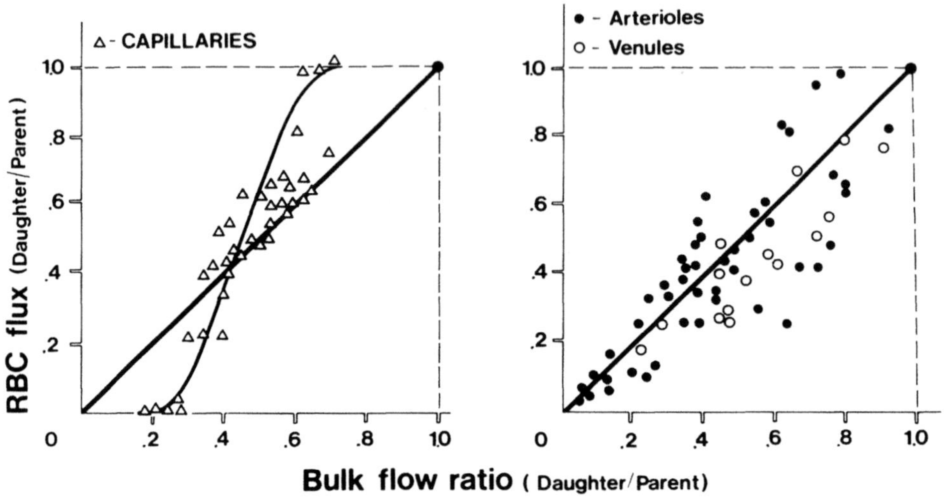

Figure 5.13. Relations between fractional flux of red cells from parent into daughter vessels and the fractional blood flow in the same vessels. Left panel: capillaries approximately 10 μm in diameter. Right panel: arterioles and venules from 20 to 90 μm in diameter. Diagonal line in each panel indicates 1:1 relationship between RBC flux and bulk flow ratios. From (58).

states and in the pesence of inflammatory agents [64,65]. The WBCs arriving at a convergence branch point tend to remain in close contact with the endothelium if there are RBCs entering simultaneously from the other branch. The more deformable RBCs would squeeze past the WBC and, in the process, exert a lateral force to displace the WBC toward the endothelial surface [66]. A similar phenomenon has been observed when a WBC enters from a capillary into a venule at right angle [67]. Finally, when the shear rate is low and RBC aggregation occurs, e.g. in venules at slow flows, the WBCs are displaced towards the vessel wall by the RBC rouleaux [19,20,68,69], and this provides another rheological mechanism by which WBCs can be brought to close vicinity of the endothelium. Therefore, rheological mechanisms involving the interaction between RBCs and WBCs lead to the radial displacement of the WBC towards the endothelial surface where the WBC tends to roll at a slow velocity. The close proximity between the WBC and the endothelium and the slow rolling velocity of the WBC would increase the probability of WBC-endothelial interactions (e.g. adhesion) and place the WBC in a strategical position, both spatially and temporally, to react to extravascular chemotactic signals.

5.1.6. Modeling of microcirculatory networks

The behavior of blood cells at branch points can be used to model cell distribution in a microvascular network. By using the anatomical features of the microvascular architecture in a capillary network, e.g. in the rabbit omentum [59], and assigning the boundary hemodynamic conditions and input Hct, the distributions of intravascular hematocrit and flow throughout the network can be computed, based on the knowledge on the relationship between RBC flux and flow at these branch points [59].

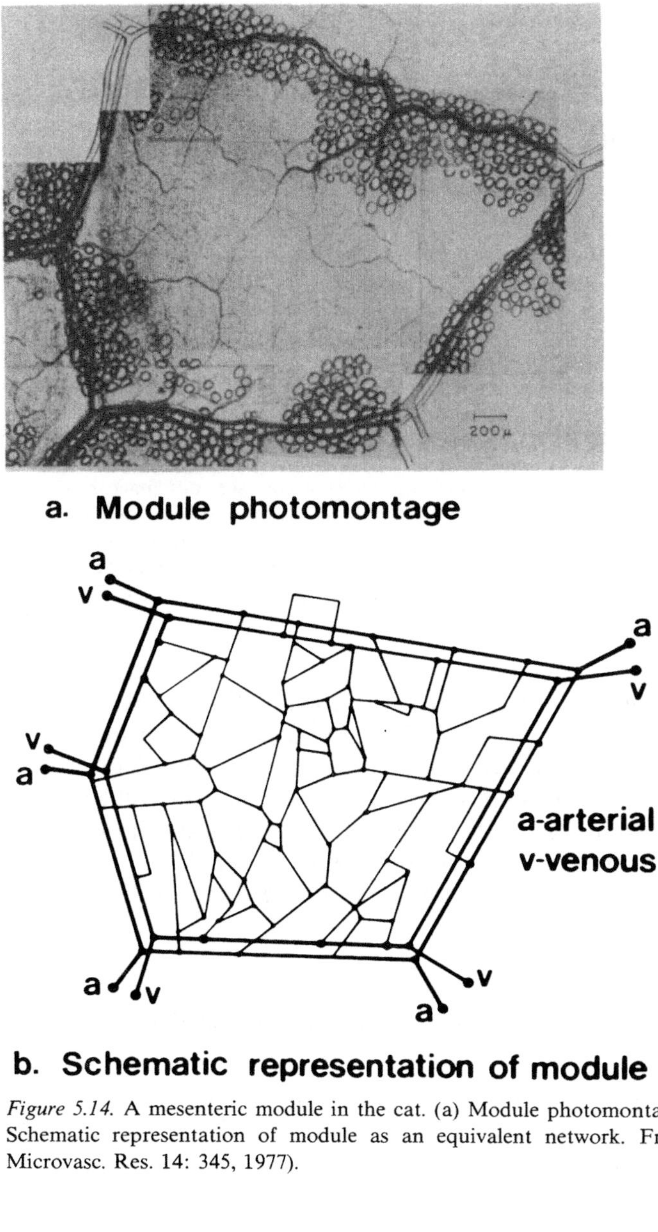

Figure 5.14. A mesenteric module in the cat. (a) Module photomontage from microphotographs. (b) Schematic representation of module as an equivalent network. From (Lipowsky and Zweifach, Microvasc. Res. 14: 345, 1977).

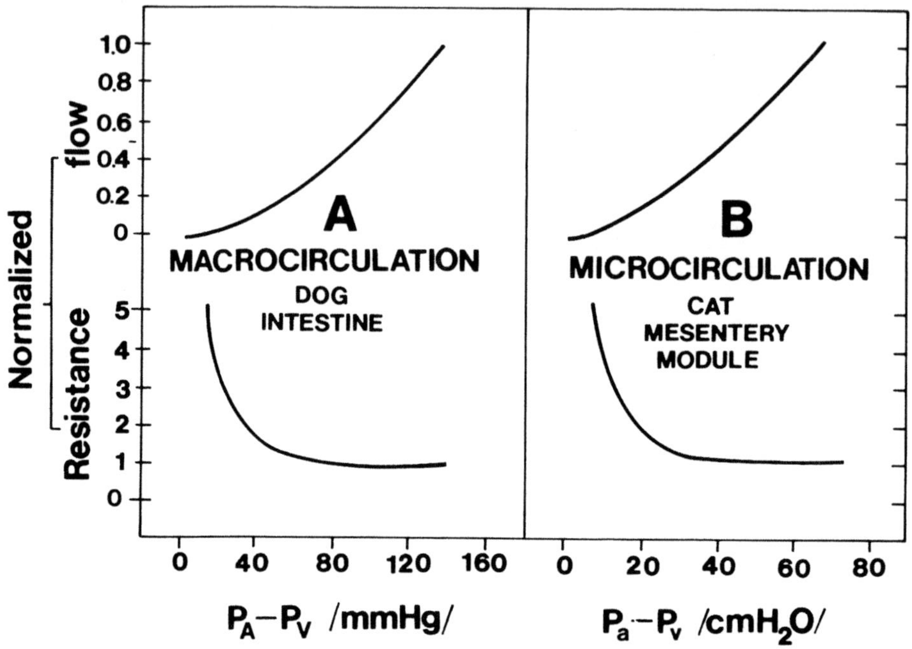

Figure 5.15. Variations of blood flow and resistance with arterio-venous pressure difference in the dog intestine (A) and a cat mesenteric module (B). In (A), the flow and resistance were normalized by dividing the data by the corresponding values obtained at an artery-to-mesenteric vein pressure difference of 140 mmHg. In (B), the flow and resistance were normalized by dividing the data by the corresponding values obtained at an arteriole-to-venule pressure difference of 70 mmHg. From (58).

With the use of the geometric features in the microvascular network and the relationship between apparent viscosity and shear rate determined in the microcirculation, the method of electrical network analysis can be applied to deduce the pressure-flow-resistance relationship in a microvascular network [70] such as the mesenteric module shown in Fig. 5.14. The steep rise in resistance at very low flow rates as predicted from such network analysis (Fig. 5.15A) is in general agreement with the experimental results on the isolated intestine [71] (Fig. 5.15b).

5.2. Circulatory consequences of pathological alterations in blood rheology

The above discussions on the role of blood rheology in governing flow resistance, oxygen delivery and transcapillary fluid shifts can be applied to considerations on clinical conditions involving hematological and cardiovascular diseases.

5.2.1. Hemorheological abnormalities in hematological disorders

As pointed out in Section 5.1.1. above, the bulk viscosity of normal blood flowing in large vessels is a function of Hct, plasma viscosity, red cell aggregation, and red cell deformability, with the last two parameters being flow dependent. In small vessels, the concentration and adhesiveness of white blood cells can also exert significant effects on flow resistance. Many hematological disorders involve abnormalities in one or more of the fundamental determinants of blood viscosity. For example, abnormal increases in hematocrit, plasma viscosity, red cell aggregation and red cell rigidity are found in polycythemia, multiple myeloma, sialic acid deficiency and sickle cell disease, respectively. The following is a brief summary of blood rheology in these conditions, with the aim of illustrating several common principles and of correlating the hemorheological data with some in vivo hemodynamic measurements. A more detailed discussion on various hematological disorders is given in Chapter 8 (Leblond).

Polycythemia

The main disturbance in polycythemia (both secondary polycythemia and polycythemia vera) is an increase in Hct. In addition to the high Hct, polycythemic patients also have slight increases in plasma viscosity and red cell rigidity. Red cell aggregation is not significantly altered. As a result of these rheological abnormalities, the blood viscosity in polycythemia is elevated at both high and

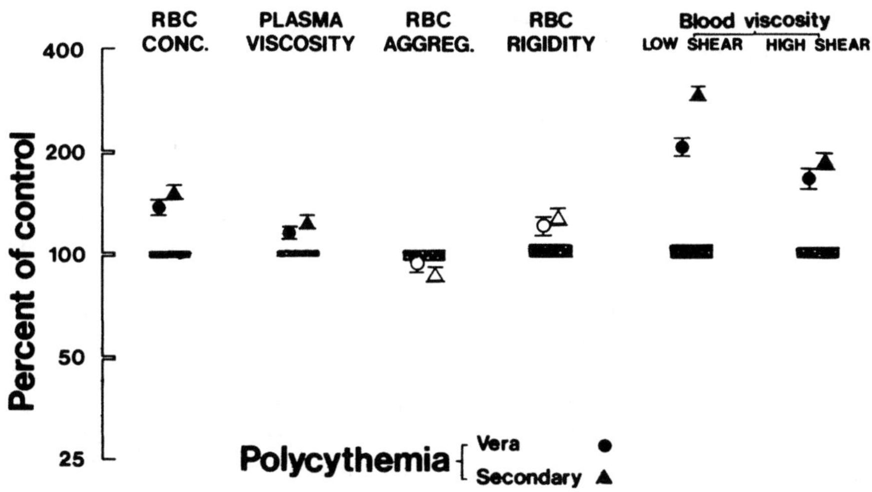

Figure 5.16. Hemorheological data (mean ± S.E.M.) in patients with polycythemia vera and secondary polycythemia, plotted as percent of control values (logarithmic scale). Shaded areas indicate mean ± S.E.M. of normal controls. Closed symbols indicate significance of difference between patient data and normal controls ($p < 0.01$). From (87).

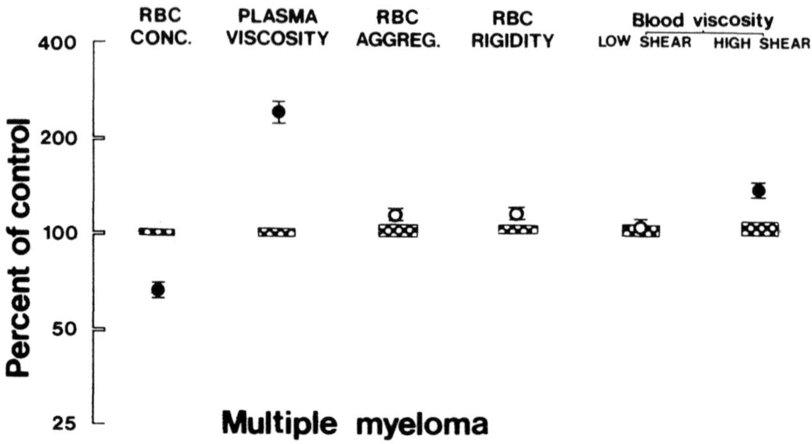

Figure 5.17. Hemorheological data in patients with multiple myeloma. See Fig. 5.16 for explanation. From (87).

low shear rates (Fig. 5.16). From in vivo measurements on cardiac output and arterial pressure [72] and in vitro determination of blood viscosity, one can compute the vascular hindrance (Z in Equation 4a). In polycythemic patients with an expanded blood volume, the increase in η_B is accompanied by a decrease in vascular hindrance (vasodilation), leading to an essentially unchanged systemic flow resistance. In polycythemic patients without an increase in blood volume, however, vascular hindrance remains normal; therefore, systemic flow resistance rises with η_B, and blood flow through the systemic circulation falls. These results indicate that an increase in vascular hindrance such as that due to arterial occlusive disease is especially dangerous in polycythemic patients.

Multiple myeloma

In multiple myeloma, the primary hemorheological disturbance is an elevation of plasma viscosity, but this is compensated by a concomitant decrease in Hct (Fig. 5.17). Red cell aggregation is not significantly enhanced, probably because the γ-globulins are too small to cause significant bridging of red cells. Red cell deformability is also not altered. As a result of the opposing changes in plasma viscosity and Hct, blood viscosity at low shear rates may be almost normal. Blood viscosity at high shear rates is elevated as the increase of plasma viscosity overrides the decrease of Hct. The low Hct of 0.20–0.25 found in these patients is just the optimum Hct computed theoretically on the basis of the elevated plasma viscosity (Fig. 5.10b). This serves to illustrate the compensatory nature of the decrease in Hct, which serves to optimize O_2 transport in the face of a rheological abnormality. When the Hct of blood samples taken from myeloma patients is artificially adjusted in vitro to the level of normal subjects (e.g., 0.45), the blood viscosity at both high and low shear rates increases markedly to several times normal, and this would be severely detrimental to O_2 delivery.

Sialic acid deficiency

As pointed out in Chapter 3, the negative surface charges on the normal human red cell membrane give rise to an electrostatic repulsive potential which counteracts the aggregation energy resulting from macromolecular bridging [73,74]. Hemorheological studies were performed on a patient with deficiencies of N-acetylneuraminic acid (sialic acid) and negative surface charge on his red cell membrane to approximately one-half normal [75]. The Hct, plasma viscosity and red cell rigidity of the patient were within normal ranges (Fig. 5.18). Red cell aggregation was enhanced, and this was accompanied by a corresponding increase in whole blood viscosity at low shear rates.

Sickle cell disease

In sickle cell (SS) disease, the primary abnormality is an increase of red cell rigidity (Fig. 5.19). Even when oxygenated at $pO_2 \geq 100$ mmHg, the SS cells have a higher degree of rigidity than the normal AA cells [76-79]. When the pO_2 is reduced to 20 mmHg, the degree of rigidity increased dramatically [80,81]. The rigidity of individual SS red cells following deoxygenation is demonstrated more clearly by the rise in relative resistance of dilute cell suspensions flowing through polycarbonate filters with a pore diameter of 5 μm [82]. The SS patients have a reduced Hct, and this serves to offset the effects of increased cell rigidity on whole blood viscosity. This low Hct is in the range of the computed optimum Hct and illustrates once again the control mechanisms which operate to provide the

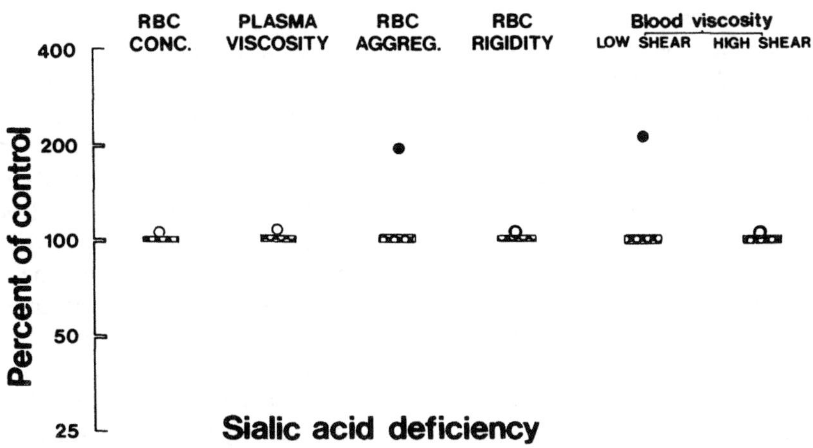

Figure 5.18. Hemorheological data in a patient with sialic acid deficiency. See Fig. 5.16 for explanation. From (87).

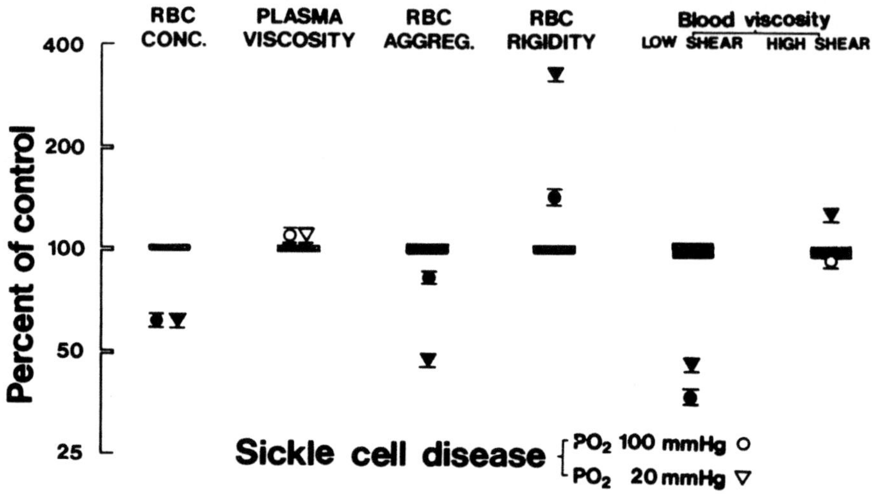

Figure 5.19. Hemorheological data at two levels of PO_2 (100 and 20 mmHg) for 15 patients with sickle cell disease. See Fig. 5.16 for explanation. From (87).

optimum Hct. The plasma viscosity is not significantly different from normal, but the degree of red cell aggregation is reduced because the rigid cells do not deform easily to form rouleaux. As a result of the combination of these factors, the viscosity of SS blood when oxygenated is essentially normal at high shear rates and lower than normal at low shear rates (Fig. 5.19). Even when deoxygenated to $pO_2 = 20$ mm Hg, the SS blood viscosity at low shear rates is still lower than normal due to the decreases in Hct and red cell aggregation. At high shear rates, when red cell aggregation is not a factor, the viscosity of deoxygenated SS blood becomes significantly higher than normal as the increased cell rigidity overrides the low Hct. When the Hct of the SS sample is adjusted in vitro to 0.45, the elevation of blood viscosity becomes markedly greater [81].

The effects of the increased rigidity of SS cells following deoxygenation on their passage through the microcirculation in vivo have been investigated by intravital microscopy in experimental animals following exchange transfusion with human SS cells [83-86]. The flow resistance and in vivo apparent viscosity in single microvessels (Equation 9) of the cremaster muscle in the mouse have been calculated from measurements of microvascular dimension, intravascular pressure and flow velocity [26]. The administration of SS cells causes an increase in resistance and an elevation of the in vivo apparent viscosity, especially following the reduction of tissue pO_2 by using deoxygenated superfusing solution (Fig. 5.20). This increase of in vivo apparent viscosity with deoxygenation is similar to the hemorheological findings in vitro [80,82]. Following the injection of SS cells labeled with rhodamine isothiocyanate, fluorescent microscopy of the cremaster

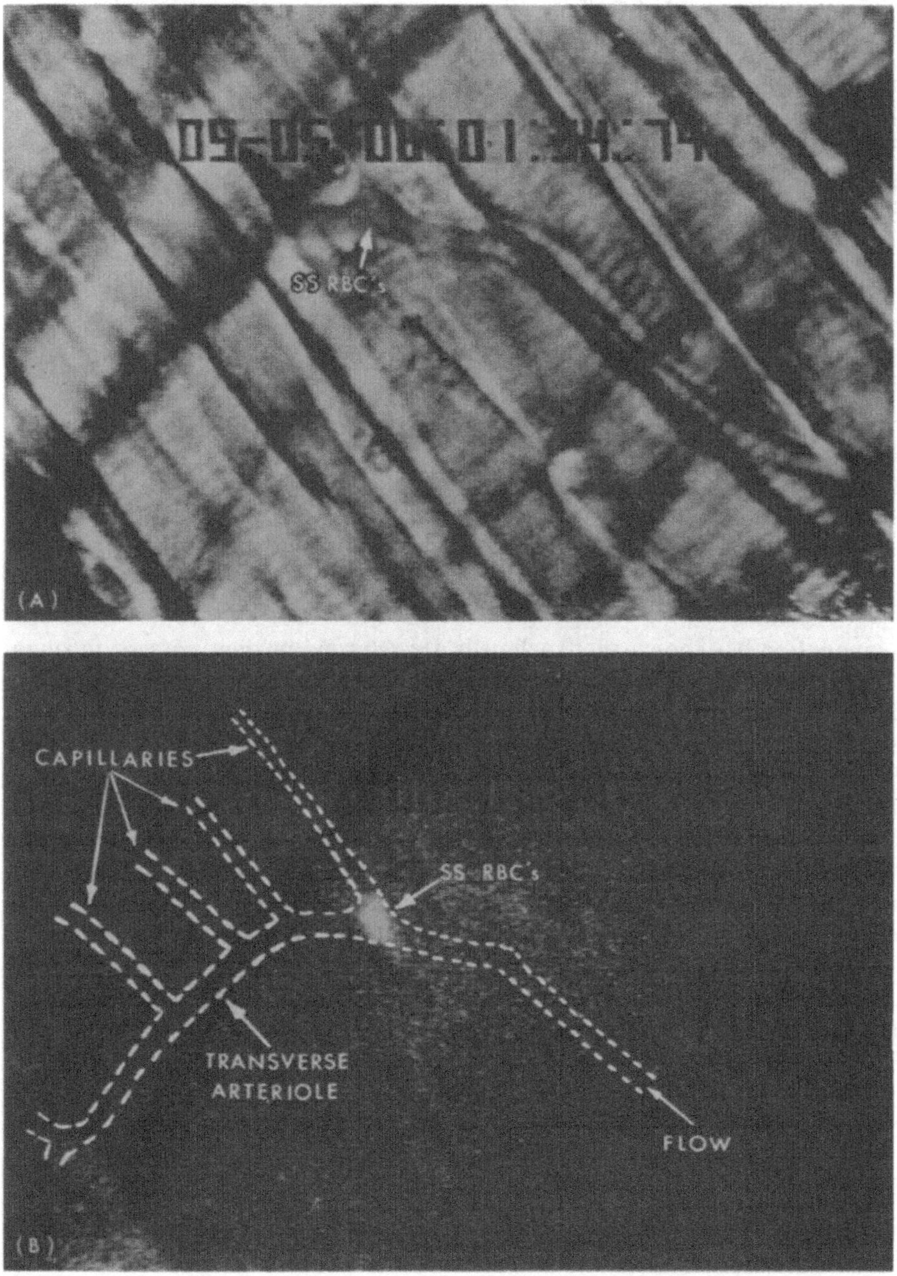

Figure 5.20. (A) SS cells (labelled with FITC) sequestered in a terminal arteriole in the cremaster muscle of the mouse, as viewed under ordinary bright-field illumination. (B) Same scene, viewed under fluorescence illumination, with the vascular walls outlined by dashed lines. From (26).

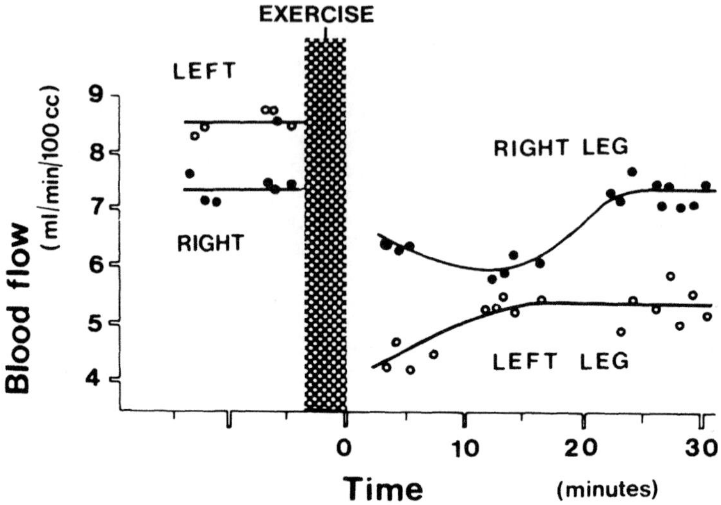

Figure 5.21. Plethysmographic blood flow measurements in a sickle cell patient. The left leg had ulcers, while the right side did not. Note the decrease in blood flow following exercise, especially in the ulcerated leg. From (87).

microcirculation has shown that such cells are retarded in their passage through, or trapped at, the branch points from terminal arterioles to capillaries [26].

The role of the rheological behavior of sickle cells in affecting blood flow in the sickle cell patient has been studied by intravital microscopy of the finger nailfold and by plethysmography of the lower extremities [86,87]. Fig. 5.21 shows the leg blood flows measured by plethysmography before and after muscular exercise. In normal AA subjects, the local metabolic changes induced by exercise cause vasodilation and an increase in blood flow through the exercising limb. In contrast, the blood flow in the SS patient (Fig. 5.16) decreased following exercise, especially in the leg that had an ulcer. This indicates that the local increase in viscous resistance of SS cells (and possibly microvascular obstruction) following deoxygenation overrides the decrease in vascular hindrance due to vasodilation, leading to a reduction of blood flow in exercise.

5.2.2. Hemorheological abnormalities in cardiovascular disease

Hemorheological abnormalities are also present in some cardiovascular disorders involving primarily myocardial dysfunction or vascular derangement. The following is a brief summary of the bulk hemorheological properties in some of these conditions, with the aim of correlating the hemorheological data with in vivo hemodynamics. More detailed discussions on these cardiovacular disorders are given in Chapters 6 (Dormandy), 10 (Barnes and Willars) and 11 (Forconi, Pieragalli and Ernst).

Myocardial infarction
Hemorheological abnormalities have been found in patients with acute myocardial infarction [88-91]. Analysis of the various hemorheological components showed that there were slight but significant increases of Hct, plasma viscosity and red cell aggregation in acute myocardial infarction [88], as compared to the normal controls (Fig. 5.22).

The increases in plasma viscosity and red cell aggregation are attributable to elevations in fibrinogen and α_2-globulin concentrations. The plasma may also contain some factor which can cause a decrease in red cell filterability [92]. The combination of these factors causes an increase in whole blood viscosity, especially at low shear rates. There were variations in the degree of elevations of blood viscosity among the patients studied; those who later developed complications (e.g., thromboembolism, shock and cerebral involvement) during the course of hospitalization had the highest viscosity upon admission. Therefore, the elevation of blood viscosity in myocardial infarction may have prognostic significance. During hospitalization, the Hct decreased gradually, but plasma viscosity and red cell aggregation continued to increase over the next few days. After approximately one week, all these hemorheological abnormalities lessened progressively, and blood viscosity returned towards normal level. Hemorheological measurements made two months after the acute infarction showed results comparable to those obtained on normal controls. Simultaneous determinations of flow resistances and blood viscosity have been made in patients with myocardial

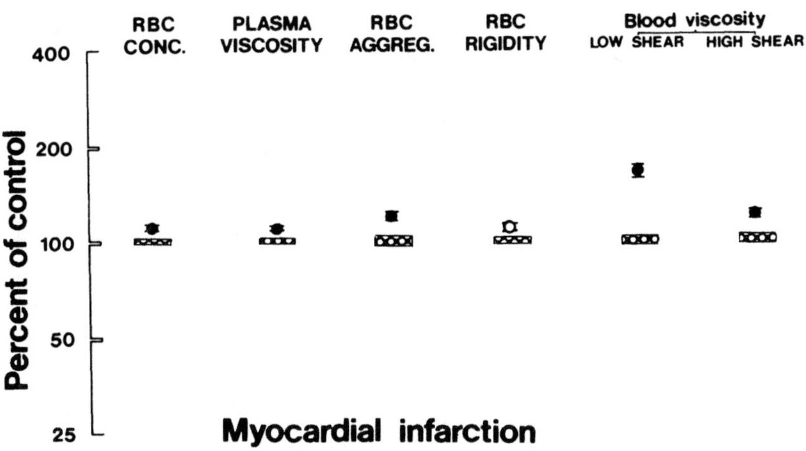

Figure 5.22. Hemorheological data in 25 patients with acute myocardial infarction (data obtained on admission). See Fig. 5.16 for explanation. From (87).

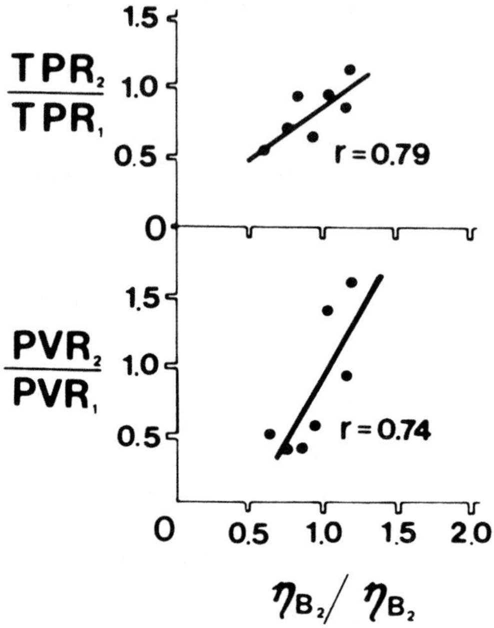

Figure 5.23. Correlation of *recovery/acute phase* ratios of total peripheral resistance in the systemic circulation (TPR_2/TPR_1, top panel) and pulmonary flow resistance (PVR_2/PVR_1, bottom panel) with the *recovery/acute phase ratio* for blood viscosity (η_{B2}/η_{B1}) in myocarial infarction patients. r is coefficient of correlation. From (87).

infarction, first upon their admission (subscript 1) and again one month later (subscript 2) during recovery [86]. Fig. 5.23 shows that the resistance ratios between recovery and acute phases for both the systemic (TPR_2/TPR_1) and the pulmonary (PVR_2/PVR_1) circulations are significantly correlated with the blood viscosity ratio over this period (η_{B2}/η_{B1}). These results indicate that variations in blood viscosity may be a significant factor in effecting the changes in flow resistance that occurred between the acute stage and the recovery phase.

Essential hypertension

In patients with essential hypertension, blood viscosity has been found to be elevated [93-96], and the degree of elevation can be correlated with both systolic and diastolic pressure levels [94]. A correlation also exists between arterial pressure and the low-shear viscosity of blood samples with hematocrit adjusted to 45%; analysis of the results indicate that both the hematocrit level and the fibrinogen concentration contribute to the observed correlations between η_B and arterial pressure [95]. The changes in blood viscosity in essential hypertension are dependent on the renin level. The abnormalities in hemorheological components and blood viscosity are found mainly in the high-renin patients (Fig. 5.24).

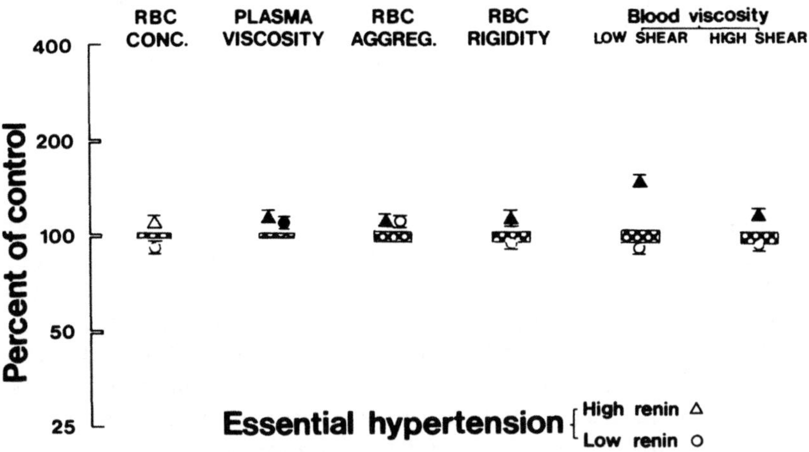

Figure 5.24. Hemorheological data in 8 patients with low-renin hypertension and 24 patients with high-renin hypertension. See Fig. 5.16 for explanation. From (87).

An interesting finding is the significant correlation between η_B and left ventricular mass in hypertensive patients [95]. Attempts to correlate the left ventricular mass with various hemodynamic parameters such as arterial pressure,

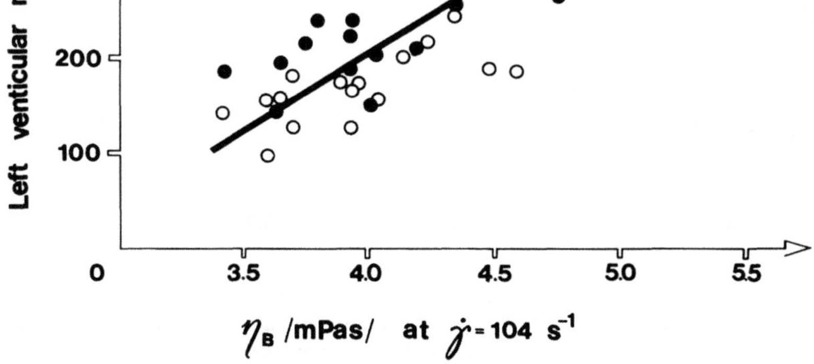

Figure 5.25. Correlation between left ventricular mass and blood viscosity (η_B) at a shear rate of 104 s^{-1} in 24 hypertensive patients (dots) and 13 normotensive subjects (open circles). The coefficient of correlation is 0.80. From (96).

cardiac output, cardiac work, tension time index, etc. have yielded coefficients of correlation less than 0.6. Blood viscosity is the only parameter that shows a coefficient of correlation of 0.8 (Fig. 5.25). These results suggest the possibility that blood viscosity may constitute a signal or initiating factor for ventricular hypertrophy in hypertension.

Low flow states
In acutely ill surgical patients [97] blood viscosity is often found to be reduced, mainly as a result of hemodilution due to transcapillary fluid influx and fluid therapy. The blood viscosity measured in vitro has been correlated with the flow resistances determined in vivo in systemic circulation and pulmonary circulation to calculate the vascular hindrances. Most of the septic patients show a decrease in systemic vascular hindrance, indicating the occurrence of vasodilation. On the other hand, most of the non-septic patients (mainly those suffering from trauma and hemorrhage) have an increase in vascular hindrance, which reflects vasoconstriction. The pulmonary vascular hindrance increases in both septic and non-septic patients.

Low flow states lead to an increase in blood viscosity at a given hematocrit (Fig. 5.2). Under these conditions O_2 delivery is better maintained at lower hematocrit levels (Fig. 5.10b). This has been verified by investigations on the effects of hematocrit variations in dogs subjected to hemorrhagic hypotension at

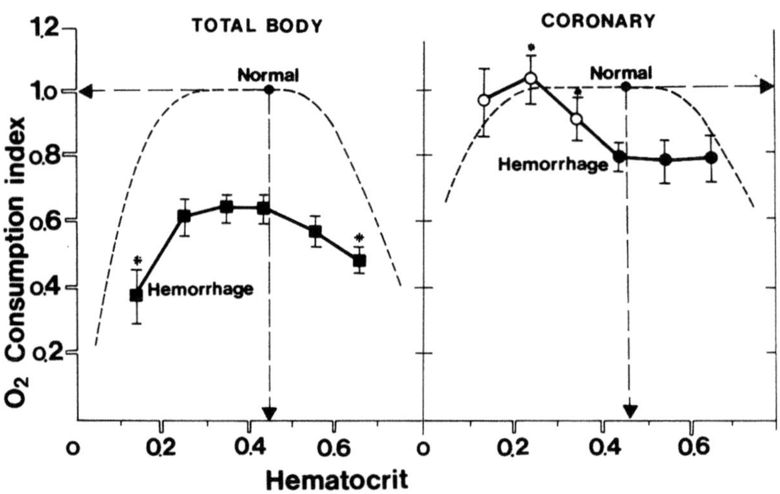

Figure 5.26. Effects of hematocrit (Hct) variations on O_2 consumption in total body (left) and in coronary (right) circulations of the dog under normal conditions (dashed lines) and following hemorrhage to mean arterial pressure = 50 mmHg (solid lines). O_2 consumption index = experimental value/value obtained at 0.45 Hct under normal conditions. Vertical bars represent S.E.M. Filled symbols indicate indices significantly different from 1.0 ($p < 0.05$). Asterisks denote significant difference from posthemorrhage value at Hct = 0.43. From (50).

Table 5.1. Effects of leukoctye adhesion on vascular hindrance in an arteriole in the cat mesentery [a]

	Control	Posthemorrhage
Measured parameters		
ΔP (mmHg)	5.3	0.81
V_{rbc} (mm/sec)	36.0	3.2
D (μm)	42.0	42.0
Hct (%)	9.5	9.5
No. WBCs adhered	0	100
Calculated parameters		
$\Delta P/L$ (dyn/cm^3)	43.6×10^3	6.6×10^3
Q (cm/sec)	32.1×10^{-6}	2.77×10^{-6}
R/L (dyn-cm^{-6}-sec^{-1})	1.39×10^9	2.40×10^9
η_a (cP)	1.06	1.06 [b]
D_{eff} (μm)	42.0	36.7

[a] L = 1.62 mm.
[b] Assumed.

an arterial pressure of 50 mmHg [50]. The range of optimum hematocrit for myocardial O_2 transport and consumption changed from 0.20–0.60 in the control state to 0.20–0.25 in the low flow state (Fig. 5.26). The reduction in Hct due to transcapillary fluid influx in acutely ill surgical patients suffering from low flow states illustrates yet another example of the control of Hct near the optimum level.

In the presence of WBC adhesion to vascular endothelium, e.g., in a microvascular preparation subjected to significant surgical trauma, the apparent viscosity (η_a) in the microvasculature calculated from Equation 1 by using the vessel diameter without taking into account the localized lumen narrowing due to WBC adhesion, is considerably higher than that obtained in the absence of WBC adhesion (Fig. 5.27). This apparent elevation of η_a actually reflects an increase in resistance due to a reduction of the luminal diameter by the adhered WBC, as illustrated by the data shown in Table 5.1 for a 42 μm mesenteric arteriole with two micropipettes inserted over a distance of 1.62 mm. In the control period before hemorrhage, there were no adhered WBCs; after hemorrhage 100 WBCs were found to adhere to the endothelium over this 1.62 mm length of arteriole. The Δp and V_{rbc} decreased after hemorrhage, but the luminal diameter (D, measured between the endothelial surfaces, ignoring the presence of adhered WBCs) and the intravascular hematocrit remained unchanged in this arteriole. If the values of D, $\Delta p/L$ and V_rbc obtained after hemorrhage were substituted into Equation 9, the η_a value would have been found to be nearly doubled, as in the curve with WBC adhesion shown in Fig. 5.27. Since the microvessel hematocrit remained unchanged and the wall shear rate in this vessel was still on the order of 500 s^{-1}, it is reasonable to assume that η_a actually did not change and that the increase in flow resistance ($R = \Delta p/Q$) was instead due to the effective narrow-

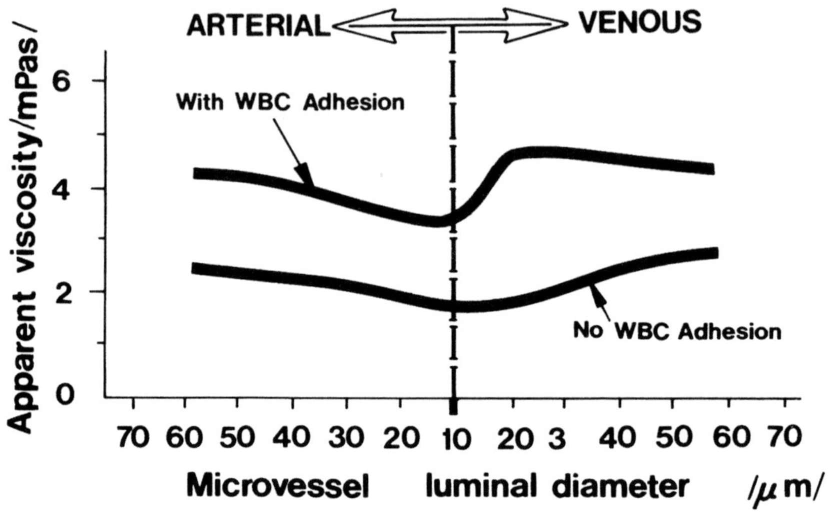

Figure 5.27. Arteriovenous distribution of apparent viscosity as a function of microvessel diameter with and without white blood cell adhesion to vascular endothelium. From (58).

ing of the lumen due to the adhered WBCs. The effective luminal diameter (D_{eff}) in the presence of WBC adhesion can be calculated from the post-hemorrhage and control data, with the assumption that the post-hemorrhage η_a remained at the control level:

$$D_{eff} = \left[\frac{Q}{Q_c} \frac{\Delta P_c}{\Delta P} \right]^{1/4} D_c \tag{18}$$

where the subscript c refers to control values. The D_{eff} was found to be 36.7 μm (Table 5.1), which is 5.3 μm smaller than the value of 42.0 μm for D (luminal diameter measured between endothelial surfaces, ignoring the adhered WBCs). Since the WBCs have a diameter of 7 μm and the number of adhered WBCs was approximately one per 16 μm vessel length, this effective narrowing of the luminal diameter by 5.3 μm is not an unreasonable estimate of the hemodynamic influence of the adhered WBCs in this case. From these considerations, the increase in flow resistance following WBC adhesion should be viewed as the result of an increase in vascular hindrance (due to vessel narrowing) rather than an elevation in apparent viscosity.

5.2.3. Compensatory adjustments to pathological alteration in blood rheology

Compensatory changes in hematocrit. When the increase in whole blood viscosity is due to an increase in plasma viscosity (e.g. multiple myeloma), red cell aggregation (e.g., Waldenström macroglobulinemia), red cell rigidity (e.g. sickle cell disease), or white cell concentration (e.g. leukemias), there is a decrease in hematocrit which serves to minimize the increase in blood viscosity. The low hematocrit level observed in these conditions is actually the optimum value for oxygen delivery under the abnormal rheological states (Fig. 5.10), and this may be viewed as a compensatory process in minimizing the curtailment of oxygen delivery caused by the hyperviscosity. Another important factor to be considered is the compensatory vasodilation of the normal vasculature in hematological disorders which can counteract the increase in blood viscosity and minimize the decrease in oxygen delivery (Equation 15).

Following hemorrhage, because of the vasoconstriction and the elevation in blood viscosity due to low shear, O_2 delivery is better maintained at lower hematocrit levels (Fig. 5.10). It is interesting that the post-hemorrhage transcapillary influx of fluid does cause a reduction of hematocrit [98].

Co-existence of vascular and rheological abnormalities. Compensatory vasodilation is an important factor in maintaining oxygen delivery when there are rheological abnormalities due to hematological or flow abnormalities. When the primary disturbance is in the vascular system, however, vascular hindrance is high and the vasculature may lose its ability to undergo compensatory vasodilation. Under these circumstances, any increase in blood viscosity would amplify the detrimental effect of the increased vascular hindrance in reducing blood flow and oxygen delivery. Therefore, the slight degree of hemorheological abnormalities in vascular diseases may have a much greater pathophysiological importance than the large changes seen in hematological disorders.

5.3. Summary and conclusions

The above discussions indicate that the rheological behavior of blood can affect flow resistance, oxygen transport and transcapillary fluid transfer. Changes in blood rheology and cardiovascular functions can compensate for each other.

Alterations in blood rheology assume greater pathophysiological significance when there are cardiovascular disorders, because of the mutual exacerbation rather than compensation. Additional work is needed to further elucidate the pathophysiological roles of rheological abnormalities in cardiovascular and hematological diseases. It is especially important to determine the in vivo hemodynamic and metabolic functions together with the rheological behavior of blood, so that the role of blood rheology can be properly interpreted in the context of the overall circulatory performance.

Clinical hemorheology is an interdisciplinary field, involving the application of knowledge derived from many disciplines of basic sciences to the understanding of the pathophysiological role and therapeutic implications of blood rheology in

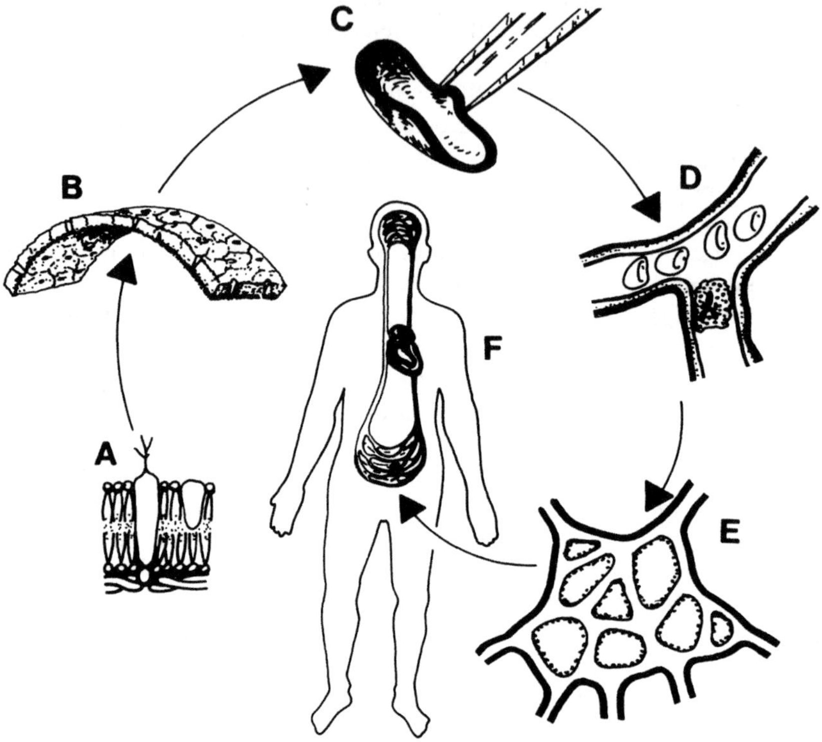

Figure 5.28. Schematic drawing showing the different levels of interdisciplinary investigations from molecular (A) and membrane (B) levels to single cells (C), microvessels (D), microcirculatory network (E) and organ circulation (F), aimed at the application of knowledge derived from many disciplines of basic sciences to the understanding of the role of blood rheology in clinical disorders. From (58).

clinical disorders (Fig. 5.28). Further advances in research on the role of hemorheology in clinical fields require an interdisciplinary approach combining efforts by basic scientists and clinical investigators.

References

1. Lamport H. 1955: Hemodynamics. In: Textbook of Physiology (17th ed.), edited by J.F. Fulton. Philadelphia, PA: Saunder, 595-599.
2. Chien S. 1975: Biophysical behavior of red cells in suspensions. In: The Red Blood Cell, 2nd edition, edited by D. MacN. Surgenor, Academic Press, N.Y., Vol. 2, pp. 1031-1133.
3. Lipowsky H.H., Kovalchek S., Zweifach B.W. 1978: The distribution of blood rheological parameters in the microcirculation of cat mesentery. Circ. Res. 43, 738-749.
4. Burton A.C. 1972: Physiology and Biophysics of the Circulation. Year Book, Chicago.
5. Schmid-Schönbein H. 1976: Microrheology of erythrocytes, blood viscosity, and the distribution of blood in the microcirculation. In: "Cardiovascular Physiology II", Vol. 9 (A.C. Guyton, A.W. Cowley, eds.), pp. 1-62. University Park Press, Baltimore.

6. Caro C.G., Pedley T.J., Schroter R.C. and Seed W.A. 1978: The Mechanics of the Circulation. Oxford Univ. Press, Oxford.
7. Benis A.M., Usami S., Chien S. 1972: Evaluation of viscous and inertial pressure losses in isolated tissue with a simple mathematical model. Microvasc. Res. 4, 81-93.
8. Fung Y.C. 1981: Biomechanics, mechanical properties of living tissues. Springer, New York.
9. Lichtman M.A. 1973: Rheology of leukocytes, leukocyte suspensions and blood in leukemia. J. Clin. Invest. 52, 350-358.
10. Chien S., Schmalzer E.A., Lee M.M.L., Impelluso T., Skalak R. 1983: Role of white blood cells in filtration of blood cell suspensions. Biorheology 20, 11-27.
11. Braide M., Amundson B., Chien S., Bagge U. 1984: Quantitative studies on the influence of leukocytes on the vascular resistance in a skeletal muscle preparation. Microvasc. Res. 27, 331-352, 1984.
12. Engler R.L., Schmid-Schönbein G.W., Pavelec R.S. 1983: Leukocyte capillary plugging in myocardial ischemia and reperfusion in the dog. Am. J. Pathol. 111, 98-111.
13. Harkness J. 1971: The viscosity of human blood plasma; its measurement in health and disease. Biorheology 8, 171-193.
14. Chien S., Usami S., Taylor H.M., Lundberg J.L., Gregersen M.I. 1966: Effects of hematocrit and plasma proteins on human blood rheology at low shear rates. J. Appl. Physiol. 21, 81-87.
15. Goldsmith H.L., Marlow J. 1972: Flow behavior of erythrocytes. I. Rotation and deformation in dilute suspensions. Proc. Soc. Lond. (Biol) 182, 351-384.
16. Fischer T.M., Stoehr-Liesen M., Schmid-Schönbein H. 1978: The red cell as a fluid droplet, tank tread-like motion of the human erythrocyte membrane in shear flow. Science 202, 894-896.
17. Goldsmith H.L., Marlow J.C. 1979: Flow behavior of erythrocytes. II. Particle motions in concentrated suspensions of ghost cells. J. Collloid Interface Sci. 71, 383-407.
18. Schultz D.L. 1972: Pressure and flow in large arteries. In Cardiovascular Fluid Mechanics (ed. D.H. Bergel), Vol. I, pp. 287-312.
19. Chien S., Usami S., Skalak R. 1984: Blood flow in small tubes. In: Handbook of Physiology, Circulation. Section on Microcirculation, edited by E.M. Renkin and C. Michel, Am. Physiol Soc., Bethesda, MD, Vol. I, pp. 217-249.
20. Fahraeus R. 1929: The suspension stability of blood. Physiol. Rev. 9, 241-274.
21. Cokelet G.R. 1976: Blood rheology interpreted through the flow properties of the red cell. In: Microcirculation (ed. J. Grayson and W. Zingg). New York: Plenum, Vol. I, pp. 9-32.
22. Lipowsky H.H., Usami S., Chien S. 1980: In vivo measurements of "apparent viscosity" and microvessel hematocrit in the mesentery of the cat. Microvasc. Res. 19, 297-319.
23. Klitzman B., Johnson P.C. 1982: Capillary network geometry and red cell distribution in the hamster cremaster muscle. Am. J. Physiol. 242, H211-H219.
24. Sarelius I.H., Duling B.R. 1982: Direct measurement of microvessel hematocrit, red cell flux, velocity and transit time. Am. J. Physiol. 243, H1018-H1026.
25. Gaehtgens P. 1980: Flow of blood through narrow capillaries: Rheological mechanism determining capillary hematocrit and apparent viscosity. Biorheology 17, 183-189.
26. Lipowsky H.H., Usami S., Chien S. 1982: Human SS red cell rheological behavior in the microcirculation of cremaster muscle. Blood Cells 8, 113-126.
27. Miller M.E., Myers K.A. 1975: Cellular deformability of the human peripheral blood polymorphonuclear leukocyte: method of study, normal variation and effects of physical and chemical alterations. Res. J. Reticuloendothel. Soc. 18, 337-345.
28. Schmid-Schönbein G.W., Sung K.L.P., Tözeren H., Skalak R., Chien S. 1981: Passive mechanical properties of human leukocytes. Biophys. J. 36, 243-256.
29. Chien S., Schmid-Schönbein G.W., Sung K.L.P., Schmalzer E.A., Skalak R. 1984: Viscoelastic properties of leukocytes. In: White Cell Mechanics: Basic Science and Clinical Aspects (eds. H.J. Meiselman, M.A. Lichtman, P.L. LaCelle), Alan R. Liss, New York. pp. 19-51.
30. Evans E.A., Kukan B. 1984: Passive material behavior of granulocytes based on large deformation and recovery after deformation tests. Blood 64, 1028-1035.

31. Lichtman M.A. 1984: The relationship of excessive white cell accumulation to vascular insufficiency in patients with leukemia. In: White cell mechanics: Basic science and clinical aspects. Alan R. Liss, New York, pp. 295-306.
32. Chien S. 1969: Blood rheology and its relation to flow resistance and transcapillary exchange, with special reference to shock. Advances in Microcirculation 2, 89-103.
33. House S.D., Johnson P.C. 1986: Diameter and blood flow of skeletal muscle venules during local flow regulation. Am. J. Physiol., in press.
34. Intaglietta M., Pawula R.F., Tompkins W.R. 1970: Pressure measurements in the mammalian microvasculature. Microvasc. Res. 2, 212-220.
35. Wiederhielm C.A., Woodbury J.W., Kirk S., Rushmer R.F. 1967: Pulsatile pressures in the microcirculation of the frog's mesentery. Am. J. Physiol. 23, 684-696.
36. Intaglietta M., Tompkins W.R. 1973: Microvascular measurements by video image shearing and splitting. Microvasc. Res. 5, 309-312.
37. Wayland H., Johnson P.C. 1967: Erythrocyte velocity measurement in microvessels by a two-slit method. J. Appl. Physiol. 22, 333-337.
38. Tompkins W.R., Monti R., Intaglietta M. 1974: Velocity measurements of self-tracking correlator. Rev. Sci. Inst. 45, 647-649.
39. Baker M., Wayland H. 1974: On-line volumetric flow rate and velocity profile measurement of blood in microvessels. Microvasc. Res. 7, 131-143.
40. Whittaker S.R.F., Winton F.R. 1933: The apparent viscosity of blood flowing in the isolated hindlimb of the dog and its variation with corpuscular concentration. J. Physiol. London 78, 339-369.
41. Levy M.N., Share L.S. 1953: The influence of erythrocyte concentration upon the pressure-flow relationships in the dog's hind limb. Circ. Res. 1, 247-255.
42. Benis A.M., Usami S., Chien S. 1970: Effect of hematocrit and inertial losses on pressure-flow relations in the isolated hindpaw of the dog. Circ. Res. 27, 1047-1068.
43. Djojosugito A.M., Folkow B., Öberg B., White S. 1970: A comparison of blood viscosity measured in vitro and in a vascular bed. Acta Physiol. Scand. 78, 70-84.
44. Fåhraeus R., Lindqvist T. 1931: The viscosity of the blood in narrow capillary tubes. Am. J. Physiol. 96, 562-568.
45. Barbee J.H., Cokelet G.R. 1971: The Fåhraeus effect. Microvasc. Res. 3, 6-16.
46. McDonald K.M. 1974: Effect of hematocrit and colloid induced changes in blood viscosity on renal hemodynamics and renin release in dogs. Circ. Res. 34, 112-122.
47. Fan F.-C., Schuessler G.B., Chen R.Y.Z., Chien S. 1980: Effect of hematocrit alteration on the regional hemodynamics and oxygen transport. Am. J. Physiol. 238, H545-H552.
48. Lipowsky H.H., Rofe S., Tannenbaum L., Firrell J.C., Usami S., Chien S. 1981: Microvessel hematocrit distributions at bifurcations. Microvasc. Res. 21, 249-250.
49. Jan K.M., Chien S. 1977: Effect of hematocrit variations on coronary hemodynamics and oxygen utilization. Am. J. Physiol. 233, H106-H113.
50. Jan K.-M., Heldman J., Chien S. 1980: Coronary hemodynamics and oxygen utilization after hematocrit variations in hemorrhage. Am. J. Physiol. 239, H326-H332.
51. Gaehtgens P., Kreutz F., Albrecht K.H. 1979: Optimal hematocrit for canine skeletal muscle during rhythmic isotonic exercise. Eur. J. Appl. Physiol. 41, 27-39.
52. Antonini E., Wyman J., Moretti R., Rossi-Fanelli A. 1963: The interaction of bromthymol blue with hemoglobin and its effect on the oxygen equilibrium. Biochem. Biophys. Acta 71, 124-138.
53. Benesch R., Benesch R.E., Yu C.I. 1968: Reciprocal binding of oxygen and diphosphoglycerate by human hemoglobin. Proc. Nat. Acad. Sci. 59, 526-532.
54. Sirs J.A. 1968: Hemorheological aspects of the respiratory function of erythrocytes. In: Hemorheology (ed. A.L. Copley), pp. 505-514. Pergamon, Oxford.
55. Zander R., Schmid-Schönbein H. 1972: Red cell rheology and oxygen transport. In: Hemodilution, Theoretical Basis and Clinical Application (ed. K. Messmer, H. Schmid-Schönbein), Karger, Basel, pp. 48-53.

56. Messmer K. 1981: Compensatory mechanism for acute dilutional anemia. Bibl. Haematologica 47, 31-42.
57. Wade J.P. 1983: Transport of oxygen to the brain in patients with elevated haematocrit values before and after venesection. Brain 106, 513-23.
58. Chien S. 1985: Role of blood cells in microcirculatory regulation. Microvasc. Res. 29, 129-151.
59. Schmid-Schönbein G.W., Usami S., Skalak R., Chien S. 1980: Cell distribution in capillary networks. Microvasc. Res. 19, 18-44.
60. Gaehtgens P. 1980: Flow of blood through narrow capillaries: Rheological mechanisms determining capillary hematocrit and apparent viscosity. Biorheology 17, 183-189.
61. Yen R.T., Fung Y.C. 1978: Effect of velocity distribution and red cell distribution in capillary blood vessels. Am. J. Physiol. 235, H251-H257.
62. Fung Y.C. 1973: Stochastic flow in capillary blood vessels. Microvasc. Res. 5, 34-48.
63. Lipowsky H.H., Rofe S., Tannenbaum L., Fiurrell J.C., Usami S., Chien S. 1981: Microvessel hematocrit distributions at bifurcations. Microvas. Res. 21, 249-250.
64. Zweifach B.W., Grant L., McCluskey R.T. 1973: The Inflammatory Process. Academic Press, New York, 2nd ed.
65. Williams T.J., Jose P.J., Forest M.J., Wedmore C.V., Clough G.F. 1984: Interactions between neutrophils and microvascular endothelial cells leading to cell emigration and plasma protein leakage. In White Cell Mechanics: Basic Science and Clinical Aspects (ed. H.J. Meiselman, M.A. Lichtman, P.L. LaCelle). Alan R. Liss, New York, pp. 195-208.
66. Schmid-Schönbein G.W., Usami S., Skalak R., Chien S. 1980: The interaction of leukocytes and erythrocytes in capillary and postcapillary vessels. Microvasc. Res. 19, 45-70.
67. Bagge U., Karlsson R. 1980: Maintenance of white blood cell margination at the passage through small venular junctions. Microvasc. Res. 20, 92-95.
68. Goldsmith H.L., Spain S. 1984: Margination of leukocytes in blood flow through small tubes. Microvasc. Res. 27, 204-222.
69. Nobis U., Fries A.R., Gaehtgens P. 1982: Rheological mechanisms contributing to WBC-margination. In White Blood Cells: Morphology and Rheology as Related to Function (ed. U. Bagge, G.V.R. Born, P. Gaehtgens). Nijhoff, The Hague, pp. 57-65.
70. Lipowsky H.H. 1982: Determinants of microvascular blood flow. The Physiologist 25, 357-363.
71. Selkurt E.E., Scibetta M.P., Cull T.E. 1958: Hemodynamics of intestinal circulation. Circ. Res. 6, 92-99.
72. Weber P.M., Pollycove M., Bacaner M.B., Lawrence J.H. 1969: Cardiac output in polycythemia vera. J. Lab. Clin. Med. 73, 753-762.
73. Jan K.-M., Chien S. 1973: Role of surface electric charge in red blood cell interactions. J. Gen. Physiol. 61, 638-654.
74. Chien S. 1980: Aggregation of red blood cells: An electrochemical, colloid chemical problem. In Bioelectrochemistry: Ions, Surfaces and Membranes. Adv. in Chemistry Series, Am. Chem. Soc., Washington, D.C., pp. 1-32.
75. Chien S., Cooper G.W., Jr., Jan K.-M., Miller L.H., Howe C., Usami S., Lalezari P. 1974: N-acetylneuraminic acid deficiency in erythrocyte membranes: biophysical and biochemical correlates. Blood 43, 445-460.
76. Chien S., Usami W., Bertles J.F. 1970: Abnormal rheology of oxygenated blood in sickle cell anemia. J. Clin. Invest. 49, 623-634.
77. Evans E., Mohandas N., Leung A. 1984: Static and dynamic rigidities of normal and sickle erythrocytes: major influence of cell hemoglobin concentration. J. Clin. Invest. 73, 477-488.
78. Nash G.B., Johnson C.S., Meiselman H.J. 1984: Mechanical properties of oxygenated red blood cells in sickle cell (HbSS) disease. Blood 63, 73-82.
79. Stuart J. 1984: Sickle-cell disease and vascular occlusion - rheological aspects. Clin. Hemorheol. 4, 193-207.
80. Usami S., Chien S., Scholz P.M., Bertles J.F. 1975: Effect of deoxygenation on blood rheology in sickle cell disease. Microvasc. Res. 9, 324-334.

81. Chien S. 1977: Rheology of sickle cells and erythrocyte content. Blood Cells 3, 283-296.
82. Usami S., Chien S., Bertles J.F. 1975: Deformability of sickle cells as studied by microsieving. J. Lab. Clin. Med. 86, 274-279.
83. LaCelle P.L. 1977: Oxygen delivery to muscle cells during capillary vascular occlusion by sickle erythrocytes. Blood Cells 3, 273-281.
84. Klug P.P., Lessin L.S. 1977: Microvascular blood flow of sickled erythrocytes: a dynamic morphological study. Blood Cells 3, 263-272.
85. Kaul D.K., Fabry M.E., Windisch P., Baez S., Nagel R.L. 1983: Erythrocytes in sickle cell anemia are heterogeneous in their rheological and hemodynamic characteristics. J. Clin. Invest. 72, 22-31.
86. Chien S. 1981: Hemorheology in disease, pathophysiological significance and therapeutic implications. Clin. Hemorheol. 1, 419-442.
87. Chien S., Lipowsky H.H. 1984: Capillary circulation in sickle cell anemia. Intern. J. Microcirc. Clin. Exp. 3, 493.
88. Jan K.M., Chien S., Bigger J.T., Jr. 1975: Observations on blood viscosity changes after acute myocardial infarction. Circulation 51, 1079-1084.
89. Dintenfass L. 1976: Rheology of blood in diagnostic and preventive medicine: an introduction to clinical hemorheology. Butterworths, London.
90. Di Perri T., Forconi S., Guerrini M., Rossi C., Pieragalli D. 1979: Blood viscosity in the different stages of ischaemic heart disease. In: Angina Pectoris and Myocardial Infarction, International Congress Series no. 491, Excerpta Medica, Amsterdam-Oxford-Princeton, pp. 348-353.
91. Lowe G.D.O., Barbenel J.C., Forbes C.D. (Ed.) 1981: Clinical Aspects of Blood Viscosity and Cell Deformability. Springer Verlag, New York.
92. Dormandy J., Boyd M., Ernst E. 1981: Red cell filterability after myocardial infarction. Scand. J. Clin. Lab. Invest. 156, Suppl. 41, 195-198.
93. Chrysant S.G., Frohlich E.D., Adamopoulos P.N., Stein P.D., Whitcomb W.H., Allen E.W., Neeler J. 1976: Pathophysiologic significance of stress or relative polycythemia in essential hypertension. Am. J. Cardiol. 37, 1069-1972.
94. Letcher R.L., Chien S., Pickering T.G., Sealey J.E., Laragh J.H. 1981: Direct relationship between blood pressure and blood viscosity in normal and hypertensive subjects: Role of fibrinogen concentration. Am. J. Med. 70, 1195-1202.
95. Devereaux R.B., Drayer J.I.M., Chien S., Pickering T.G., Letcher R.L., DeYoung J.L., Sealey J.E., Laragh J.H. 1984: Whole blood viscosity as a determinant of cardiac hypertrophy in systemic hypertension. Am. J. Cardiol. 54, 592-595.
96. Dintenfass L. 1981: Hyperviscosity in Hypertension. Pergamon Press, New York.
97. Scholz P.M., Karis J.H., Gump F.E., Kinney J.M., Chien S. 1975: Correlation of blood rheology with vascular resistance in critically ill patients. J. Appl. Physiol. 39, 1008-1011.
98. Chien S. 1967: Role of the sympathetic nervous system in hemorrhage. Physiol. Rev. 47, 214-288.

6
Cardiovascular diseases

John A. Dormandy
St. James' and St. George's Hospitals, Sarsfeld Road, London SW12, United Kingdom

6.1. Introduction

Looking back over the whole area of cardiovascular diseases during the past three decades, the most striking impression is one of almost total failure to solve the basic problems. The incidence, course or outcome of hypertension, angina, myocardial infarction, cerebrovascular accidents or limb ischemia have remained largely unaltered; despite continuing research effort both in the laboratory and in hospitals. The principal pathological process underlying all these common diseases is atherosclerosis; and although a number of primary risk factors for atherosclerosis have been recognized and attempts made to treat or abolish some of them, atherosclerosis and diseases of the cardiovascular system remain the foremost killers. This is perhaps not altogether surprising as the mechanism of action of most of these risk factors, for instance smoking and heredity, remain speculative.

The laboratory and clinical evidence amassed on cardiovascular diseases has been concerned with histological studies of the vessel wall, biochemistry of the blood and to a lesser degree of the vessel, investigation of clotting factors and studies of platelets and prostaglandins. Most of these investigations were carried out under static conditions and rarely was any effort made to simulate the flow conditions of blood under which atherosclerosis in fact develops. It is only in the last decade that flow properties of blood and the effects of blood flow on the individual constituents of blood and the vessel wall have begun to be studied seriously. The results are detailed in the earlier sections of this book, where the various laboratory techniques available for assessing the rheological properties of blood are described. In this chapter the application and relevance of the results of these techniques to cardiovascular diseases are considered. Whilst the rheological approach will not solve all the problems of cardiovascular pathology, it will certainly increase our understanding of it.

In 1877 Robert Koch formulated his criteria for linking particular bacteria to particular diseases. Similarly, criteria can be postulated for linking an abnormal laboratory finding to the pathophysiology of a particular disease of the circulation. A possible set of such criteria for meaningfully linking a hemorheological abnormality to a circulatory disease would be the following:

1. The hemorheological abnormality should be shown to be a primary risk factor in the development of the disease.
2. The hemorheological abnormality should be more common in the patients suffering from that disease than in the normal population.
3. The magnitude of the hemorheological abnormality should be related to the severity of the disease, its prognosis and the possible development of complications.
4. Normalizing the hemorheological abnormality should improve the clinical state of the patient.

Whilst these criteria are clearly fulfilled in some clinical states like polycythemia, in many of the common cardiovascular conditions only partial evidence is so far available to answer some of these criteria. It is this evidence that will be presented in this chapter.

The interdependence of whole blood viscosity, plasma viscosity, plasma proteins, red cell concentration, red cell and white cell rheology, red cell aggregability and the prevailing shear stress has been considered in earlier chapters. Such a galactic view of hemorheological determinants is illustrated in Fig. 6.1. Therefore

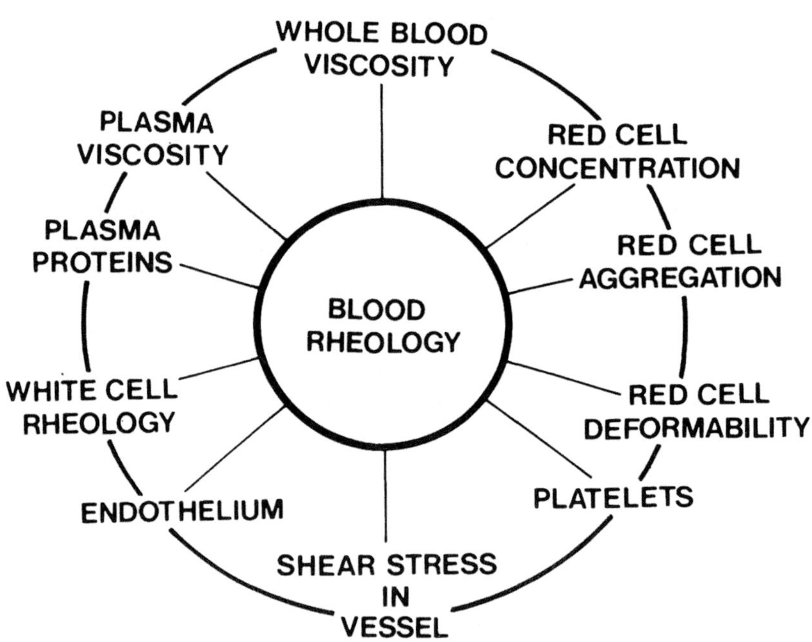

Figure 6.1. Diagramatic representation of the interdependance of a larger number of hemorheological determinants.

the evidence linking hemorheological abnormalities to cardiovascular diseases should be evaluated not only in terms of studies where blood viscosity or blood cell rheology were measured directly, but also in studies where other primary determinants of hemorheology were measured. The general principles and the various modalities of hemorheologically based treatment are considered in detail in Chapter 12 and here only the evidence directly bearing on cardiovascular diseases will be considered. These diseases will be discussed under the headings of myocardial ischemia, hypertension, cerebral ischemia, ischemia of the legs and Raynaud's phenomenon.

6.2. Myocardial ischemia

6.2.1. Epidemiological evidence

Unfortunately direct clinical measurement of blood viscosity has only become possible in the last 20 years. Over this period it has been shown repeatedly that by far the most important determinant of whole blood viscosity is the red cell concentration. It is equally generally accepted that after the hematocrit the plasma fibrinogen concentration is the most significant determinant of whole blood viscosity. There is virtually no doubt left that an increase in red cell or plasma fibrinogen concentration must be associated with an increase in whole blood viscosity, except possibly in some cases where there is a compensatory change in some other factor affecting whole blood viscosity, such as red cell deformability. It is therefore reasonable to consider long term epidemiological studies where the red cell or plasma fibrinogen concentrations have been measured even though the whole blood viscosity was not determined directly.

The original Framingham Study published in 1970 did not demonstrate a relationship between initial hematocrit and subsequent coronary heart disease [1]. The Stockholm Study of risk factors for myocardial infarction showed that in subjects aged under 60, those with a hemoglobin in the top quintile had twice the incidence of new coronary events compared with the remaining 80% [2]. More recently in the Puerto Rico Study of 8700 men followed for eight years clinical evidence of myocardial ischemia was more than double in the high hematocrit (over 0.49) than the low hematocrit group (under 0.42) [3]. A similar result was found in a study of 8000 Japanese men followed for 10 years [4]. A sixfold increase in mortality was also recorded by Burge in patients with a hematocrit of over 0.50 [4]. However, these results have not so far been confirmed in the more recent, and therefore shorter, Northwick Park Study [6]. The Stockholm Study also showed that the erythrocyte sedimentation rate (ESR) was a good prognostic indicator of future myocardial ischemic disease. The raised ESR was most probably due to an increased red cell aggregability associated with a raised plasma fibrinogen. A plasma fibrinogen over 4 g/l was also shown to increase the

Table 6.1. Clinical evidence that a high red cell concentration may be a primary risk factor in cardiovascular diseases.

	Threshold point red cell concentration	Ratio of incidence
Increased risk of cerebrovascular accident		
– Framingham Study (9), for men and women	15g% and 14g%	2:1
– Lowe *et al.* (61)	Hct 50%	2:1
– Tohgi *et al.* (10)	Hct 51%	3:1
Increased risk of myocardial ischemia		
– Burch *et al.* 1962 (12)	Hct 50%	
– Stockholm study (2)	Top quintile	2:1
– Puerto Rico study (3)	42% vs 49%	2:1
– Honolulu study (11)	Top quintile	2:1
Increased risk of hypertension		
– Framingham study (9), for men and women:	16g% and 15g%	2:1
Overall mortality		
– Burge *et al.* (5)	Hct 50%	6:1

risk of cardiac disease in a group of diabetics [7]. The Northwick Park Study also showed that a high fibrinogen level was a greater risk for cardiovascular death than a high cholesterol [6]. Finally, in a $13\frac{1}{2}$ years follow-up of almost 800 men, Wilhelmsen and colleages found that the fibrinogen level was significantly raised in subjects who subsequently developed a myocardial infarction and was a better predictor than smoking [8].

Table 6.1 lists some of the studies relating a high red cell concentration to a risk of serious cardiovascular disease. In most, the threshold point beyond which the red cell concentration becomes a hazard is around 0.50. The ratio of the incidence of cardiovascular complications for hematocrit values above to below this level is approximately two to one. Indeed it would seem that the cardiovascular complication rate in these subjects, with a high normal hematocrit supposedly without disease, is higher than in patients with polycythemia vera receiving standard treatment. Whether these patients represent a separate pathological entity or merely one end of a normal spectrum is largely academic, the fact is that they are much more likely to develop cardiovascular complications and die. On the contrary, most groups believed to have a relatively low risk of cardiovascular disease, such as pre-menopausal women, undernourished, vegetarians and sportsmen, also have a relatively low hematocrit, as well as possibly other favourable hemorheological factors. Some of the resistance to recognizing a high red cell concentration as dangerous and worthy of medical attention, stems from the reluctance to accept that the normal range of any physiological variable is not optimal. This is an evolutionary, philosophical and teleological argument. Biological evolution is very slow and was not designed to cope with the very rapid rate of human evolution. As a consequence, there are a number of so-called diseases of civilization, ranging from atherosclerosis to alcoholism, which evolution has not yet had time to select out. The danger to the cardiovascular system of our ancestors, for millenia, was traumatic hemorrhage, and in the absence of blood transfusions a relativey high initial red cell mass would confer benefit in surviving massive hemorrhage. It is only very recently that the danger to our cardiovascular system has been narrowing of the arteries and ischemia; atherosclerosis being a modern disease in evolutionary terms, whilst hemorrhage is one of the few conditions we have learnt to treat effectively. It is therefore althogether conceivable that the inherited normal range of red cell concentration is no longer optimal for surviving vascular rather than hemorrhagic ischemia. It is surely in the essence of natural biological selection that the average or normal lags behind the optimal. Nature has also provided us with a surplus of virtually all tissues: nephrons, alveoli, plasma clotting factors or endocrine cells. Undoubtedly the red blood cells are also subject to nature's extravagance. Whilst in many cases, as in the case of alveoli or nephrons, a large safety margin is beneficial and carries no risk, this is not true in the case of the plasma fibrinogen or red cell concentration, where a massive accidental loss is now very rare but an excess can be dangerous.

6.2.2. Established myocardial ischemia

All hemorheological factors are abnormal in patients with established myocardial ischemia, as indeed is virtually everything else measureable in blood. The increased level of plasma fibrinogen is the principal cause for the increased plasma viscosity and red cell aggregability. Since Burch first pointed out in 1961 [12] the increased hemoglobin concentration in patients with clinical myocardial ischemia compared to apparently healthy controls, many others have confirmed this finding. Blood cell filterability has also been shown to be abnormal [13,14]. Thus an abnormality in all three primary determinants leads to significant increase in whole blood viscosity at all shear rates; although as usual the differences are most marked at the lowest shear rates [15]. Whether these changes are primary or secondary to the ischemia is still uncertain, but by their effect on the flow properties of the blood they would be expected to increase the ischemia of the myocardium. Changes in the flow properties of the blood would be particularly critical in the presence of coronary artery disease where there is little reserve in terms of reflex vasodilatation and the myocardial perfusion pressure is decreased. Indeed there is evidence that patients with extensive coronary artery disease on angiography also have more pronounced hemorheological abnormalities [16]. Thus myocardial ischemia is associated with pathological flow properties of the blood.

A particularly interesting finding has been the hemorheological defect in patients with so-called "non-coronary angina", that is in patients who have clinical and electrocardiographic evidence of ischemia in the absence of any demonstrable coronary artery or arteriolar defects [17]. Such rheological abnormalities may play a primary role in this subgroup of patients.

Although there have been no longitudinal studies of patients with established myocardial ischemia to assess the importance of hemorheological changes in the precipitation of an acute ischemic episode, patients with unstable angina have significantly more severe abnormalities than patients with stable angina [18]. A deterioration in various hemorheological determinants has also been recorded immediately preceding an acute infarction [13]. The Siena school has described acute changes in whole blood viscosity and blood filterability during attacks of angina, which reversed when nitroglycerine stopped the pain [19,15]. The link between hemorheological abnormalities and arterial thrombosis, considered in detail in Chapter 7, may also be relevant in the precipitation of myocardial infarction.

6.2.3. Changes associated with acute myocardial ischemia

The hemorheological changes which take place at the time of an acute myocardial infarction have been well documented and are illustrated in Fig. 6.2. Once the clinical syndrome of myocardial infarction has begun the principal hemorheological changes are hemoconcentration, increased plasma fibrinogen concentration and decreased blood cell filterability. These changes all tend to cause an increase in blood viscosity, although the time scales are different [20].

There is agreement that plasma fibrinogen rises after myocardial infarction, as it does in a number of chronic and acute illnesses. After infarction there is usually an interval of 1 or 2 days before the fibrinogen level increases, reaching a peak on approximately the fourth day. The α_2-macroglobulins have a weaker effect on plasma viscosity than fibrinogen, but increase similarly following infarction. This again is a nonspecific reaction seen in many pathologic states. It is not unexpected that most workers report a parallel rise in the plasma viscosity [21,22]. It reaches its maximum around day three and thereafter decreases slowly, but has been found to be slightly elevated even 60 days later [23]. Similarly the altered plasma protein pattern will increase red cell aggregation [23,24], which in turn will be responsible for the increase of blood viscosity at low flow rates, which may exist in the marginal tissues around the necrotic area.

Three groups of workers have found a decreased blood filterability after myocardial infarction [20,24,25]. In one study, normal values were found immediately after the onset of pain and the time course of the subsequent changes was described in detail. The lowest values (28% of normal) were found approximately 12 hours after the first symptoms of infarction. After 24 hours, the red

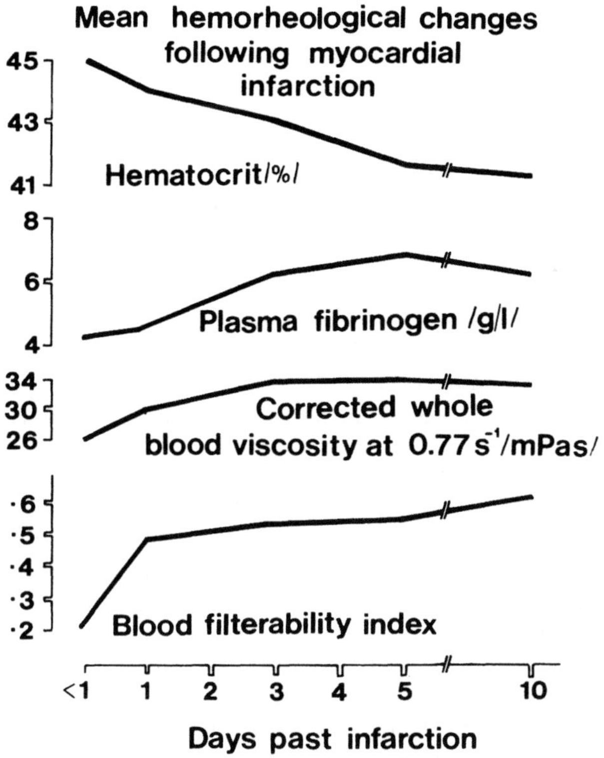

Figure 6.2. Changes in hemorheological determinants associated with an acute myocardial infarction.

cell filterability had returned to near normal values. This temporary but dramatic decrease in red cell filterability was thought to be secondary to changes in the plasma [20]. In the last year or two the emphasis has begun to shift from the red to the white cell as the more important potential cause of microcirculatory ischemia under pathological circumstances. Although the red cells are much more numerous, it is almost invariably a white cell which is seen to obstruct a capillary, causing a train of red cells to pile up behind it. Many of the earlier blood filtration tests believed to be looking at red cell deformability were probably principally influenced by the behavior of the "contaminating" white cells. Recent animal experiments suggest that granulocytes play a crucial role in determining the extent of infarction in the myocardium [26]. Fig. 6.3 shows the results of the first attempt to assess granulocyte rheology specifically in a group of patients following myocardial infarction [27]. The "clogging" produced by a standardized number of granulocytes increased rapidly after a myocardial infarction. This finding of a marked acute qualitative rheological change in white blood cells brings a new emphasis to the association between myocardial ischemia and the

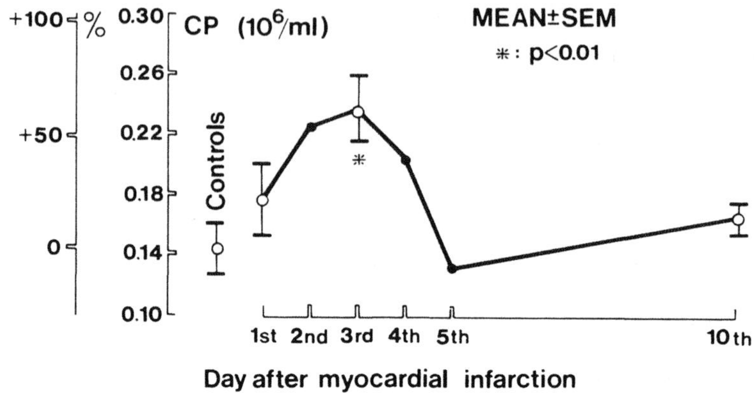

Figure 6.3. Changes in the rheological properties of granulocytes following acute myocardial infarction.

total white cell count. In a preliminary report of the Caerphilly Study, after age, the white cell count showed the closest association with myocardial infarction, much closer for instance than smoking habit [28]. A number of other epidemiological studies had reported such a correlation between white cell count and myocardial ischemia for some years, although the reports had largely remained unnoticed [29,30,31].

The hematocrit is the most important determinant of whole blood viscosity and many studies report a high hematocrit immediately after myocardial infarction. This is followed by a slow decline of the hematocrit during the first week of treatment [20,21,32,33,34]. The presence of an elevated hematocrit and dehydration following infarction has long been recognized and is probably due to fluid restriction and increased perspiration, resulting possibly in a reduction of plasma volume [35]. The subsequent fall in hematocrit can be attributed to the body's autoregulation as well as to the administration of intravenous fluids. The epidemiological evidence that a relatively high hemoglobin concentration, even within the so-called normal range, is a risk factor for myocardial infarction has already been mentioned. Similarly, it is a general clinical impression that myocardial infarction is rare in patients with severe anemia. As the viscosity of whole blood is principally governed by the hematocrit, the measured viscosity is often "corrected" to a standard hematocrit, attempting to eliminate the effects of different hematocrits. However, the problem is more complex: the hematocrit varies physiologically within the vascular bed, and neither the corrected viscosity nor the measured viscosity of blood taken from a peripheral vein can give reliable information about the situation in other parts of the circulation. A new approach has been suggested to partially overcome the problem by expressing measurements as a ratio of hemoglobin level divided by the measured blood viscosity. This ratio would reflect the oxygen delivery to peripheral tissues. Fig. 6.4 illustrates the value of this ratio in some typical diseases.

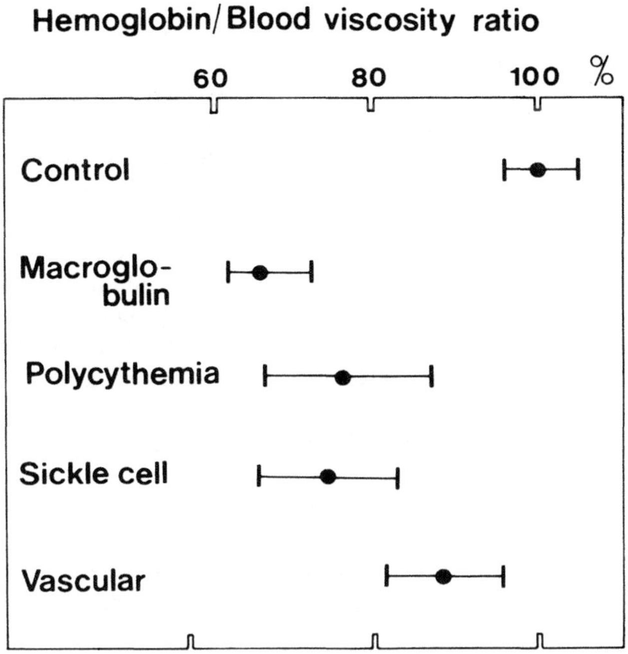

Figure 6.4. The hemoglobin over measured blood viscosity in some diseases, reflecting the oxygen delivering capacity of the blood.

All factors so far considered affect whole blood viscosity. The methodological difficulties already described here and in preceding chapters, plus the fact that different shear rates were used in different studies, make a comparison difficult. Nevertheless, each study on its own gives valid information and leaves no doubt that the blood viscosity rises beyond the normal range as a consequence of myocardial infarction [20,23,21,22,24]. It would seem reasonable to assume that the changes in the flow properties of blood during the evolution of a myocardial infarction may play a role in its pathological and clinical outcome. Chien described a direct correlation between changes in blood viscosity and changes in the resistance of the systemic and pulmonary circulations during the first month after myocardial infarction [36]. Indeed there is clinical evidence that the severity of the earliest changes does relate to subsequent prognosis. Direct evidence comes from studies on experimental animals. After ligation of a coronary artery, the size of the resulting necrosis depended on the viscoity of the blood, which was altered by changing the hematocrit [37].

It could also be demonstrated that the apparent yield shear stress, which reflects the rheological properties of blood near zero flow, was closely correlated to the size of experimentally induced infarction in dogs. Prospective clinical studies are obviously difficult and none have so far been reported. However, there have been many studies correlating the clinical course of the myocardial infarction with the hemorheologic changes observed. The severity of clinical symptoms and occurrence of complications were found to correlate with plasma viscosity, whole blood viscosity [23], and blood filterability [20,24]. In one study the 12 patients out of 25 studied who developed an arrhythmia, shock, or who died had a blood viscosity above 48 mPas at 0.52 s^{-1}. Only two patients above this level did not develop a complication [23]. Patients with a fibrinogen concentration above 4 g/l after myocardial infarction had a higher incidence of serious complications such as death, shock or re-infarction [38]. Similarly, in a study of red cell deformability in 51 patients, the mean filterability index of the 32 patients who did not develop complications was 0.47 (S.D. $\pm$ 0.05) compared to 0.22 ($\pm$0.07) in patients who subsequently developed pulmonary edema, and 0.11 ($\pm$0.04) in those who developed cardiogenic shock [20].

A possible explanation for the apparent predictive value of the hemorheological changes associated with myocardial or any form of ischemia is that these changes are both the consequence and the cause of ischemia. A vicious cycle may be envisaged where the local metabolic and other changes in the ischemic tissues cause a hemorheological deterioration which in turn perpetuates or extends the area of ischemia. Such a vicious cycle may spiral towards recovery or necrosis, a choice that may be a logical point for therapeutic intervention.

6.2.4. Therapeutic implications

Using the analogy with Koch's postulates, the fourth criterion for attaching clinical importance to hemorheology in a particular group of diseases is that improving the rheological properties of blood by various therapeutic maneuvers should be of demonstrable benefit to patients with those diseases. The various therapeutic techniques available are described in Chapter 12, where their theoretical justification and experimental basis are also detailed. Clinically, very few of these techniques have been applied to patients with either acute or chronic myocardial ischemia. There has been one limited study using a defibrinogenating enzyme in patients with unstable angina which appears to have been beneficial [39]. Streptokinase is now widely used in the treatment of acute myocardial infarction with the principal aim of dissolving a recent thrombus. It does also have the additional effect of lowering plasma fibrinogen and therefore blood viscosity very rapidly.

Hemodilution in ischemic heart disease, based on rheological considerations, rather than just part of the ancient but widespread medical practice of venesection, was probably first described by Burch in 1965 [40]. The largest study used low molecular weight dextran infusion immediately after an acute infarct to reduce both the red cell and the fibrinogen concentration. After a ten year period up to 1972 the conclusion of the studies was that there was a significant improvement in both short and long term survival [41]. Nevertheless the current view of the majority of proponents in normovolemic hemodilution is that it is potentially unsafe in patients with diminished myocardial reserve [42]. Plasmapheresis and other rheologically orientated treatments have not been used in acute myocardial infarction.

In the near future the therapeutic implications of the changes described in patients at risk or with overt myocardial ischemia are likely to be in the area of primary and secondary prevention. The evidence already presented suggests that it would be reasonable to treat patients at risk of myocardial ischemia who had a hematocrit or plasma fibrinogen in the upper range of normal with a view to decreasing these concentrations and eliminating what appears to be a significant risk factor. This suggestion has to be seen against the background where the only risk factors whose elimination has reduced the incidence of this disease are smoking and hypertension.

6.3. Hypertension

It is of course possible that any danger of myocardial or cerebral ischemia from a high red cell concentration is in fact due to an indirect effect of the red cell concentration on other cardiovascular risk factors, in particular hypertension. Gaisbock originally described in 1905 an association between hypertension and raised red cell count [43]. By definition, in essential hypertension none of the classical causes for a high blood pressure, such as renal or arterial disease, can be found. The normal heart, when faced with an increased peripheral resistance offered by hyperviscous blood, can only maintain cardiac output by increasing the perfusion pressure. The high blood pressure could be compensating at least in part for the increased blood viscosity. In the 1950's and 1960's there were a number of reports of significantly increased red cell concentration, often due to contracted plasma volume, in patients with essential hypertension [44]. (A decreased circulating volume is the very opposite of what is found in most forms of secondary or malignant hypertension.) The Framingham data show that subjects with an initial hemoglobin over 15 g/l for women and 16 g/l for men subsequently developed a diastolic pressure above 90 mm of mercury approximately twice as often as subjects with a hemoglobin concentration below these levels [9]. Chien and his colleagues have demonstrated a close correlation between arterial blood pressure in hypertensives and raised blood viscosity, due to a combination of elevated red cell and fibrinogen concentrations [45]. Subsequently they showed that the left ventricular mass correlates better with blood viscosity than with arterial pressure, cardiac output or cardiac work [46]. An interesting type of hypertension, where an increased red cell concentration has recently been implicated as a possible causal factor, is the hypertension of pre-eclampsia, where Heilman has shown a fascinating individual correlation between blood pressure and red cell concentration [47].

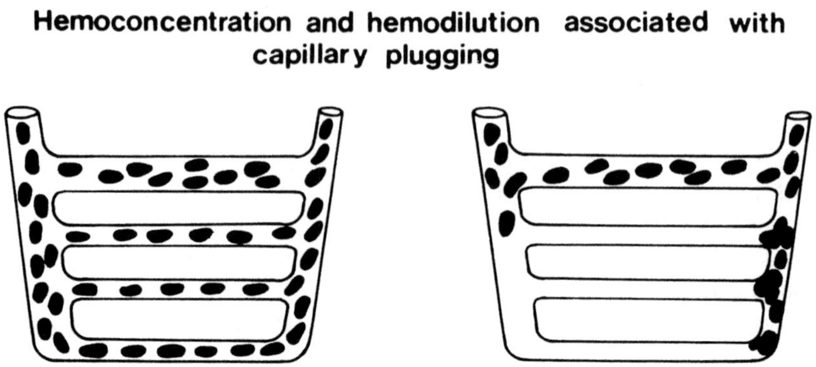

Figure 6.5. Plugging of some capillaries may result in increased plasma trapping and a raised central circulating hematocrit, a possible explanation for the hemoconcentration often seen in ischemic disease and the lowering of the hematocrit associated with relief of the ischemia.

Smoking, a well-known risk factor for hypertension, also increases the red cell mass, without altering the plasma volume, thus increasing the viscosity of the blood. An increase in red cell concentration may not be the only cause of increased peripheral resistance due to hyperviscosity. Chien has shown an increase in plasma viscosity in all patients with essential hypertension, although the hematocrit was only raised in those with a normal or high renin activity [32].

A significant alteration in the filterability of the blood, originally ascribed to decreased red cell deformability, has been described in patients with essential hypertension [48,49] and malignant hypertension [50]. The techniques used in these studies were almost certainly sensitive to white cells and the changes in blood filterability may have been due to an abnormality in white cell rheology. Increased plugging of the microcirculation, albeit temporary, would increase total peripheral resistance and thus predispose to hypertension. Matrai has also put forward the interesting concept, illustrated in Fig. 6.5, which suggests that increased capillary plugging would tend to increase the central hematocrit and blood viscosity. This could also explain the hemoconcentration observed in a number of chronic and acute ischemic states. It is interesting in this context to note that a new serotonin antagonist, which has recently been shown to be an effective antihypertensive agent has also been found to significantly decrease white cell clogging [51].

6.4. Cerebral ischemia

6.4.1. Physiological and epidemiological evidence

On an evolutionary time scale the greatest danger to the blood supply of the brain arose from ischemia due to hemorrhage and the consequent hypotension, or long term severe anemia. Autoregulation of the cerebral circulation, which attempts to protect the brain from both these stresses, may perhaps be inappropriate when the danger is from atherosclerosis, thrombosis and associated hemorheological abnormalities. There is a continuing controversy as to whether the viscosity of blood has a primary direct effect on cerebral blood flow. On the one hand several workers have confirmed the original findings of Gottstein [52] and the Queen Square group [53] that there is an inverse relationship between cerebral blood flow and hematocrit or blood viscosity [14]. The control by viscosity theory has been strengthened by the significantly decreased cerebral blood flow in patients with anemia accompanied by a paraproteinemia, which increased their blood viscosity [54]. The opposite view, that the viscosity of blood has little influence on the cerebral circulation because of the overwhelming autoregulation by oxygen, is supported by the finding of an increased cerebral blood flow despite a high red cell count in patients whose hemoglobin has an abnormally low oxygen releasing capacity [55]. It is also supported by the unchanged cerebral blood flow of patients in whom the blood viscosity was substantially lowered by plasma exchange [56]. A recent study of cerebral blood flow in patients with increased plasma viscosity due to paraproteinemia also suggests that autoregulation maintains normal cerebral blood flow and oxygen transport despite increased blood viscosity [57]. It may be that the oxygen tension and the viscosity of the blood are independent variables.

Epidemiologically, of all the viscosity factors a raised red cell concentration, albeit within the normal range, is the most solidly documented in the pathogenesis of cerebral ischemia. In the study from Framingham over 5,000 subjects free of cerebrovascular diseases at entry were followed for 16 years. The risk of cerebral infarction in both sexes was found to be proportional to the hemoglobin concentration: men with a hemoglobin value over 15 g% and women over 14 g% had twice as many cerebral infarcts as those with lower values [9]. In a retrospective study Tohgi looked back at the records of 432 consecutive autopsies, 76 of whom died of cerebral infarction. He found a very close correlation between the incidence of cerebral infarction as the cause of death and a high hematocrit during life; a remarkable 50% of deaths were due to infarction in patients with a hematocrit above a modest 46% [10]. Finally it is a well recognized clinical fact that even severely anemic patients do not show neurological symptoms [58]. In Wilhelmsen and colleagues' 13½ years follow up of nearly 800 men a raised plasma fibrinogen was a better predictor of subsequent stroke than even hypertension [88]. Although the blood filterability has been shown to be reduced in patients with clinical cerebral ischemia [59,60], so far there have been no longitudinal studies to see if these microrheological abnormalities are related to future progress.

6.4.2. *Role in the evolution of cerebral infarction*

Indirect evidence that the red cell concentration does play some role in cerebral perfusion are the studies showing its effect on the progression of infarction. For instance, Lowe and colleagues published an analysis of possible predictive factors in 320 patients admitted with acute cerebrovascular accidents, approximately half of whom died during that admission. They found that if the red cell concentration was over 0.50 in patients under 75 years of age, the mortality was more than twice that in patients with a red cell concentration below 0.50 [61]. In a clinical study the size of cerebral infarction, measured by computerized axial tomography, has been related to the patient's red cell concentration [62]. In an experimental gerbil model the size of non-perfused area of brain, as mortality, were improved if the red cell concentration was below 0.51 [63]. The plasma fibrinogen concentration has also been related to the prognosis of patients with acute cerebral ischemia [64].

Since the development of a clinically applicable technique to assess blood filterability, a number of studies have been carried out in patients with recent cerebral infarction to investigate the microrheology of blood. Several hundred patients have been studied after acute cerebral ischemia and the blood filterability has been found to be decreased by 30% to 70% compared to healthy controls. Two large studies are of interest, because they followed patients longitudinally and could therefore comment on the prognostic and predictive value of blood filterability tests. In the first study on 52 patients following acute cerebrovascular accident, 34 of the 37 patients who died within thirty days had the worst filterability results immediately on admission. The difference in filterability between these and the 15 patients who survived for thirty days was highly significant. In another larger study performed by Boisseau and his colleagues on 152 patients, it was shown that cerebral hemorrhage did not influence blood filterability, but that patients with cerebral thrombosis who subsequently died had a blood filterability approximately 60% of those patients who survived [65]. As in the case of myocardial infarction, it would seem that significant microrheological alterations occur at the time of infarction and play a role in the pathology of the evolution of the infarct and therefore clinical progress.

6.4.3. *Therapeutic implications*

The cerebral circulation is the area where therapeutic hemodilution has gained most popularity and hence also most controversy. The role of normovolemic hemodilution in the cerebral circulation is promising. Fig. 6.6 compiled by Henriksen and colleagues summarizes the changes in cerebral blood flow brought about by different degrees of hemodilution in a number of clinical studies. It can be seen that the benefit in terms of blood flow and oxygen delivery is greatest if the initial red cell concentration is near the upper end of the normal range.

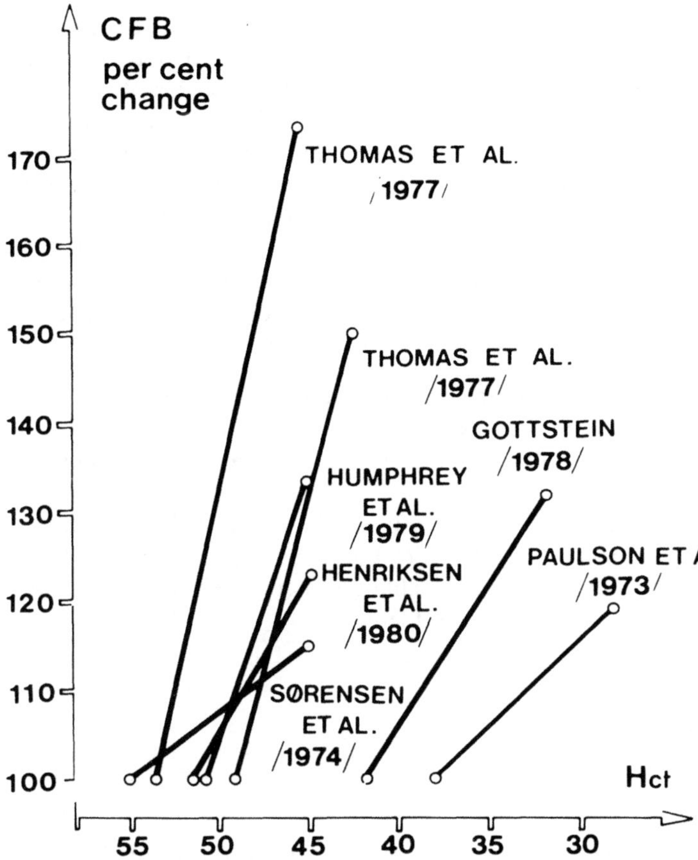

Figure 6.6. Summary of various trials of therapeutic hemodilution to improve cerebral blood flow. From Henniksen et al (17).

Gottstein has been the main proponent of hemodilution in the treatment of acute strokes and has summarized the considerable clinical experience from this and other groups showing a very definite improvement associated with significantly longer survival [58]. Patients' alertness has also been shown to improve with lowering of the hematocrit [66]. An interesting study by Wood and colleagues demonstrated a significant increase in the regional blood flow of the affected area of the brain following acute hemodilution [67].

There have only been isolated reports of plasma exchange or pharmacological normalization of elevated plasma fibrinogen [68] and it is not possible yet to assess the potential of these two new modalities in the treatment or prophylaxis of cerebral ischemia. But abnormalities in blood filterability are often secondary to a plasma defect and therefore plasma exchange may well be effective in situations where specific abnormalities in blood filterability can be demonstrated. A number of pharmacological agents said to improve red cell deformability have been used in the treatment of cerebral ischemia; most clinical experience has been reported with pentoxifylline [41]. However, neither with pentoxifylline nor with any other agent has clinical efficacy been directly related to improvement in the rheological properties of blood cells on a patient to patient basis.

In conclusion, although the hemorheological approach to the pathology and treatment of cerebral ischemia has already resulted in significant advances and is likely to produce further improvement in the management of these patients in the future, a number of questions still remain to be answered:

1. What are the correct selection criteria for normovolemic hemodilution?
2. What is the optimal hematocrit for oxygen delivery to the ischemic brain?
3. Is there any vascular autoregulation in response to changes in blood cell rheology?
4. Which of the hemorheological drugs currently available are of definite clinical benefit, and is this benefit directly related to the hemorheological effect?
5. To what extent are the hemorheological changes associated with acute and chronic cerebral ischemia a cause or an effect?

6.5. Ischemia of the leg

6.5.1. Pathological role

Basic hydrodynamic consideration would suggest that the viscosity of the blood must be related in an inverse fashion to total leg blood flow, but there is little direct evidence to prove this in humans. Fig. 6.7 shows one series of experiments carried out in sedated patients with clinically normal peripheral circulation [69]. It shows that the percent change in calf blood flow is two to three times greater than the percent change in viscosity. (This ratio depends on the shear rate at which the viscosity is measured.) A fundamental objection to all such studies is that whatever technique is used for artificially changing blood viscosity it could itself have a direct effect on blood flow rather than through an effect on the viscosity of the blood. Several studies have been reported in the last decade, comparing the whole blood viscosity of groups of intermittent claudicants and normal controls, all showing a significant 10 to 25 percent increase in the mean values for the claudicants with some overlap of individuals [70,71,72]. The difficulty of proving that an apparently asymptomatic control does not have subclinical arterial disease makes the difference between patients and so-called normal controls all the more significant. The studies of acute or chronic ischemia carried out by the Siena school are particularly fascinating [73]. Sampling venous

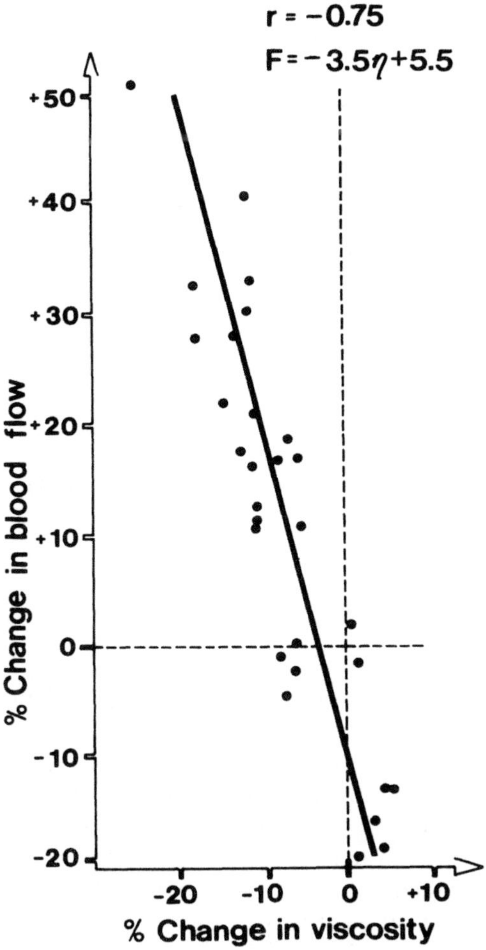

Figure 6.7. Correlation between change in calf blood flow in normal subjects and change in blood viscosity brought about by acute change in the hematocrit.

blood draining acutely ischemic limbs, they have shown that changes in viscosity can occur very rapidly in ischemia and that such acute changes are reversible. Furthermore, artificially induced ischemia by arterial occlusion only brought about these changes in patients who had atherosclerotic disease.

All three primary determinants of whole blood viscosity are changed in patients with leg ischemia: red cell concentration, plasma viscosity and blood cell rheology. There is a slight but significant degree of hemoconcentration, as well as a raised plasma fibrinogen concentration [70]. The latter is responsible for an increased plasma viscosity and increased red cell aggregability. The role of an abnormality in the rheology of the cellular components of blood is more

Table 6.2. Blood filtration studies in leg ischemia.

	n	method	chage compared to controls	Reference
1. Reid et al. '76	44	A	−30%	78
2. Angelkort et al. '79	25	A	−35%	79
3. Angelkort et al. '81	65	A	−40%	80
4. Di Perri et al. '81	80	A	−30%	81
5. Perego et al. '81	45	A	−20%	82
6. Alderman et al. '81	68	A	−30%	83
7. Ernst et al. '81	88	B	−35%	84
8. Winkenwerden et al. '82	43	B	−10%	85
9. Jouve et al. '83	70	A	−25%	86
		B	−16%	
10. Stuart et a. '82	–	C	N.S.	87
11. Bareford et al. '82	64	C	N.S.	88
12. Matrai et al. '84	44	D	N.S.	89

Methods: A = Whole blood technique
B = Removing buffy coat
C = Removing all white cells
D = New technique

controversial. Table 6.2 summarizes the results of early filtration studies. The abnormalities reported using whole blood (Method A) may have been due to white cell clogging of the filter pores. Efforts to remove most of the white cells and platelets (Method B) however still gave abnormal filtration results. Complete removal of all white cells (Method C) seemed to abolish the dramatic differences in filtration rates reported earlier [74]. The now obvious conclusion that it is the rheology of the white cells which is deranged seemed only just to have been appreciated. The most recent techniques of filtration (Method D) can distinguish between changes in cell transit time and pore clogging, and it would seem that in blood from patients with leg ischemia the red cells are characterized only by a slightly decreased transit time; more importantly the white cells are involved in increased clogging [75]. A shift in the balance of clogging and unclogging by white cells has also been described in animal models of muscle ischemia [76]. A series of studies from Siena suggest that changes in whole blood or red cell filterability may be determined by the activation of white cells and platelets. Rheological abnormalities in patients with ischemic disease may be largely dependant on an increase in such activation [79]. Changes in white cell rheology have only recently been measured in the blood of patients with leg ischemia. One of the commonest drugs used to improve the rheological properties of the blood in patients with intermittent claudication has recently been shown to have most marked effects on white cell clogging [11]. Theoretically, abnormal white cell clogging can be due to increased rigidity or adhesiveness. The evidence at the moment suggests that the former is the more important in leg ischemia, as the white cells are probably not normally activated as they traverse the microcirculation.

6.5.2. Clinical significance

Primary or secondary polycythemia, myelomatosis or other paraproteinemias and leukemia may all present clinically with leg ischemia in the absence of any significant vessel disease. Strong clinical suspicion will be aroused by the presence of distal pulses confirmed by a normal arm-to-ankle systolic pressure gradient. These cases are rare but must be recognized as specific treatment of the underlying cause is often successful.

There are a few longitudinal trials of intermittent claudicants, where the clinical progress over a year or more has been related to the initial levels of various rheological risk factors. Increased values of hematocrit, fibrinogen and

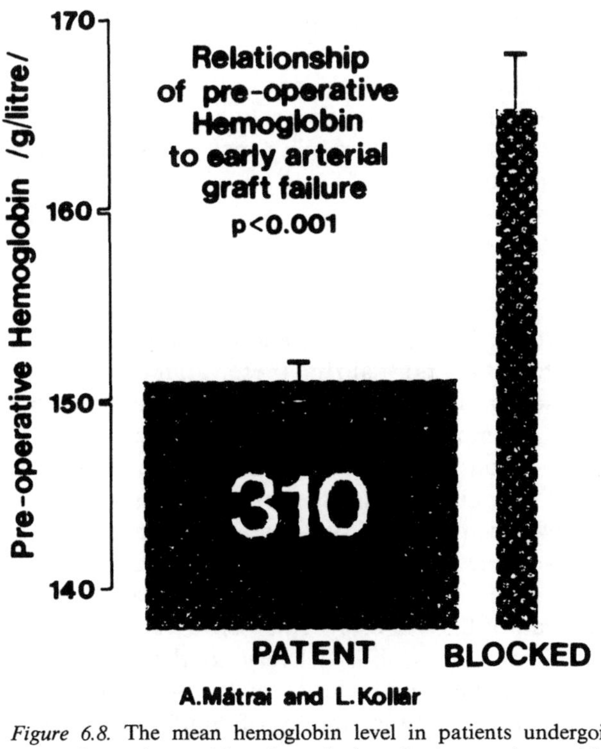

Figure 6.8. The mean hemoglobin level in patients undergoing femoro-popliteal arterial bypass, comparing patients with early graft thrombosis to patients with patent grafts. [93]

whole blood viscosity [90] and decreased blood filterability [78] have all been shown to be significant indicators of poor prognosis in terms of increasingly severe claudication, development of rest pain or gangrene and, finally, the need for surgery. This is true not only with regard to the natural history of the disease or for patients under medical treatment, but also for surgical patients undergoing reconstructive arterial procedures or distal amputations [91]. A possible pathological basis for this prognostic effect may be the viscous vicious spiral mentioned earlier in relation to myocardial ischemia.

The harmful effect of what used to be considered a high normal hematocrit in terms of failure of arterial reconstructions is particularly striking and tends to go against what used to be the traditional surgical teaching. This rather surprising clinical observation was already made ten years ago [92]. Fig. 6.8 illustrates the results of a recent study in patients undergoing femoro-popliteal arterial reconstructions. The pre-operative hemoglobin level was very much higher in patients with early post-operative failures than in those whose reconstructions remained patent [93].

Assessment of blood cell rheology may have a significance quite apart from the purely physical one of affecting capillary blood flow. The red cell membrane is one type of cell membrane readily sampled in a patient and it may be a convenient way of assessing pathological metabolic processes in cellular membranes in general. Although the red cell membrane is very different from the endothelial surface, nevertheless certain pathological processes may take place simultaneously in both. For instance, the abnormal absorption of proteins on its surface. It is possible that changes in red cell filterability may reflect abnormal processes also affecting the endothelium.

6.5.3. Therapeutic implications

If abnormally high fibrinogen or red cell concentration and decreased blood cell filterability are significant risk factors, then normalizing these variables may have a therapeutic benefit in leg ischemia. Unfortunately the evidence that such maneuvres are clinically useful is incomplete, and at times contradictory.

The experimental evidence in favour of hemodilution is quite strong. In subjects with apparently normal leg circulation, the improvement in blood viscosity and calf blood flow outweighed the disadvantage of decreased oxygen carrying capacity in acute normovolemic hemodilution down to a hematocrit of around 0.40 [70]. However in a group of polycythemic subjects, without leg ischemia, hemodilution from a mean of 0.57 to 0.47 hematocrit over a period of weeks, reduced resting and maximal hemoglobin delivery to the leg [94]. In animal models of leg ischemia, similar benefits in terms of leg blood flow have been demonstrated. In a well controlled animal model of hindlimb ischemia, hemodilution from a mean hematocrit of 0.48 to 0.35 was shown to completely normalize the healing of the ischemic skin [95]. However, the evidence for a clinical benefit in patients with ischemia is less clear. In terms of the non-surgical treatment of leg ischemia, some uncontrolled studies showed a definite objective, as well as subjective, improvement in claudication [96,97]. A controlled trial in more severe ischemias with rest pain was negative. An interesting phenomenon is the wide variation in response to hemodilution which seems to be a feature of most trials on claudication. Some patients seem to derive a very dramatic improvement, but so far it has proved impossible to predict these good responders in terms of any practical pre-treatment assessment. The actual morphology and anatomy of the underlying vascular abnormality may well be the important determinant but until the recent advent of digital substraction angiography it has been impossible to investigate this routinely. This is supported by preliminary results of the first double-blind, placebo-controlled, cross-over trial of normovolemic hemodilution in patients selected on the basis of the morphological abnormality in their leg arteries [98].

There has been a definite shift in the surgical practice towards aiming at a low hematocrit prior to reconstructive arterial operations, in some cases employing the regular use of preoperative normovolemic hemodilution. This changing attitude is taking place despite the absence of any properly controlled clinical trial showing a decrease in the high incidence of complications following this type of surgery, although there is again good evidence from controlled studies in animal models. For instance using a model of narrow prosthetic arterial grafts with a poor distal "run-off" a dramatic improvement in early patency rate was achieved by per-operative hemodilution (Fig. 6.9) [99].

Defibrinogenation is theoretically much more attractive than hemodilution. Lowering plasma fibrinogen not only improves many measureable rheological properties of blood, but it is also generally accepted that the circulating plasma fibrinogen concentration can be lowered to at least 30% of the normal without any risk whatsoever. Controlled defibrinogenation should therefore be a useful technique even in patients whose initial fibrinogen concentration is within the normal range. A major practical problem has been that the only really effective defibrinogenating therapy available at the moment is the use of purified enzymes from snake venoms, which have to be given by injection and after a few weeks become inactivated by antibodies. Furthermore, fibrin degradation products may be as harmful as fibrinogen rheologically [100]. Again, a number of uncontrolled or open studies showed definite subjective and objective improvement [101,102], whilst a controlled double-blind study showed no consistent benefit [103] (see Chapter 12). There seems a clear need for an effective and safe oral preparation which can significantly lower plasma fibrinogen concentration. Plasma exchange has not produced any convincing results in ischemia of the legs [104].

Although it seems logical to accept that the flow properties of the individual blood cells must affect total blood flow and tissue perfusion, the exact mechanisms involved are still controversial and are discussed in detail in Chapters 4

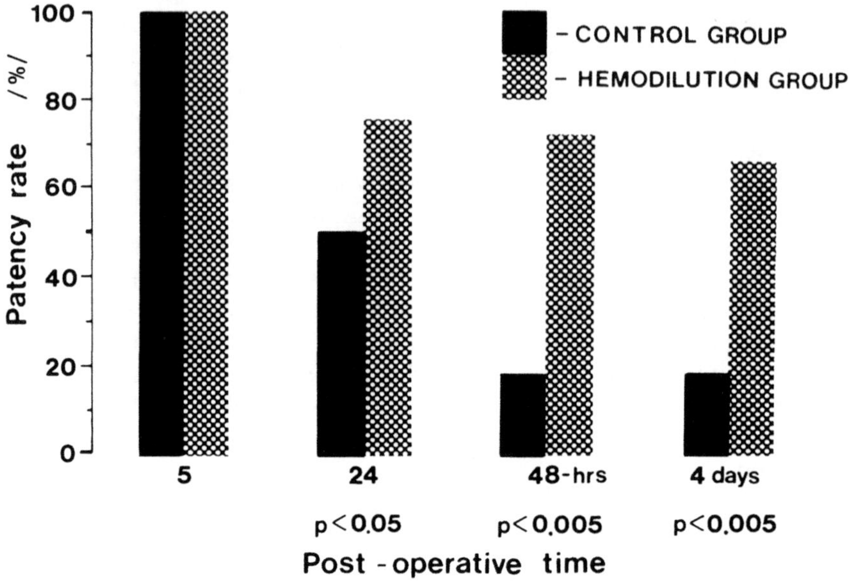

Figure 6.9. Patency of 3 mm diameter prosthetic grafts inserted in the rabbit aorta with artificially decreased distal "run-off". The effect of pre-operative hemodilution.

and 5. Deleterious changes in the physical properties of blood cells may take the form of decreased deformability, decreased surface charge, and increased aggreability of the red cells, or increased rigidity or adhesiveness of the white cells. A variety of pharmacological agents have been shown to correct such abnormalities in various systems. The type of evidence available in relation to different medications is described in detail in Chapter 12.

The present situation could be summarized by saying that many drugs improve the microrheological properties of blood in vitro, some also in vivo and a few have been shown to have some clinical benefit [105]. But in no case has a direct relationship been demonstrated between rheological and clinical improvement on a patient-to-patient basis. This does not mean that these newer hemorheologically acting substances are ineffective, but rather that the case has not yet been proven. Unfortunately, in most trials either the hemorheological or the clinical effects have been studied; rarely both. The most extensive clinical trials have been carried out using Pentoxifylline [106], a drug which recently has also been shown to have an effect on white cell rheology in vitro [11] and in vivo [107]. A more detailed description of the clinical trials which have been carried out using possibly hemorheologically active drugs can be found in Chapter 12. An assessment of the clinical effectiveness of hemorheologically active medications in the treatment of leg ischemia must be reviewed in the context of the practicalities of the problem: Firstly, it is extremely difficult to design and carry out a really convincing clinical trial in intermittent claudication. Secondly, at the moment there is no pharmacological therapy of proven efficacy for the large majority of the patients who are unsuitable for surgical reconstruction. Thirdly, most of the hemorheological agents are safe, devoid of significant side effects and their proposed mechanism of action is at least logical. For these reasons their use in claudicants is perfectly acceptable as an adjunct to other aspects of total mangement such as weight reduction, treatment of coexisting disease, elimination of smoking and other risk factors and the pursuit of a regular exercise program.

In summary, if a claudicant fails to respond to the usual general measures and some form of pharmacological treatment is thought to be warranted, then the use of a drug with demonstrable in vivo hemorheological effect is justified. At least the approach is logical and likely to be safe. If a patient's condition is more severe, with crippling claudication or rest pain, as an alternative to surgery it may be reasonable to try one of the techniques which have a more rapid and profound rheological effect, albeit more complicated and less safe. The order of preference may be: normovolemic hemodilution, controlled defibrinogenation and plasma exchange. As yet, the possible dangers of using any of these modalities long term is not known. Although it will become clinically apparent within a few days whether any of these techniques is effective in a particular patient, it would be easier to monitor their effect with some form of objective assessment of blood flow, tissue perfusion or walking distance under controlled circumstances.

6.6. Raynaud's phenomenon

6.6.1. Pathological role

The effect of temperature on blood viscosity has been well studied. Both whole blood and plasma viscosities increase when the temperature is lowered. The effect of temperature on blood filterability has been studied less and most of the existing evidence is summarized in the second Proceedings of the Royal Society of Medicine Red Cell Filterability Workshop [19]. The Siena school regularly carry out all their clinical hemorheological measurements at 37°C and some of the most exciting clinical results, widely referred to in this book, come from this centre.

It is logical to look for possible abnormalities in relation to the temperature effects in patients with Raynaud's phenomenon. In some studies whole blood viscosity has been shown to increase abnormally as the temperature is lowered [108]. In the absence of cryoproteins this may be associated with the increased plasma fibrinogen concentration described by some authors. It would seem, though, that whilst an increase in plasma or whole blood viscosity may be factors in precipitating an attack in some patients, it is unlikely to be a common etiological factor. However, they must be an important component in the pathological processes during the attack. The temperature of the blood in the typical white finger is 15 to 30°C lower than the central blood temperature. Plasma and whole blood viscosities as well as the rheological properties of the blood cells are considerably worsened at these lower temperatures. Capillary plugging by individual cells and the increase in low shear viscosity of the blood in the larger vessels are particularly relevant. During a Raynaud's attack, there is no flow in the affected digit and although there is a considerable decrease in the blood contained within the finger, hence the white color, there must be some static blood at least in the digital arteries. For the attack to come to an end, the low shear viscosity of this static column of blood must be exceeded. An abnormal increase in the yield stress of blood would tend to prolong the duration of an attack and may determine the amount of irreversible tissue damage. Capillary plugging by blood cells, which may become abnormally rigid at low temperatures, may have a similar effect. One group of workers described a significant increase in the viscosity of the blood coming from the hand during the ischemic phase, which partly reversed when the Raynaud's attack came to an end [109].

Decreased red cell filterability has been described in the blood of Raynaud's patients even at the same temperature as the controls. The differences would of course be even greater if the blood of the patients were at a lower temperature than that of the healthy controls. The plasma fibrinogen is one of the most important rheological factors determining the low shear blood viscosity and has been described as increased in Raynaud's patients by several workers. The hematocrit is the other important determinant of low shear blood viscosity, but the usually measured central hematocrit cannot be equated with the concentration of the red cells in the involved finger vessels.

6.6.2. Therapeutic implications

Part of the screening of patients presenting with Raynaud's phenomenon should be the exclusion of gross rheological abnormalities such as paraproteinemia, leukemia, cryoglogulinemia or marked hyperfibrinogenemia. The results of pharmacological therapy of Raynaud's phenomenon has been notoriously varied; many types of medications have an apparently beneficial effect in some patients, while not in others, possibly a reflection of the heterogeneity of the underlying disorder. Similarly, none of the medicines with a hemorheological effect has been shown to be consistently effective in this condition. The therapeutic scene is much more hopeful when considering plasma exchange. Plasma exchange has a marked hemorheological effect by lowering plasma fibrinogen in the short term and by increasing blood filterability for several weeks. These changes have been particularly impressive in Raynaud's patients and are presumably due to the presence of some plasma factor which secondarily affects the rheology of the blood cells [110]. These rheological changes have been shown to be accompanied by a marked parallel clinical improvement, both subjectively and objectively [111].

6.7. Conclusions

Hemorheology, like all new disciplines, follows a typical pattern of development; a phase of early excitement merging into a plateau of conflicting enthusiasm and skepticism aroused by all new ideas. Suddenly the new concepts become fashionable and there is widespread interest and work hoping that they will answer all the old existing problems. At the present time hemorheology is probably some way along this third phase. We probably have yet to reach the last phase of its development, where hemorheology will be seen as just one of the aspects of cardiovascular disease of greater or lesser importance in different aspects of these diseases. Whilst at the moment it is difficult to predict what the final level of importance will be, it is possible to look at the existing evidence and to try to evaluate it in terms of the four criteria for linking hemorheological abnormalities to circulatory diseases listed at the beginning of this chapter.

Both in terms of primary and secondary risk, there is good evidence that hemorheological factors are important in the coronary and cerebral circulation. Their precise role in precipitating infarction is unclear and involves consideration of all the mechanisms which may link hemorheological phenomena to thrombosis considered elsewhere in this book (Chapter 7). However, once the initial ischemic accident has taken place the extent of damage and therefore the clinical progress of the patient seems to be closely related to the magnitude of the hemorheological changes observed immediately after myocardial or cerebral infarction. It is in the treatment of cerebral ischemia that there has also been greatest experience with the use of normovolemic hemodilution. The technique of plasma exchange, by contrast, has become best established in the treatment of Raynaud's phenomenon. The long-term answer to hemorheological treatment probably lies with the development of the second generation of hemorheologically active oral medications. It is an approach which has already gained widespread clinical acceptance in the area of leg ischemia. Further progress will have to be linked to a better understanding of which particular component of hemorheological factors, such as the red cell, white cell or plasma, is most critical and susceptible to pharmacological improvement.

At be beginning of this chapter allusion was made to the little progress made during the last three decades in solving the problem of atherosclerotic cardiovascular disease. While hemorheology alone is unlikely to be the key to unlock this problem, it is very likely to be a part of the combination lock.

6.8. References

1. Kannel W.B., Gordon T. 1970: The Framingham Study - an epidemiological investigation of cardiovascular disease. Washington D.C., R.V.S. Gort, Printing Office.
2. Bottiger L.E., Carlson L.A. 1973: The Stockholm Prospective Study. 2. Skandia Int. Symposia "Early phases of coronary heart disease", 158-181. Nordinska Bokhandelns Forlag, Stockholm.
3. Sorlie P.D., Garcia-Palmieri M.R., Costas R., Havlik R.J. 1981: Hematocrit and risk of coronary heart disease: The Puerto Rico Heart Health Program. Amer. Heart Jour. 101, 456-461.
4. Carter C., McGee D., Reed D., Yano K., Stemmermann G. 1983: Hematocrit and the risk of coronary heart disease: The Honolulu Heart Program. Amer. Heart J. 105, 674-679.
5. Burge P.S., Johnson W.S., Prankerd T.A.J. 1975: Morbidity and mortality in pseudopolycythemia. Lancet 1, 1266-1269.
6. Meade T.W., North W.R.S., Chakrabarti R., Stirling Y., Haines A.P., Thompson S.G., Brozovie M. 1980: Haemostatic function and cardiovascular death: early results of a prospective study. The Lancet 1, 1050-1054.
7. Wardle E.N., Piercy D.A., Anderson J. 1973: Some chemical indices of diabetic vascular disease. Postgrad. Med. J. 49, 1-9.
8. Wilhelmsen L., Svardsudd K., Korsan-Bengtsen K., Larsson B., Welin L., Tibblin G. 1984: Fibrinogen as a risk factor for stroke and myocardial infarction. N. Engl. J. Med. 311, 501-505.
9. Kannel W.B., Gordon T., Wolf P.A., McNamara, P. 1972: Haemoglobin and the risk of cerebral infarction: The Framingham Study. Stroke 3, 409-420.
10. Tohgi H., Yamanouchi H., Murakami M., Kameyama M. 1978: Importance of the hematocrit as a risk factor in cerebral infarction. Stroke 9, [4], 369-374.
11. Schmalzer E.A., Chien S. 1984: Filterability of subpopulations of leukocytes: effect of Pentoxifylline. Blood, 64, 542-546.
12. Burch G., DePasquale N.: Erythrocytosis and ischemic heart disease. Amer. Heart J. 62, 139.
13. Volger E. 1984: Rheological aspects of coronary artery and coronary small blood vessel diseases (Syndrome X). Clin. Hemorheol. 4, 209-221.
14. Di Perri T. 1981: The hyperviscous vicious circle. Viscositas, 1, 4-5.
15. Di Perri T., Forconi S., Guerrini M., Rossi C., Pieragalli D. 1979: Blood viscosity in the different stages of ischemic heart disease, angina pectoris and myocardial infarction. International Congress Series No. 491, Excerpta medica, 348-353.
16. Lowe G.D.O., Drummond M.M., Lorimer A.R., Hutton I., Forbes C.D., Prentice C.R.M., Barbenel J.C. 1980: Relation between extent of coronary artery disease and blood viscosity. Br. Med. J. 280, 673-674.
17. Johnsson R., Frick M.H., Valle M., Vuopio P., Tarssanen L. 1981: Red cell flexibility and oxygen affinity in patients with angina pectoris and normal coronary arteries. Annals of Clin. Res. 131, 77-80.
18. Fuchs J., Weinberger I., Rotenberg Z., Erdberg A., Davidson E., Joshua H., Agmon J.: Plasma Viscosity in ischemic heart disease. Amer. Heart J.. 108, 435-349.
19. Dormandy J. 1983: Red cell deformability and filterability. Ed. J. Dormandy. Published by Martinus Nijhoff. The Hague.
20. Dormandy J.A., Ernst E., Matrai A., Flute P.T. 1982: Hemorheologic changes following acute myocardial infarction. Am. Heart J. 104, 1364-1367.
21. Kellog F., Goodman J.R. 1960: Viscosity of blood in myocardial infarction. Circ. Res. 8, 972.
22. Bondoli A. et al: Changes in blood viscosity and plasma proteins in myocardial infarction. Resuscitation, 5 [3], 175-181.
23. Jan K.M., Chien S., Bigger B.T. 1975: Observations on blood viscosity changes after acute myocardial infarction. Circulation 51, 1079-1084.
24. Volger E., Ostner K., Klein J., Wirtzfeld A. 1979: Changes in red cell aggregation and deformability after acute myocardial infarction. Microvasc. Res. 17, 153.

25. Drummond M.M., Lowe G.D.O., Belch C.D., Barbanel J.C., Forbes C.D. 1980: An assessment of red cell deformability using a simple filtration technique. J. Clin. Path. 33, 373-376.
26. Dahlgren M.D., Peterson M.A., Engler R.L., Schmid-Schönbein G.W. 1984: "Leukocyte rheology in cardiac ischemia" In: White cell mechanics. Basic science and clinical aspects. Ed. by H.J. Meiselman, M.J.Y. Lichtman, P.L. LaCelle. Published by Alan Liss, New York, p. 271-283.
27. Dormandy J. 1985: Changes in blood cell rheology following myocardial infarction. Proc. 4th Europ. Conf. Clin. Hemorheol., Siena.
28. Yarnell J.W.G., Sweetnam P.M., Elwood P.C. Eastham R., Gilmour R.A., O'Brien J.R., Etherington M.D. 1985: Haemostatic factors and ischaemic heart disease. The Caerphilly study. Brit. Heart J. 53, 483-487.
29. Friedman G.D., Klatsky A.L., Siegglaub A.B. 1974: The leukocyte count as a predictor of myocardial infarction. N. Engl. J. Med. 290, 1275-8.
30. Zalokar J.B., Richard J.L., Claude J.R. 1981: Leukocyte count, smoking and myocardial infarction. N. Engl. J. Med. 304, 465-468.
31. Prentice R.L., Szatrowski T.P., Fujikura T., Kato H., Mason M.W. and Hamilton H.M. 1982: Leukocyte count and coronary heart disease in a Japanese. Amer. J. Epidemiol. 116, 496-509.
32. Chien S. 1981: Haemorheology in clinical medicine. Rec. Adv. Cardiovasc. Dis. 11, 21-26.
33. Burch G., DePasquale N. 1963: Phlebotomy: in patients with erythrocytosis and ischaemic disease. Arch. Int. Med. 3, 687.
34. Hershberg P.I., Wells R.E., McGandy R.B. 1972: Haematocrit and prognosis in patients with acute myocardial infarction. JAMA 219, 855-860.
35. Sedziwy L., Shillingford J., Thomas M. 1968: Some observations on haematocrit changes in patients with myocardial infarction. Brit. Heart Journal 30, 344.
36. Chien S. 1981: Hemorheology in disease, pathophysiological significance and therapeutic implications. Clin. Haemorheol. 1, 419-442.
37. Tucker W.Y., Bean J., Vandevanter S., Cohn L.H. 1980: The effect of haemodilution on experimental myocardial infarct size. Eur. Surg. Res. 12, 1-11.
38. Cristal N., Slonim A., Bar-Ilan I., Hart A. 1983: Plasma fibrinogen levels and the clinical course of acute myocardial infarction. Angiology 34, 693-698.
39. Sputl von F., Pimminestorfer E., Froschaver J. 1978: Therapeutic defibrination by Arvin in unstable angina pectoris combined with hyperfibrinogenaemia. Wien. Klin. Wschr. 22, 792-796.
40. Burch G.E., DePasquale N.I. 1965: Haematocrit, viscosity and coronary blood flow. Dis. Chest 48, 225.
41. Hopkins R.W., Fratianne R.B., Rao K.V., Damewood C.A. 1974: Effects of haematocrit and viscosity on continuing haemorrhage. Trauma 14, 482-493.
42. Messmer K. 1981: Compensatory mechanisms for acute dilutional anemia. Bibl. Hematologica 47, 31-42.
43. Gaisböck F. 1905: Die Bedeutung der Blutdruckmessung für die {rztliche Praxis. Dtsch. Arch. Klin. Med. 83, 363-365.
44. Tarazi R.C., Fröhlich E.D., Dustan H.P. 1968: Plasma volume in men with essential hypertension. N. Engl. J. Med. 278, 762-765.
45. Letcher R.L., Chien S., Pickering T.G., Sealey J.E., Laragh J.H. 1981: Direct relationship between blood pressure and blood viscosity in normal and hypertensive subjects: Role of fibrinogen and concentration. Am. J. Med. 70, 1195-1202.
46. Devereaux R.B., Drayer J.I.M., Chien S., Pickering T.G., Letcher R.L., Deyoung J.L., Sealey J.E., Laragh J.H. 1984: Whole blood viscosity as a determinant of cardiac hypertrophy in systemic hypertension. Amer. J. Cardiol. 54, 592-595.
47. Heilmann L., Siekmann U., Schmid-Schönbein H., Ludwig H. 1981: Hemoconcentration and pre-eclampsia. Arch. Gynecol. 231, 7-21.

48. Freitas J., Braz-Nogueira J., Nogueira da Costa J., Martins e Silva J. 1983: Erythrocyte filtrability and oxyhemoglobin dissociation in hypertensive patients. Acta Medica Portuguesa, Supp. 4, 77-78.
49. Coccheri S. 1982: Blood viscosity and red blood cell deformability changes in health and disease. Microcirculation, Clinical Experimental 1, No. 3, 204.
50. Isles C., Lowe G.D.O., Drummond M.M., Forbes C.D., Kennedy A.C., Lever A.F. 1981: Blood rheology in malignant phase hypertension. Scand. J. Clin. Lab. Invest. 41, Suppl. 156, 175-176.
51. Dormandy J. unpublished results.
52. Gottstein V. 1965: Physiologie und Pathophysiologie des Hirnkreislaufs. Med. Welt 15, 715-726.
53. Thomas D.J. 1982: Whole blood viscosity and cerebral blood flow. Stroke 13, 285-7.
54. Humphrey P.R.D., Du Boulay C.M., Marshall J., Pearson T.C., Russell R.W., Slater N.G.P., Symon L., Wetherley-Mein G., Zilkha E. 1980: Viscosity, cerebral blood flow and hematocrit in patients with paraproteinaemia. Acta. Neurol. Scand. 61, 201-209.
55. Wade J.P.H., Du Boulay G.H., Marshall J., Pearson T.L., Russell R.W., Shirley J.A., Symon L., Wetherley-Mein G., Zilkha E. 1980: Cerebral blood flow, haematocrit and viscosity in subjects with a high oxygen affinity hemoglobin variant. Acta Neurol. Scand. 61, 210-215.
56. Brown M.M., Marshall J. 1982: Effect of plasma exchange on blood viscosity and cerebral blood flow. Brit. Med. J. 284, 1733-1738.
57. Brown M.M., Marshall J. 1985: Regulation of cerebral blood flow in response to changes in blood viscosity. The Lancet 1, 604-609.
58. Gottstein U. 1984: Evaluation of isovolemic hemodilution. Clinical Hemorheology 4, 133-149.
59. Ott E., Lechner H. 1982: Hemorheologic and hemodynamic aspects of cerebrovascular disease. Pathol. Biol. 30, 611-614.
60. Sakuta S., Takamatsu S., Satoh K. et al 1979: Deformability of erythrocytes in cerebrovascular disorders. Acta Neurol. Scand. 60 (72), 641-645.
61. Lowe G.D.O., Jaap A.J., Forbes C.D. 1983: Relation of atrial fibrillation and high haematocrit to mortality in acute stroke. The Lancet 1, 784-786.
62. Harrison M.J.G., Kendall B.E., Pollock S., Marshall J. 1981: Effect of haematocrit on carotid stenosis and cerebral infarction. The Lancet 1, 114-115.
63. Pollock S., Tsitsopoulos P., Harrison M.J.G. 1982: The effect of haematocrit on cerebral perfusion and clinical status following carotid occlusion in the gerbil. Stroke 13, 167-170.
64. Pilgeram L.O. 1974: Abnormalities in clotting and thrombolysis as a risk factor for stroke. Thromb. Diath. Haemorrh. 31, 245-264.
65. Boisseau M.R., Lorient-Roudaut M.F., De Connink L., Doutremepuich C., Le Rebeller M.J., Bricaud H. 1983: Troubles hemorheologiques et alterations de la filtrabilite erythrocytaire au cours des maladies vasculaires. Acta Med. Port. Supp. 4, 37-45.
66. Willison J.R., Thomas D.J., Du Boulay G.H., Marshall T., Paul E.A., Pearson T.C., Russell A.W., Symon L., Wetherley-Mein G. 1980: Effect of high hematocrit on alertness. Lancet 1, 846-848.
67. Wood J.H., Polyzoidis K.S., Epstein C.M., Gibby F.L., Tindall G.T. 1983: Improvement in cerebral blood flow and power spectral EEG after isovolemic hemodilution in stroke patients. J. Cereb. Blood Flow and Metab. 3, 588-589.
68. Grotta J., Ackerman R., Correia J., Fallick G., Chang J. 1982: Whole blood viscosity parameters and cerebral blood flow. Stroke 13, 296-301.
69. Dormandy J.A. 1971: Influence of blood viscosity on blood flow and the effect of low molecular weight dextran. Brit. Med. J. 4, 716-719.
70. Dormandy J.A., Hoare E., Colley J., Arrowsmith D.E., Dormandy T.L. 1973: Clinical, haemodynamic, rheological and biochemical findings in 126 patients with intermittent claudication. Brit. Med. J. 4, 576-581.
71. Forconi S., Guerrini M., Ravelli P., Rossi C., Ferrozzi G., Pecchi S., Biasi G. 1979: Arterial and venous blood viscosity in ischaemic lower limbs in patients affected by peripheral obliterative arterial disease. J. Cardiovasc. Surg. 20 (4), 379-384.

72. Stuart J., George A.J., Blunt R.J., Strachan C.J.L., Hurlow R.A. 1979: Hyperviscosity and coagulation activation in peripheral vascular disease. Thrombosis and Haemostasis 42, 348.
73. Di Perri T. 1979: Rheological factors in circulatory disorders. Angiology 30 (7), 480-486.
74. Stuart J., Kenny M.W., Aukland A., George A.J., Neumann V., Shapiro L.M., Cove D.H. 1983: Filtration of washed erythrocytes in atherosclerosis and diabetes mellitus. Clin. Hemorheol. 3, 23-30.
75. Matrai A., Bogar L., Flute P.T., Dormandy J.A. 1984: Comparison of four blood filtration techniques. Clin. Hemorheol. 4 (6), 513-523.
76. Bagge U., Amundson B., Lauritzen C. 1980: White blood cell deformability and plugging of skeletal muscle capillaries in haemorrhagic shock. Acta Physiol. Scand. 108, 159-163.
77. Di Perri T., Forconi S., Guerrini M., Laghi Pasini F., Acciavatti A., Pieragalli D., Ceccatelli L., Pasqui A.L., Del Bigo C., Franchi A., Martelli G. 1983: Evidence of interrelationship among blood cells and whole blood filterability changes in man. Clin. Haemorheol. 3, 253.
78. Reid H.L., Dormandy J.A., Barnes A.J., Lock P.F., Dormandy T.L. 1976: Impaired red cell deformability in peripheral vascular disease. Lancet 1, 666-668.
79. Angelkort B., Maurin N., Boateng K. 1979: Influence of Pentoxifulline on erythrocyte deformability in peripheral occlusive arterial disease. Curr. Med. Res. Opin. 6, 255-258.
80. Angelkort B., Kiesewetter H. 1981: Influence of risk factors and coagulation phenomena on the fluidity of blood in chronic arterial occlusive disease. Effects of pentoxifylline. Scand. J. Clin. Lab. Invest. 41, Suppl. 156, 185-187.
81. Di Perri T., Forconi S., Guerrini M., Pecchi S., Cappelli R. 1981: Modificazioni Emoreologiche Nelle Arteriopatie. Giorn. Geront. XXIX, 487.
82. Perego M.A., Sergio G., Artale F. 1981: Haemorheological aspects relative to pathophysiology and clinical treatment of peripheral occlusive arterial disease. La Ricerca Clin. Lab. 11, Suppl. 1, 281-291.
83. Alderman M.S., Ridge A., Morley A.A., Ryall R.G., Walsch J.A. 1981: Effect of total leucocyte count on whole blood filterability in patients with peripheral vascular disease. J. Clin. Pathol. 34, 163-166.
84. Ernst E., Flute P., Dormandy J. 1981: Red cell filterability in peripheral vascular disease. Clin. Hemorheol. 1, 472.
85. Winkenwerder W., Adams K., Lineberger T., Johnson G. (Jr.). 1982: Blood filtration in patients with peripheral vascular disease. Clin. Hemorheol. 2, 201-207.
86. Jouve R., Juhan-Vague I., Arnaud C., Sambuc R., Billerey M., Mercier C., Serradimigni A. 1983: Erythrocyte deformability and acute phase reactant proteins in atherosclerosis obliterans patients. Clin. Haemorheol. 3, 481-489.
87. Neumann V., Cove D.H., Shapiro L.M., George A.J., Kenny M.W., Meakin M., Stuart J. 1983: Effect of Ticlopidine on platelet function and blood rheology in diabetes mellitus. Clin. Haemorheol. 3, 13-21.
88. Bareford D., Lucas G.S., Caldwell N.M., Stone P.C.W., Baar S., Stuart J. 1985: Erythrocyte deformability in peripheral occlusive arterial disease. J. Clin. Pathol. 38, 135-139.
89. Matrai A., Ernst E., Flute P.T., Dormandy J.A. 1984: Blood filterability in peripheral vascular disease: Red cell deformability or cell sticking. Clin. Hemorh. 4, 311-325.
90. Dormandy J.A., Hoare E., Khattab A.H., Arrowsmith D.E., Dormandy T.L. 1973: Prognostic significance of rheological and biochemical findings in patients with intermittent claudication. Brit. Med. J. 4, 581-583.
91. Bailey M.J., Johnston C.L.W., Yates C.J.P., Somerville P.G., Dormandy J. 1979: Preoperative hemoglobin as predictor of outcome of diabetic amputations. Lancet 2, 168-170.
92. Bouhoutsos J., Morris T., Chavatzas D., Martin P. 1974: The influence of hemoglobin and platelet levels on the results of arterial surgery. Brit. J. Surg. 61, 984-986.
93. Matrai A., Kollar L. 1987. Importance of the preoperative hemoglobin concentration in arterial surgery. Europ. Surg. Res. 19, 1-5.

94. Milligan D.W., Tooke J.E., Davies J.A. 1982: Effect of venesection on calf blood flow in polycythaemia. Brit. Med. J. 284, 619-620.
95. Parker M.C. 1984: Haemodilution in peripheral vascular surgery. Arch. of Emergency Medicine 1, Suppl., 31-37.
96. Yates C.J.P., Berent A., Andrews V., Dormandy J.A. 1979: Increase in leg blood flow by normovolemic haemodilution in intermittent claudication. Lancet 2, 166-168.
97. Rudofsky G., Meyer P., Strohmenger H.U. 1981: Effect of hemodilution on resting flow and reactive hyperemia in lower limbs. Biblt.. Haemat. 47, 157-164.
98. Ernst E., Matrai A., Kollar L. 1986: A randomized, double blind, placebo-controlled, cross-over trial on hemodilution in claudicants - preliminary results. Clin. Hemorheol. 6, 297-302.
99. Mahir M.S., Hynd J.W., Flute P.T., Dormandy J.A. 1985: The effect of normovolaemic haemodilution on the early patency rate of small calibre vascular prostheses. Europ. Surg. Res. 17, Suppl. 1, 15.
100. Rampling M.W., Whittingstall R., Linderkamp O. 1984: The effects of fibrinogen and its plasmin degradation products on the rheology of erythrocyte suspensions. Clin. Hemorheol. 4, 533-543.
101. Goyle K.B., Reid H.L., Dormandy J. 1977: Treatment of severe intermittent claudication by controlled defibrination. Lancet 1, 625.
102. Ehrly A.M. 1984: Evaluation of enzymatic defibrinogenation. Clin. Hemorheol. 4, 151-159.
103. Lowe G.D.O., Dunlop D.J., Lawson D.J., Pollock J.G., Watt J.K., Forbes C.D., Prentice C.R., Drummond H.N. 1982: Double-blind controlled clinical trial of Ancrod for ischaemic rest pain of the leg. Angiology 33, 46-50.
104. Walker R.T., Matrai A., Dormandy J.A., Flute P.T. 1985: Hemorheological and functional changes in intermittent claudication following plasmapheresis with haemaccell. Clin. Hemorheol. 5, 99-106.
105. Lowe G.D.O. 1984: Evaluation of rheological therapy by orally administered drugs. Clin. Hemorheol. 4, 159-175.
106. Porter J.M., Cutler B.C., Lee B.Y., Reich T., Reichle F.A., Scogin J.T., Strandness D.E. 1982: Pentoxifylline efficacy in the treatment of intermittent claudication: multicenter controlled double-blind trial with objective assessment of chronic occlusive arterial disease patients. Am. Heart J. 104, 66-72.
107. Matrai A., Ernst E. 1985. Pentoxifylline improves white cell rheology in claudicants. Clin. Hemorheol. 5, 483-492.
108. Goyle K.B., Dormandy J.A. 1976: Abnormal blood viscosity in Raynaud's phenomenon. Lancet 1, 1317-1318.
109. Forconi S., Guerrini M., Rossi C., Pecchi S. 1979: Local increase of blood viscosity during cold induced Raynaud's phenomenon. VASA 8, 116-120.
110. Dodds A.J., O'Reilly M.J.G., Yates C.J.P., Cotton L.T., Flute P.T., Dormandy J.A. 1979: Haemorheological response to plasma exchange in Raynaud's syndrome. Brit. Med. J. 2, 1186-1187.
111. O'Reilly M.J.G., Talpos G., Roberts V.C., White J.M., Cotton L.T. 1979: Controlled trial of plasma exchange in treatment of Raynaud's syndrome. Brit. Med. J. 1113-1115.

7
Thrombosis and hemorheology

G.D.O. Lowe
University Department of Medicine, Royal Infirmary, Glasgow G31 2ER, United Kingdom

7.1. Introduction

The potential importance of hemorheology in altering blood flow and oxygen delivery has been considered in Chapter 5 of this book. In Chapter 6, the contribution of rheological factors to ischemia of the heart, brain and limbs was discussed. The present chapter reviews the contribution of hemorheology to thrombosis. This is a young field, for only in recent years have rheology and thrombology come together. However, it is already apparent that rheological phenomena are potentially of considerable importance in thrombogenesis and in the pathophysiology of the tissue infarction which follows arterial thrombosis.

7.1.1. Sites of thrombosis

The importance of hemorheological factors in thrombogenesis is strongly suggested by the localisation of both venous and arterial thrombi at characteristic sites in the vascular tree. While epidemiologists and biochemists investigating the causes of thrombosis have concentrated on systemic factors, these do not provide any explanation for the focal distribution of thrombi. Many clinical and laboratory "risk factors" have been defined for *venous thromboembolism* [1], yet persons with such systemic risk factors develop venous thrombi only at characteristic sites. Sevitt [2] studied the distribution of thrombi in the deep veins of the lower limb at necropsy, and showed that thrombi occurred at sites of flow disturbance, where vortex formation might result in areas of stasis and recirculation of flow. Such flow disturbance presumably localizes the influence of the systemic prothrombotic factors.

In *arterial disease*, Mitchell [3] has pointed out that "we must avoid confusion between markers which can predict the risk of clinical events such as myocardial or cerebral infarction, and factors which actually cause vessel wall lesions. Many so-called risk factors such as smoking, hypertension and hyperlipidemia are systemic problems, whereas the striking feature of arterial plaques is their focal distribution. The carotid sinus is a severely affected segment, yet one centimetre distally the internal carotid, perfused by the same lipid laden, carbon monoxide containing, high pressure blood is virtually disease free". Again, local flow disturbance presumably localises not only atherosclerotic plaques, but also the superadded thrombosis which precipitates infarction of the heart, brain or leg.

7.1.2. Structure of thrombi

The different structures of venous and arterial thrombi further suggest the importance of flow in their formation. Venous thrombi formed *in vivo* consist largely of red cells trapped in a fibrin network, with small clumps of platelets and leukocytes [2]. Dintenfass [4] showed that similar thrombi are formed *ex vivo* in the rotational viscometer under the low shear conditions which may be expected in veins. Arterial thrombi formed *in vivo* contain relatively few red cells and are relatively rich in platelets and leukocytes: they form near arterial stenoses where shear rates are high, and similar thrombi are formed *ex vivo* under high shear conditions in the rotational viscometer [4]. It seems likely therefore that the different shear conditions in veins and arteries determine these different structures, although one must beware of over-simplification [5].

Since platelets and fibrin appear to be the important "building-blocks" in thrombi, the effects of rheological factors on platelet behavior, coagulation and fibrinolysis will first be considered. We shall then deal in turn with thrombosis in veins, the heart, the arteries, and the microcirculation.

7.2. Rheology and platelets

7.2.1. Platelets and hemostasis

The major physiological role of platelets is in hemostasis. It is useful to consider hemostasis initially, since thrombosis may be "hemostasis in the wrong place" [6]. When small blood vessels are severed, as in the skin bleeding time test, platelets adhere to subendothelial collagen and then aggregate to seal the leaking vessel with a platelet plug. Platelets which have been activated by collagen degranulate, secreting from their storage granules adenosine diphosphate (ADP), serotonin, and other substances promoting platelet aggregation; they also form thromboxane A_2 which is a potent inducer of platelet aggregation. In the presence of normal platelet function, there is an inverse correlation between the bleeding time and platelet count in the range 10-100 x 10^9/l [7]. No fibrin is observed in or behind the hemostatic plug for 10-30 minutes after injury [8], and there is only slight prolongation of the bleeding time in hemophiliacs or anticoagulated patients (see Chapter 1).

Studies of platelet rheology in the microcirculation *in vivo* have been limited by difficulties in visualising these small (2-4 μm diameter) and transparent cell fragments. Recently, Tangelder [9] stained platelets selectively with the dye, acridine red, allowing the study of their flow behavior in small arterioles in the rat mesentery. Tangelder found that the concentration distribution of platelets was non-uniform, with twice the mean platelet concentration near the vessel wall compared to the center of the vessel. Furthermore the orientation of the disc-shaped platelets was non-random: they tended to align with their long axes in the planes of shear, and this alignment increased from the vessel centre towards the wall [9]. These observations *in vivo* may be explained by the *ex vivo* studies of blood flow in small tubes previously performed by Goldsmith and colleagues, and recently reviewed by Goldsmith and Karino [10]. The flexible red cells tend to migrate away from the wall, and are centralized and packed in the axial stream. The concentration of red cells in the center of the tube and the interactions between red cells result in lateral displacement of platelets, which frequently collide with the vessel wall and with each other. Since shear stresses are highest near the vessel wall, platelets nearest the wall experience maximal alignment in flow.

Teleologically, the concentration of red cells towards the centre of arterioles, and of platelets towards the vessel wall, seems favorable for their respective functions. The red cells in the axial stream travel more rapidly than plasma, resulting in a lower dynamic hematocrit (the Fåhraeus effect, Chapter 4), and this is one mechanism for the physiological dilution of blood in the microcirculation [11]. The resulting low apparent blood viscosity in arterioles reduces systemic peripheral arterial resistance and facilitates oxygen delivery to tissues via nutritional capillaries. At the same time, the rheological positioning of platelets near the vessel wall facilitates their interaction with exposed subendothelium in hemostasis. Platelets near the vessel wall are more likely to collide with the wall and with each other, and also to produce an increased concentration of platelet-secreted substances near the wall. They should also scavenge any substances released by the vessel wall more effectively, and in the event of vessel wall damage would be more likely to encounter the released chemical activators (e.g. collagen), especially when maximally aligned with one of their flat sides (with its greater surface area) close to the endothelium [9]. Finally, platelets near the vessel wall are exposed to the highest shear stresses (which may activate them) and have the lowest flow velocities (and hence the greatest time to adhere to injured areas of the vessel wall).

7.2.2. Effects of red cells on platelets in hemostasis

The role of red cells in hemostasis was suspected by Duke in his classic paper of 1910 [12] on the contribution of platelets to bleeding and to the skin bleeding time. Duke noted that the bleeding time was prolonged in anemia, and that transfusion reduced the bleeding tendency in thrombocytopenia even after the platelet count had fallen to the pretransfusion level. Hellem and colleagues [13] showed that the bleeding time in anemia was shortened by transfusions of washed red cells, an effect also shown by Livio et al [14] in anemic uremic patients.

To determine whether an increased hematocrit was associated with a shortened bleeding time, we studied the relationships between bleeding time, hematocrit and platelet count in a group of anemic, normal and polycythemic subjects, all of whom had normal platelet count and renal function [15]. An inverse correlation was observed between bleeding time and hematocrit, consistent with an effect of red cells on platelet-vessel wall interaction. Interestingly, we also observed an inverse correlation between hematocrit and platelet count [15]. It is possible that high hematocrits promote increased platelet-vessel wall interaction and hence reduced platelet survival, although animal studies suggest that this may only occur at hematocrits greater than 0.75 [16]. Alternatively, it is possible that hemostasis of the platelet-vessel wall interaction requires increased platelet production in anemia and decreased production when the hematocrit is high. A third possibility is that the decrease in platelet count at higher hematocrit may be explained by hemodilution in the larger blood volume [16].

We have also suggested that the longer bleeding time in women may reflect their lower hematocrit compared to men, while the shorter bleeding time in patients with arterial disease may reflect their higher hematocrit [15]. Consistent with the effect of hematocrit on the bleeding time is the report of Challoner et al [17] that bleeding time increased following reduction of the hematocrit by serial venesection in men with high hematocrit.

Since platelet adhesion and platelet aggregation are two distinct processes in hemostasis and thrombosis, we shall now consider the effects of shear forces and of red cells on these two processes in turn.

7.2.3. Platelet adhesion

Platelet adhesion has been defined as the direct attachment of platelets to the vessel wall [18]: the subsequent, indirect attachment of platelet aggregates, which are added onto the direct platelet attachment, is more properly termed *platelet cohesion* [18], and is considered below under platelet aggregation. Early experimental work on platelet adhesion was conducted in columns packed with glass beads, or on artificial surfaces. These methods measure both adhesion and aggregation and depend critically on the type of surface and on flow conditions: hence they show poor reproducibility and are no longer in common use [19]. However, studies using these methods were able to show effects of hematocrit, ADP, shear rate and von Willebrand factor [19].

Most recent studies of specific platelet adhesion to subendothelium have been performed using the Baumgartner perfusion chamber model, and these have recently been reviewed by Turitto and Baumgartner [18]. In this model, a segment of a rabbit aorta, which has been de-endothelialized by using a balloon catheter, is everted and mounted on a rod in a perfusion chamber. Rabbit or human blood (citrated or fresh) is perfused through the chamber, and the numbers of contacted, attached, spread, bound, and aggregated platelets are then each quantitated morphometrically. The wall shear rate is varied by altering the dimensions of the perfusion chamber, rather than the flow rate [18]. Studies performed over the past 10 years have shown that platelet adhesion in this model is dependent on vessel wall factors, the plasma level of the large molecular weight protein complex called von Willebrand factor which links platelets to subendothelium and which is deficient in von Willebrand's disease, the platelet membrane glycoprotein Ib which interacts with von Willebrand factor and which is deficient in Bernard-Soulier disease, and prostacyclin which may be an endothelial defence mechanism against platelet thrombosis [18].

Rheological factors, particularly blood flow and platelet diffusion, also have a pronounced influence on platelet adhesion in the Baumgartner system. *Blood flow* provides a continuing supply of fresh platelets to replace those depleted by interaction with the vessel wall. Platelet adhesion increases with flow rate, and specifically with *wall shear rate*. This shear-dependency is observed at shear rates below 600-800 s^{-1} (typical for flow in large veins and arteries), but not at higher shear rates. *Platelet diffusion* due to intercellular collisions in flowing blood is dependent on shear rate and also *hematocrit*. Platelet adhesion increased 50-fold with whole blood (hematocrit 0.40] compared to platelet-rich plasma. At lower shear rates the physical effects of red cells could explain this difference, but at higher shear rates (above 2600 s^{-1}) and at higher hematocrits (above 0.40) chemical effects of red cells on platelets (e.g. release of ADP, which will be considered later) may be more important [18,20].

Platelet adhesion appears to depend not only on hematocrit, but also on red cell size and deformability. Aarts and colleagues [21] found that the hematocrit dependence of platelet adhesion was absent in goat blood (MCV 25 fl, mean diameter 3 μm), present at hematocrits up to 0.40 in rabbit blood (MCV 70 fl, diameter 6 μm) and marked in human blood (MCV 95 fl, diameter 8 μm) at hematocrits up to 0.60. Studies in human blood have shown a positive correlation between platelet adhesion and mean red cell diameter [21], and also between platelet adhesion and red cell rigidity when the latter was altered by drugs or by treatment with cholesterol-loading or diamide [22]. Whether these red cell effects are physical or chemical is not yet known.

7.2.4. Platelet aggregation and secretion

Platelet aggregation occurs when a stimulus interacts with a specific platelet receptor and produces a series of events which require metabolic energy and which result in a change in the platelet membrane such that platelets adhere to each other: fibrinogen and divalent cations are required as cofactors [23]. Platelet aggregation *ex vivo* has usually been studied in stirred platelet-rich plasma from anticoagulated blood (usually sodium citrate) utilising the changes in light transmission (wavelength 600 nm) which occur during aggregation [24,25]. Platelet secretion *ex vivo* can be assessed concurrently by measurement of adenosine triphosphate (ATP), using luciferase [23].

A variety of chemical stimuli may promote platelet aggregation, including ADP, collagen, thrombin, platelet aggregating factor (PAF) and thromboxane A_2 (or its precursor, arachidonic acid). ADP-induced aggregation has been most studied. ADP induces a shape change in the platelets, and makes available a fibrinogen-binding site on the platelet membrane, which is a complex of membrane glycoproteins IIb and IIIa, and calcium. Glanzmann's thrombasthenia (abnormality of glycoproteins IIb and IIIa) and afibrinogenemia are congenital bleeding disorders with prolonged bleeding time and decreased aggregation to ADP. In the presence of physiological concentrations of ionised calcium, however, ADP does not cause the secretion of platelet granule constituents, nor the formation of thromboxane A_2. Collagen causes secretion of granule contents as well as thromboxane A_2 formation; thrombin and PAF can induce aggregation and secretion through other mechanisms. Serotonin and adrenaline act synergistically with other aggregating agents, but are not themselves strong inducers of secretion and aggregation [23].

Physical factors also influence platelet aggregation and secretion. Aggregation in platelet-rich plasma with added ADP does not occur in the absence of flow, which brings platelets into contact. Aggregation *ex vivo* varies with temperature and with speed of stirring in conventional aggregometers [26]: 37°C and 1,100 r.p.m. are commonly used [19,23]. The effects of hydrodynamic factors have been studied *ex vivo* in platelet-rich plasma and in whole blood, both in tube flow and in rotational viscometers. High shear stresses induce changes in platelet reactivity in tube systems: for example, Yu et al [27] observed increased platelet aggregation in washed platelet suspensions following oscillatory flow. However, as discussed in Section 7.2.1., the concentration of platelets in tube flow varies with the distance from the wall and with the effects of red cells, hence measurements in tube systems can only be semi-quantitative. Rotational viscometers achieve a more homogeneous distribution of defined, adjustable shear forces throughout the sample [28]. However, many studies using rotational viscometers have subjected platelets to high shear stresses for several minutes [e.g. 29,30], whereas *in vivo* local high shear stresses only occur for milliseconds [28,31], and high shear stresses are encountered in *ex vivo* artificial organs for a few seconds.

More recent studies have therefore exposed platelet-rich plasma or whole blood to high shear stresses in rotational viscometers for fractions of a second or a few seconds. Wurzinger et al [28] exposed heparinised platelet-rich plasma to shear rates up to 21,000 s^{-1} for 7-700 ms in a Couette viscometer. They found that high shear forces resulted in platelet activation, damage, and microaggregate formation within milliseconds, the magnitude of shear stress being more effective than the duration of exposure time. The parameter most sensitive to increasing shear stress was platelet factor 3 activity, i.e., the procoagulant activity of platelets which is attributed to platelet phospholipids in the membrane and granules. It is relevant that Zwaal and colleagues [32] found that lysis of less than 1% of platelets caused increased platelet factor 3 activity. In contrast to previous studies using longer shear-exposure times, release of beta-thromboglobulin from platelet granules did not occur until platelets were lysed, as detected by release of lactic dehydrogenase [28].

The mechanisms by which platelets in platelet-rich plasma are activated by shear stress (other than lysis) are not known, but may include release of ADP. Anderson et al [29] found impaired platelet aggregation to exogenous ADP following shear exposure, possibly due to ADP exposure during shearing, following which platelets become refractory to ADP. Yung and Frojmovic [33] showed that ADP-stimulated platelets aggregate at relatively low shear rates (circa 30 s^{-1}). Moritz and colleagues [34] concluded that shear-release of ADP from platelets was the principal mediator of shear-induced aggregation in platelet-rich plasma. Previous experiments with aspirin, which inhibits platelet synthesis of thromboxane A_2, suggested that thromboxane A_2 played no major role in shear-induced aggregation, but that thromboxane A_2 synthesis was associated with shear-induced secretion [30].

7.2.5. Effects of red cells on platelet aggregation

Jen and McIntire [35] recently studied platelet aggregation in whole blood (heparinised and citrated), exposed to shear rates up to 18,000 s^{-1} for 6-300 s in a cone-plate viscometer. Aggregate size distribution curves were measured using a Coulter Counter/Channellyzer and computer. Shear-induced aggregates increased with shear rate and shear time, and could develop within 6 seconds above a donor-specific shear rate threshold (2,000-3,000 s^{-1}). Heparinised blood was more sensitive to shear than citrated blood. Such exposure times and shear rates in heparinised blood would occur during cardiopulmonary bypass and hemodialysis.

Jen and McIntire [35] found that whole blood was more sensitive to shear than platelet-rich plasma, and suggested four possible reasons. First, it could reflect the higher viscosity of blood compared to plasma, if shear stress rather than local shear rate stimulates aggregation. Secondly, increased platelet diffusivity in the presence of red cells could promote inter-platelet collisions (Section 7.2.3). Thirdly, shear-induced leukocyte damage might promote platelet-leukocyte aggregation [36]. Finally, ADP release from red cells during subhemolytic shearing could be responsible. A variety of previous studies support this last possibility.

As previously discussed (Section 7.2.3.), platelet retention in glass bead columns measures both platelet adhesion and platelet aggregation (or cohesion) [19]. Hellem [37] showed that platelet retention in whole blood depended on the hematocrit, and that if platelet-rich plasma was used, few platelets were retained unless ADP was added [38]. Harrison and Mitchell [39] abolished the difference in platelet retention between blood and platelet-rich plasma by adding the pyruvate kinase system, which removes ADP. Born [31] and Schmid-Schönbein et al [40] proposed that sheared red cells liberated ADP, which promoted shear-induced aggregation. Reimers and colleagues [41] measured shear-release of sufficient radio-labelled adenine nucleotides from red cells to account for the potentiation of platelet aggregation by red cells. Jen and McIntire [35] reduced both sensitivity to, and stability of, shear-induced aggregation in whole blood by adding the creatine phosphokinase system, which again removes ADP.

In a series of studies, Born and colleagues have studied shear release of ADP as a mechanism for hemostasis in whole blood flowing in narrow tubes. Apyrase, which removes ADP, increased the bleeding time in artificial vessels [42] and in isolated rat mesenteries [43]. *In vivo*, the bleeding time in rat and rabbit mesenteries was prolonged by the creatine phosphokinase and pyruvate kinase systems [44]. One source of the released ADP may be red cells, since chlorpromazine, in concentrations which stabilise the red cell membrane but which have no direct antiplatelet effect, increases the bleeding time in artificial vessels [45] and in man [46].

Recent studies suggest that platelet aggregation may be induced by ADP released from red cells even under low shear stresses. Aursnes et al [47] incubated whole blood and plasma at 37°C without stirring, and showed formation of formalin-fixable aggregates in parallel with release of ADP. Release of ADP was not observed in platelet-rich plasma, and no secretion of serotonin or beta-thromboglobulin from platelets was found. Aursnes and Vikholm [48] also showed activation of platelets by ADP released from red cells during centrifugation to prepare platelet-rich plasma. Reimers and colleagues [41] measured shear-release of radio-labelled adenine nucleotides even under low shear stresses. We have measured "spontaneous" platelet aggregation in citrated whole blood and platelet-rich plasma, gently rotated in a tube at 37°C on a roller mixer, and found that about 50% of single platelets aggregated in whole blood, compared to only a few % in platelet-rich plasma. Incubation with three ADP-removing enzyme systems greatly reduced this difference between whole blood and platelet-rich plasma [49]. We then showed that this "spontaneous" aggregation in whole blood is strongly dependent on the hematocrit, in reconstitution experiments in which the platelet count was kept constant [50] (Fig. 7.1). Burgess-Wilson et al [51] confirmed that such "spontaneous" aggregation depended on the hematocrit in a population study, even after multivariate analysis. Such effects of hematocrit are also observed on platelet cohesion to subendothelium in the Baumgartner model [52].

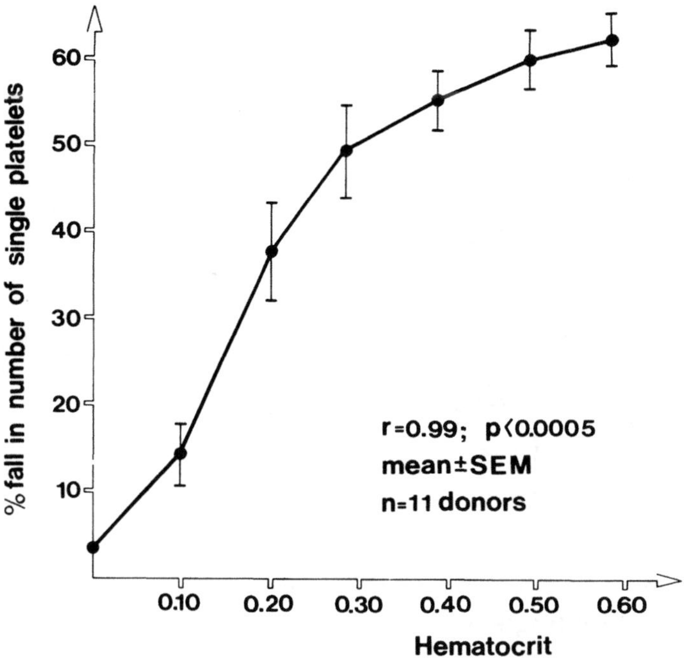

Figure 7.1. Effect of hematocrit on "spontaneous" aggregation of platelets in citrated whole blood, measured as the percentage fall in the number of single platelets. Samples from 11 donors were each reconstituted to give varying hematocrits but constant platelet count. Reproduced from (50), by permission of the Lancet.

Platelet aggregation in whole blood may depend on red cell deformability as well as hematocrit, since release of ADP may occur more readily when rigid red cells are sheared. Juhan et al [53] associated decreased red cell deformability (blood filtration) with increased whole blood aggregation (formalin-fixable platelet aggregates) in diabetics: both phenomena were reversed by insulin *ex vivo* and *in vivo*.

7.2.6. Effects of fibrinogen on platelet behavior

The plasma fibrinogen level has important effects on blood rheology, increasing plasma viscosity and red cell aggregation, and hence apparent blood viscosity. These effects are reversible *ex vivo* by defibrination with snake venom enzymes [54]. Fibrinogen also has important effects on platelet behavior. *Platelet adhesion* to artificial surfaces is greatly promoted by adsorption of fibrinogen to the surface [55]. Increasing fibrinogen levels within the human normal range are

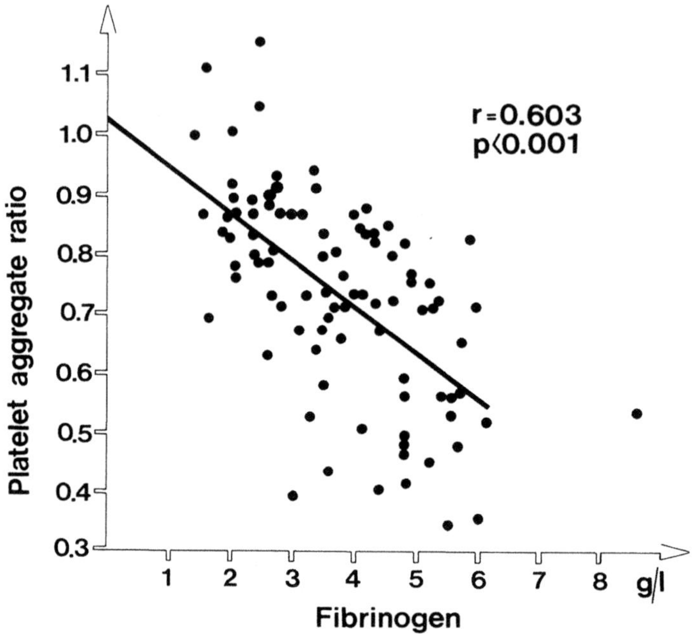

Figure 7.2. Relationship of plasma fibrinogen level to extent of whole blood platelet aggregation. Whole blood platelet aggregation was measured as the ratio of platelet count in edetic acid-formalin (which fixes aggregates) to platelet count in edetic acid. Platelet aggregation therefore increases with fibrinogen concentration. Reproduced from (58), by permission of Pergamon Press.

associated with increased adhesion to glass [56] and collagen [57]. Afibrinogenemia did not affect platelet adhesion to subendothelium in the Baumgartner model [18], but the effects of increased fibrinogen levels have not yet been studied in this model.

It has been mentioned that fibrinogen is an important cofactor in *platelet aggregation*, which is defective in afibrinogenemia. Correlations have been described between increasing plasma fibrinogen levels and both formalin-fixable platelet aggregates in whole blood [58] (Fig. 7.2) and "spontaneous" platelet aggregation in whole blood [51]. Furthermore, in a large population study, Meade and colleagues [59] confirmed a highly significant correlation between fibrinogen levels and ADP-induced platelet aggregation in platelet-rich plasma. A direct role of fibrinogen in platelet activation and aggregation seems likely, since defibrination therapy reduced ADP-induced platelet aggregation [60], ADP-induced electrophoretic mobility responses [61], and formalin-fixable platelet aggregates in whole blood [58]. In an *ex vivo* system for study of thrombus formation in dog whole blood, Schultz et al [62] related the plasma fibrinogen concentration to the platelet content of the thrombus.

7.3. Rheology, coagulation and fibrinolysis

Rheological factors (shear forces, red cells, and fibrinogen levels) are clearly important in platelet adhesion, activation and aggregation. However, platelet aggregates are initially unstable, friable structures which may be dislodged and disrupted by shear forces in flowing blood, unless they are stabilised by fibrin, which greatly increases their stability against dispersion by flow [5].

Shear forces also appear to influence blood coagulation and its endpoint, fibrin formation. Coagulationists have long appreciated that blood and plasma clotting times are affected by the frequency and technique of sample mixing by tilting clotting tubes. Dintenfass [4] found that the clotting time of blood in a rotational viscometer shortened with increasing shear rates. These results were recently confirmed by Ernst and colleagues [63], using viscometers with siliconised blood-contacting surfaces and controlled shear stress as well as shear rate. Shear-induced platelet activation seems the most likely cause for this acceleration of fibrin formation, particularly as Wurzinger et al [28] found that the procoagulant activity of platelets (platelet factor 3) was most sensitive to shear activation. However, other factors must also be considered, including increased sample mixing and hence collision frequency of coagulation factors and cofactors, decreased blood viscosity after shearing which would also promote such interactions, and increasing surface contact with increasing shear [4,63].

Hematocrit and fibrinogen levels may also promote fibrin formation. Schultz et al [62] related the fibrin content of thrombi formed in dog whole blood *ex vivo* to hematocrit and to fibrinogen levels. Increasing fibrinogen levels also increase the weight of thrombi formed in human blood *ex vivo* in the Chandler loop [64], and prolong the lysis time of plasma euglobulin clots [65]. However, increased fibrinogen concentrations lengthen clotting times *ex vivo*, possibly due to complexing of fibrinogen with soluble fibrin, which prevents fibrin polymerisation [66].

The rheology of layers of fibrinogen and fibrin may also be relevant to thrombogenesis. Copley [67] proposed that a thin layer of fibrinogen/fibrin lines the inner surface of the endothelium of blood vessels: the endoendothelial fibrin lining (EEFL). Recent investigations support the existence of this layer and Copley has given a detailed account of the evidence for its existence and of its possible functions in health and disease [67]. The latter include repeated adsorption of plasma proteins such as fibrinogen, which aggregate and gel to form a layered thrombus, termed "fibrinogenin", before the occurrence of platelet activation or thrombin generation. Such processes can be explored by rheological measurements of surface viscous and elastic moduli of layers of purified fibrinogen, or of fibrinogen in plasma. Recent studies show that some low molecular weight heparins and dextrans cause marked decreases in surface viscoelasticity [68]. In view of current interest in the use of low molecular weight heparins and dextrans in prevention of thrombosis (especially in veins), these findings suggest that clinical investigations of surface rheology of plasma and plasma protein may be a useful addition to blood rheology studies in the future.

Further basic work on the rheology of coagulation and fibrinolysis is clearly required. There is also a need for epidemiological studies on the relationship of rheological variables to markers of activation of platelets, coagulation and fibrinolysis.

7.4. Venous thromboembolism

7.4.1. Flow conditions and leg vein thrombosis

As mentioned in the introduction, venous thrombi occur most commonly at particular sites in the deep veins of the lower limb. Sevitt (2) has defined these as the dilated sinuses of the soleal veins, the pockets of large venous valves, the posterior tibial veins where they are compressed by the soleus muscle, and the proximal veins as sites where flow is disturbed. At these sites of flow disturbance, vortex formation can result in areas of stasis and recirculation of blood cells. Karino and Motomiya [69] have recently studied the microrheology of flow through venous valves, using isolated transparent dog saphenous veins and cinemicrographic techniques. Under physiological flow conditions, large paired vortices were present in each valve pocket. Microspheres continually entered the valve pockets out of the mainstream, and spent long periods of time spiralling towards the centre of the vortex before joining the mainstream. When concentrated red cell suspensions were perfused, a second, smaller, counter-rotating, secondary vortex was formed deep in each valve pocket, driven by the large primary vortex. In this secondary vortex, the red cell concentration was reduced, and very low flow velocities created a very low shear field which allowed red cell aggregation [69].

Karino and Motomiya [69] concluded that the design of venous valves allowed exchange of fluid and particles between the primary vortex and the mainstream, hence minimizing stagnation. However, stagnation was observed deep within the pocket, where the secondary vortex produced a low hematocrit which might favour hypoxia. Hamer and colleagues [70] measured hypoxemia in the venous valve pockets of dogs and man during immobility, and showed endothelial damage and valve thrombosis after only two hours of non-pulsatile flow. Hypoxic endothelial damage might conceivably release procoagulant substances, or result in decreased production of endothelial antithrombotic mechanisms such as prostacyclin or tissue plasminogen activator. We have recently shown that the application of graduated pressure elastic stockings, previously shown to prevent leg vein thrombosis, caused washout of hypoxic blood from the legs of immobile patients [71].

The secondary vortex might promote valve thrombosis not only by promoting hypoxia, but also by acting as an automatic trap for cellular aggregates [69].

Aggregates of red cells and platelets tend to centralise and grow within model vortices, as previously shown by Goldsmith and Karino [10], and the low-shear conditions in the secondary vortex could promote formation of such aggregates and their sedimentation towards the deepest portions of the valve pockets [69]. In human necropsy studies, Sevitt [2] examined apparently empty valve pockets in femoral veins by serial histology, and observed condensed foci of red cells, white cells or platelets. Sevitt suggested that these aggregates might have been deposited into the valve pockets by flow disturbance, and might act as the initial nidus from which some valve pocket thrombi could grow [2].

Rheological factors may promote not only the initiation of thrombi in the deep veins, but also their extension. The prevalence and extent of deep vein thrombosis in the lower limbs increase with the duration of bedrest [2]. A role for stasis in venous thrombosis is also suggested by the association of many "risk factors" (age, immobility, surgery, pregnancy, use of oral contraceptives, hemiplegia, paraplegia) with slow blood flow in leg veins; and also by the ability of various physical devices which increase leg blood flow to prevent postoperative leg vein thrombosis [72]. The lowest shear rates in the circulation occur in the veins [73]. Slow venous blood flow with low shear stresses allows red cell aggregation by fibrinogen molecules, which increases red cell sedimentation and local blood viscosity in low shear areas. These factors would tend to favour continued stasis and growth of thrombi, since any activated platelets, thrombin or nascent fibrin would be protected against dispersion and dilution by the blood stream [74].

Sevitt [2] showed that young thrombi have a laminar structure: large amounts of red cells trapped in a fibrin network alternating with clumps of platelets. A rheological explanation has been suggested for this layered structure [75]. The red cell-fibrin masses may have been red cell-fibrinogen aggregates, forming in low-shear areas and encouraging further stasis with the local accumulation of activated platelets and thrombin formation. This in turn may have resulted in bursts of irreversible platelet aggregation, forming the platelet clumps, while thrombin converted the fibrinogen to fibrin. It would be expected that a developing thrombus would cause (a) further flow disturbance, and (b) release of activated products: the recirculation of activated products in further vortices could then result in a self-propagating thrombus. When this thrombus occludes the vein, low shear rates should result both proximally and distally, leading to red cell aggregation, further flow reduction, fibrin deposition [18], and the growth of "red thrombi" composed mainly of red cells and fibrin [4]. Necropsy studies have confirmed the retrograde and anterograde extensions of red-cell-rich thrombi following thrombotic venous occlusion [2].

It is possible that physical devices such as elastic stockings reduce the incidence and extent of leg vein thrombi by altering venous flow conditions. Washout of hypoxic blood from leg veins by the application of graduated pressure elastic stockings may reflect reduced stagnation of blood in venous valve pockets, and may explain their efficacy in reducing the incidence of thrombosis [71]. Since elastic stockings also produce an increase in linear flow in leg veins [76], this effect may reduce extension of thrombi under low-shear conditions, which would be consistent with the efficacy of elastic stockings in reducing the prevalence of pulmonary embolism at necropsy [77].

7.4.2. Hematocrit and leg vein thrombosis

In the large veins, hematocrit is higher than in other blood vessels. Hematocrit increases further in the leg veins, due to leakage of fluid from plasma in the microcirculation [78]. This high leg-vein hematocrit might be expected to promote local increases in blood viscosity, red cell aggregation, and platelet adhesion and aggregation.

Extremes of systemic hematocrit appear related to the incidence of venous thromboembolism. In primary proliferative polycythemia, the risk of venous thrombosis increases markedly with increase in hematocrit [79], and is reduced by normalising the hematocrit prior to surgery [80]. Conversely, pulmonary thromboembolism appears to be an uncommon cause of death in anemic patients [81,82]. However, the results of studies relating postoperative venous thrombosis to hematocrits within the normal range have been conflicting [75].

Perioperative intravenous infusions of dextrans appear to reduce the incidence of pulmonary embolism [72]. This may be due in part to hemodilution and increased leg blood flow [83], although dextrans have several other potentially antithrombotic effects [72].

7.4.3. Fibrinogen and leg vein thrombosis

Increased systemic plasma fibrinogen levels, resulting in increased plasma and blood viscosity, have been associated with many "risk factors" for leg vein thrombosis, e.g. age, obesity, varicose veins, malignancy, heart failure, myocardial infarction, stroke, pregnancy, use of oral contraceptives, the nephrotic syndrome, trauma, and surgery; for references see [75]. However, neither smokers [84] nor diabetics [85] have an increased risk of leg vein thrombosis, despite their hyperfibrinogenemia. Moreover, the results of prospective studies relating fibrinogen, plasma viscosity, or blood viscosity levels to subsequent leg vein thrombosis have been conflicting: preoperative levels of these variables appear more consistently related to non-thrombotic illnesses (e.g., malignant disease) than to thrombosis [75,84]. However, the systemic levels of fibrinogen and viscosity in arm-vein blood may differ from levels in hemoconcentrated leg-vein blood. In one study, foot-vein plasma protein concentration rose by 38% during sitting for 50 minutes, while plasma oncotic pressure rose by 74% [78].

To test specifically the hypothesis that hyperfibrinogenemia might promote venous thrombosis, we have performed two double-blind, placebo-controlled trials of postoperative defibrination, using subcutaneous injections of the snake venom enzyme, ancrod. In patients with hip fracture, ancrod significantly reduced postoperative levels of fibrinogen, plasma viscosity and blood viscosity, and also decreased both the incidence and extent of deep vein thrombosis [86]. In patients undergoing elective hip replacement, ancrod did not reduce the incidence of total deep vein thrombosis, but did reduce the incidence of major thrombi in the femoral vein, from which most significant pulmonary emboli arise [87]. These results suggest that increased fibrinogen levels and blood viscosity may promote initiation and extension of venous thrombosis after hip surgery, although defibrination might also have an antithrombotic effect by partial anticoagulation.

The rheological effects of defibrination may also be beneficial in pulmonary embolism [88] and in established deep vein thrombosis of the leg [75]. Further controlled clinical trials are required to establish whether or not reduction in

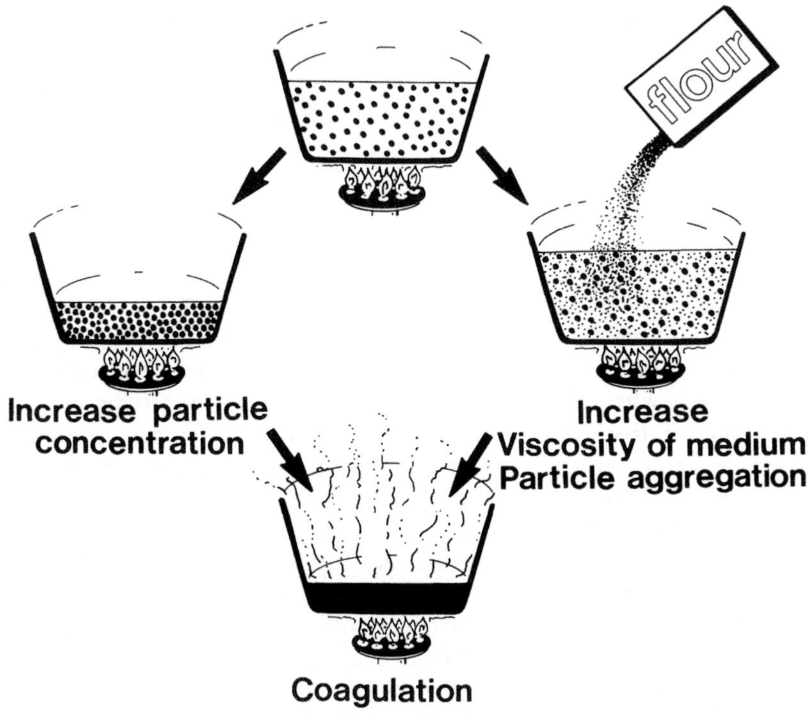

Figure 7.3. Promotion of coagulation in a solution of minced meat particles by increased particle concentration and by flour, which increases particle aggregation and the viscosity of the suspending medium. An analogy for the possible effects of hematocrit and fibrinogen on thrombosis in venous valve pockets (see text).

plasma fibrinogen levels reduces the incidence of pulmonary embolism or the postphlebitic syndrome [75]. Conventional anticoagulants (heparin and warfarin) do not reduce fibrinogen or blood viscosity levels in patients with venous thrombosis [75].

The controlled trials of hemodilution with dextran, and defibrination with ancrod, lend some support to the hypothesis that increased hematocrit and fibrinogen levels may promote venous thrombosis by their rheological effects in the leg veins. Fig. 7.3 shows this hypothesis by analogy. A traditional item of Scottish cooking is minced beef (called simply "mince"), which is boiled in salted water in a saucepan. The meat particles circulate in vortices in the saucepan, like the blood cells in a venous valve pocket. At a particle concentration of about 50%, the meat particles circulate freely and the gas-flame of the cooker (prothrombotic stimulus in the valve pocket) does not produce coagulation. All good Scottish cooks know that there are two ways to burn the mince. Firstly, excessive evaporation of fluid increases the particle concentration ("meatocrit") and hinders particle mobility at the bottom of the saucepan, resulting in coagulation. Secondly, the addition of flour as a thickening agent produces the same effect by increasing the viscosity of the medium and by aggregation of particles: hence flour should only be added near the end of the cooking period, and the mixture must then be stirred continuously to avoid burning. Fibrinogen can be compared to flour: it increases plasma viscosity and the aggregation of red cells and platelets.

7.4.4. Retinal vein thrombosis

After the leg, the second most common site for spontaneous venous thrombosis is the retina. Low flow conditions again occur at the common sites of thrombosis: arteriovenous crossings where the veins are compressed by the overlying arteries, and at the lamina cribrosa where the veins turn at right angles. Increased intraocular pressure, and defective control of intraocular pressure and systemic arterial pressure, are also risk factors which may operate by promoting low flow conditions where rheological processes may favour thrombogenesis [75].

Retinal vein abnormalities and thrombosis are common in polycythemias and plasma hyperviscosity syndromes, and several other "risk factors" (age, hypertension, hyperlipidemia, diabetes, and use of oral contraceptives) have been associated with abnormal systemic blood rheology [75]. Three series of consecutive patients with retinal vein thrombosis have documented increases in systemic blood viscosity, hematocrit and fibrinogen [89-91], and these rheological abnormalities appear to be associated with post-thrombotic microvascular complications [90,91]. Favourable clinical results have been reported for treatment of acute retinal vein thrombosis by hemodilution, defibrination, or streptokinase, but further placebo-controlled trials are required to establish their overall benefit and to test the importance of rheological factors [75].

7.5. Arterial thromboembolism

Acute arterial occlusion in the heart, brain or limbs may be due to thrombosis *in situ* (usually superimposed on a ruptured or ulcerated atheromatous plaque) or to embolism. Emboli can originate from thrombi on more proximal atheromatous plaques; from the heart; or, rarely, from venous thrombi via a patent foramen ovale (paradoxical embolism). Thus we must consider two basic types of pathology: thrombosis on atheromatous plaques, and thrombosis in the heart which subsequently embolises.

7.5.1. Cardiac thromboembolism

Cardiac thromboembolism rarely causes coronary occlusion, but is a common cause of stroke and limb gangrene. Emboli may arise from mural thrombosis after myocardial infarction; from the left atrium in rheumatic heart disease or non-rheumatic atrial fibrillation, from prosthetic heart valves, or from heart valves damaged by rheumatic heart disease or endocarditis [92]. Anticoagulant drugs are conventionally used for prevention and treatment of cardiac thromboembolism, but there is little evidence that they are beneficial [92].

While endocardial damage and prosthetic valve surfaces presumably trigger thrombosis, it seems likely that rheological factors also play a role in the formation of cardiac thrombi and perhaps also in embolism. Disturbance of intracardiac blood flow patterns would be expected in those patients who are likely to develop mural thrombi after myocardial infarction, e.g., those with left ventricular dysfunction [93]. Stagnation and vortex formation would be expected within the fibrillating left atrium. Damaged or prosthetic heart valves can result in flow disturbance and in high shear stresses which might activate platelets either directly or via red cell damage: mechanical hemolysis was a common complication of early artificial heart valves [94]. Further studies are required to model the flow disturbances produced by these cardiac disorders, and to examine prospectively the predictive value of rheological factors for thromboembolic events. For example, it would be interesting to know whether low normal hematocrits are protective because of low blood viscosity and platelet activation, or whether they confer increased risk because of increased turbulence.

7.5.2. Arterial thrombosis and atherogenesis

Arterial thrombosis usually occurs on atherosclerotic plaques. It therefore seems appropriate to consider first the rheology of atherogenesis, particularly as there is much evidence that recurrent subclinical arterial thrombosis contributes to atherosclerosis [95]. As previously mentioned, the striking feature of atheromatous plaques is their focal distribution [3]. Lesions tend to occur near bifurcations and bends: for example at the carotid sinus, terminal internal carotid, common and internal iliacs, and 2-4 cm from the ostia of the three major coronary vessels [95]. Such localisation of lesions, as well as the association of arterial blood pressure with extent of atherosclerosis, suggests that hemodynamic factors may be important in their formation. However, different workers have interpreted these facts quite differently, suggesting a variety of hemodynamic mechanisms: increased or decreased lateral pressures, increased or decreased shear stresses, and turbulence or flow separation: "a dazzling array of contradictions" [95]. Another possible mechanism is that shear forces tend to deform endothelial cells and alter their permeability to macromolecules [96].

In the last 10 years there has been much interest in the interaction of platelets with the damaged endothelium of the arterial wall. Recurrent platelet thrombosis may contribute to atherosclerosis. The "response to injury" hypothesis suggests that endothelial injury and platelet adhesion result in release of growth factors (derived from platelets, endothelial and other cells) into the arterial subendothelium. These growth factors stimulate proliferation of smooth muscle cells, which migrate from the media into the intima, synthesize collagen, and accumulate lipid to form atheromatous plaques [97]. The possible importance of platelet deposition on the endothelium in atherogenesis suggests the importance of a microrheological analysis of blood flow in models of arterial bifurcations or expansions, with emphasis not only on platelets but also on red cells (whose important effects on platelets were considered earlier).

There is current interest in the phenomena of flow separation and platelet-vessel wall interactions at stagnation points. In areas of flow separation, fluid circulates in an eddy or vortex between the mainstream and the vessel wall. Flow separation results in stagnation points downstream of arterial branchings and stenoses [98], points where platelet-rich thrombi had previously been observed in extracorporal shunts [99,100]. Goldsmith and Karino [10] have studied the microrheology of flow in vessel expansions and bifurcations. Red cells and platelets in vortices following a vessel expansion travel at varying velocities, and tend to migrate spirally outwards into the mainstream. However, aggregates of red cells and platelets tend to centralize and grow within the vortices. Some platelet thrombi were observed to adhere to the vessel wall when studies were performed with whole blood, but not with platelet-rich plasma. Platelet adhesion was found to occur within the vortex and just downstream of the reattachment point, and increased considerably with increase in hematocrit. In T-branch models, Müller-Mohnssen [101] found that red cells adhered in stagnation regions near the reattachment points, whereas platelets adhered upstream. It appears that areas of flow separation promote interactions of red cells, platelets and the vessel wall and that such interaction may encourage platelet deposition and its atherogenic consequences.

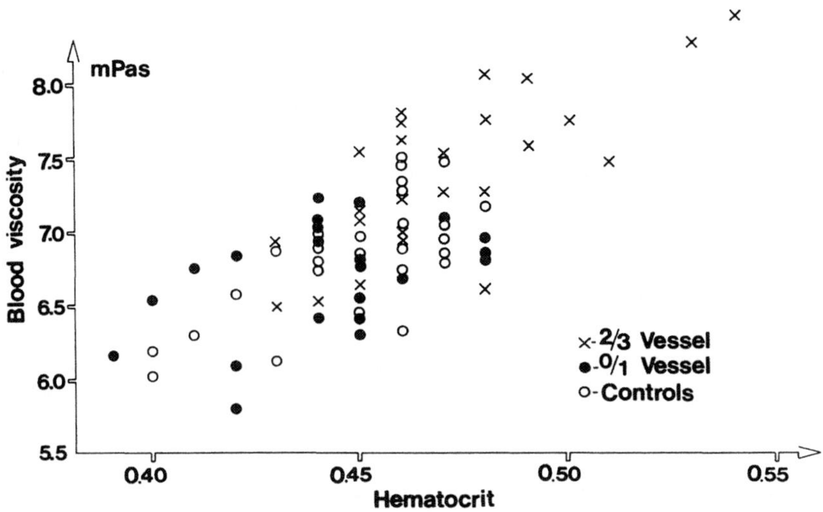

Figure 7.4. Relationship of apparent blood viscosity and hematocrit to angiographic coronary artery disease. [○] controls; [●] patients with no stenosis or stenosis of one vessel only; [×] patients with stenosis of two or three vessels. Reproduced from (102), by permission of the British Medical Journal.

In a study of 50 men undergoing coronary arteriography [102], we correlated the extent of coronary atherosclerosis with the hematocrit, and hence blood viscosity (Fig. 7.4). We have since confirmed this association in a further study of 200 men (G.D.O. Lowe and M. Kenicer, unpublished). In necropsy studies, hematocrit correlated with the extent of coronary atherosclerosis [103] and cerebral atherosclerosis [104]. In an angiographic study, Harrison and colleagues found that hematocrit was not related to narrowing of the internal carotid artery, but was higher in patients with carotid occlusion [105]. These associations of hematocrit with atherosclerosis could conceivably result from a rheological effect of red cells on atherogenesis mediated by their interactions with the endothelium and/or platelets.

In the same study on 50 men undergoing coronary arteriography [102], we also found an association of the plasma fibrinogen level with the extent of coronary atherosclerosis, and this has been confirmed in a further study of 100 men (G.D.O. Lowe and M. Small, unpublished). This association may reflect effects of fibrinogen on atherogenesis via its actions on rheology, platelets, or fibrin formation as previously discussed. Alternatively, increased fibrinogen levels may promote infiltration of fibrinogen into developing arterial lesions, of which fibrinogen is a major (but neglected) component [106,107].

Copley [108] has suggested that the endothelial lining of fibrinogen/fibrin (EEFL) may be of importance in atherogenesis. Low density lipoproteins (LDL) may either adsorb to the EEFL, or else be taken up by a layered thrombus of fibrinogen aggregates or gel (fibrinogenin). The latter pathway was suggested as a result of rheological findings that LDL - fibrinogen surface layers *in vitro* are poorly structured. Hence it was proposed that such structures *in vivo* might permit increased uptake of LDL and fibrinogen into the arterial wall [108].

A correlation between the white cell count and the extent of coronary atherosclerosis has recently been described [109]; whether this has any rheological significance is unknown.

7.5.3. Occlusive arterial thrombi on atherosclerotic plaques

Thrombi arising on coronary atherosclerotic plaques are now believed to occur in most cases of acute coronary events, whether sudden coronary death, myocardial infarction, or unstable angina [110-112]; thrombosis in cases of sudden coronary death may have been missed in previous studies due to intense fibrinolytic activity [113]. The coronary atherosclerotic plaques have usually caused stenosis and are ruptured or ulcerated [111,114]. Thromboembolism causing transient ischemia or major infarction of the brain or limbs usually arises, if not from a cardiac source, from stenosing and/or ulcerated atheromatous lesions in the supplying arteries [115-117].

The mechanisms causing an occlusive thrombus to occur on a stenosing lesion are not understood. Ulceration obviously exposes blood to subendothelium containing collagen, lipids and cell debris, all of which might activate platelets and coagulation. Furthermore, subendothelium and especially atherosclerotic plaques are deficient in the platelet inhibitor, prostacyclin. However, the factors which produce ulceration or rupture of arterial plaques are also poorly understood.

High shear stresses may be expected at critical arterial stenoses, and it is possible that these might promote mechanical ulceration and/or platelet activation. Dintenfass [4] suggested that stenoses, with their high shear stresses, could act like machine-guns, shooting platelet aggregates into the distal circulation. Platelet microaggregates have indeed been found distal to arterial stenoses in necropsy studies of the heart [118]. Born and Wehmeyer [45] suggested that high shear stresses might liberate ADP from red cells at stenoses and also during plaque rupture, promoting platelet activation and thromboses. Furthermore, activated platelets and products released from such high shear areas could recirculate and contact the vessel wall in areas of flow separation distal to the arterial stenoses, favouring post-stenotic thrombosis. Figure 7.5 shows this sequence of possible rheological effects [5].

Several epidemiological studies [119-133] have shown that high-normal levels of hematocrit (or hemoglobin), plasma fibrinogen (or erythrocyte sedimentation rate, ESR), and white cell count are primary risk factors for sudden coronary death, myocardial infarction, unstable angina, or stroke (Table 7.1). These

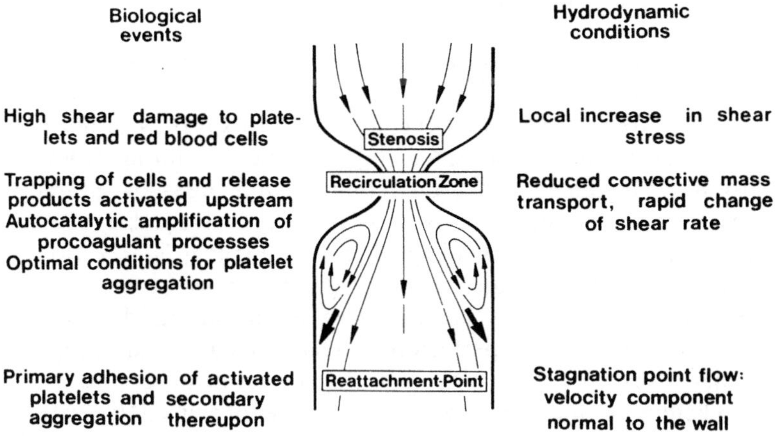

Figure 7.5. Hydrodynamic conditions at an arterial stenosis, and the possible biological consequences in blood which may promote arterial thrombosis. Reproduced from (5), by permission of H. Schmid-Schönbein and Schattauer-Verlag.

associations might conceivably result from rheological effects promoting thrombosis.

Primary prevention studies are required to investigate causal roles for these factors. A primary prevention study using clofibrate, which lowers plasma fibrinogen levels as well as lipids, reduced the incidence of non-fatal myocardial infarction but increased total mortality, for reasons which are still unexplained [134].

Table 7.1. Primary risk factors for coronary events and stroke.

	Coronary events	Stroke
Hematocrit/hemoglobin level	Elwood et al. 1974 (119)	Heyman et al. 1971 (130)
	Dawber et al. 1977 (120)	Kannel et al. 1972 (131)
	Bottiger & Carlson 1980 (121)	Kagan et al. 1980 (132)
	Sorlie et al. 1981 (122)	
	Carter et al. 1983 (123)	
White cell count	Friedman et al. 1974 (124)	Prentice et al. 1982 (133)
	Zalokar et al. 1981 (125)	
	Prentice et al. 1982 (126)	
Fibrinogen/E.S.R.	Bottiger & Carlson 1980 (121)	Wilhelmsen et al. 1984 (129)
	Meade et al. 1980 (127)	
	Stone & Thorp 1983 (128)	
	Wilhelmsen et al. 1984 (129)	

7.5.4. Outcome of occlusive arterial thrombosis

Further epidemiological studies have shown that some rheological factors, measured on admission to hospital, have prognostic significance in stroke or myocardial infarction. It is therefore possible that rheological factors influence not only thrombosis, but also the extent of ischemia and infarction resulting from the thrombotic occlusion. It is generally accepted that around areas of infarcting brain [135] or myocardium [136] there is a potentially salvageable area of ischemia. It is quite conceivable that rheological factors might influence flow in these areas of borderline viability. Vascular autoregulation may be impaired in acute ischemia, rendering rheological factors more important in determining flow. Moreover, the abrupt fall in perfusion pressure distal to an occlusive thrombus may render it insufficient to overcome rheological obstructions.

Experimental ischemia of the brain or heart can be produced by arterial occlusion: following relief of the occlusion return of flow in some areas may be delayed or absent, i.e. the so-called *no-reflow phenomenon* [137,138]. Various explanations have been proposed for this phenomenon, including swelling of tissue cells or endothelial cells or hemorrhage. However, it is also possible that *no-reflow* might result from rheological occlusions, such as platelet aggregates [117,118], red cell aggregates which would be reversed by hemodilution [136,137] or white cell plugging of capillaries [139,140]. In a retrospective study of 316 cases of acute paretic stroke admitted to our medical unit, we found that hospital mortality was associated with increased admission levels of hematocrit, mean red cell volume, white cell count, ESR and serum globulin, and decreased levels of serum albumin [141]. Eleven percent of patients had hematocrits of 50% or more on admission: in younger patients, mortality was doubled at hematocrit of 50% or more (Fig. 7.6). We later found that similar relationships of mortality to hematocrit and white cell count had been observed in a large American study, although their significance had escaped comment [142]. The increased ESR in patients who died implies increased red cell aggregation, which was partly explained by the increased ratio of serum globulin to albumin [141]. However, it probably also reflected increased fibrinogen levels, which have been associated with increased mortality in stroke by Fletcher et al [143] and subsequently by ourselves (G.D.O. Lowe, unpublished).

A causal role for increased hematocrit and mortality in stroke is suggested by the experiments of Pollock et al [144], who showed that increasing the hematocrit in a gerbil stroke model increased infarct size, and doubled the mortality at hematocrits over 50%, this can be compared with the results in our younger stroke patients (Fig. 7.6). Harrison et al [105] also associated hematocrit with infarct size in stroke patients, while Grotta et al [145] showed inverse relationships between cerebral blood flow and both hematocrit and fibrinogen in patients with cerebral ischemia. As a result of all these studies, it seems reasonable to suggest that increased levels of hematocrit, fibrinogen and the serum globulin/al-

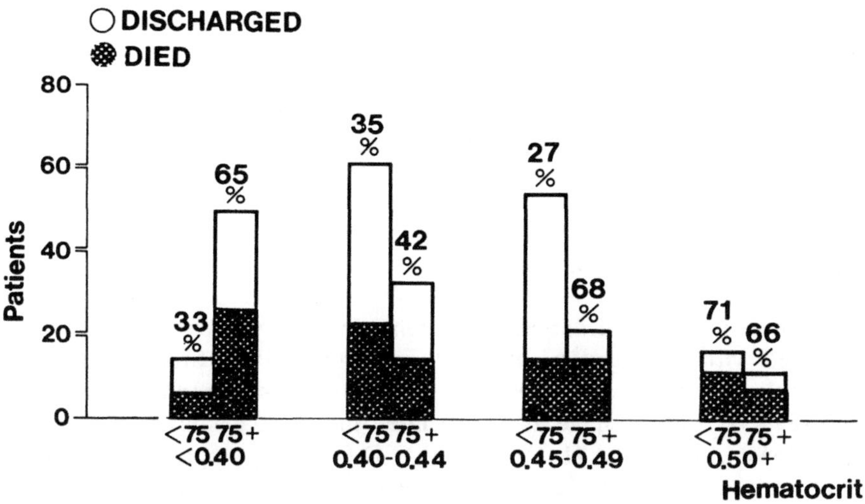

Figure 7.6. Mortality in acute stroke related to the hematocrit on admission, in patients younger than 75 years, and 75 or more. Note the doubled mortality in younger patients when hematocrit is 50% or more. Reproduced from (141), by permission of the Lancet.

bumin ratio increase red cell aggregation and blood viscosity. These rheological changes could reduce cerebral blood flow, particularly in ischemic areas with low perfusion pressures and disturbed autoregulation, resulting in increased infarct size and mortality (either directly from raised intracranial pressure from increased infarct size and ischemic edema, or indirectly from infection or pulmonary embolism in patients increasingly disabled as infarct size increases). Some support for this hypothesis comes from clinical trials of hemodilution [146] or defibrination [147] in acute stroke, although further controlled trials are required, possibly using oxygen-carrying fluids for hemodilution [136].

Our finding that increased white cell count predicted mortality in stroke [141] may reflect the contribution of white cell capillary plugging to cerebral ischemia [148]. The recent observations that pentoxifylline may improve cerebral ischemia [149] and white cell filtration [150] suggest that pharmacological improvement of white cell rheology may allow future testing of this hypothesis.

In acute myocardial infarction, increased hematocrit on admission does not appear predictive of mortality [151], whereas increased levels of white cell count and fibrinogen do appear of prognostic value [152]. Again, these associations may be due to adverse effects of white cell plugging [139] and the rheological effects of fibrinogen. Streptokinase reduces mortality as well as systemic and pulmonary arterial pressures in acute myocardial infarction, effects which might be due to reduction in fibrinogen and viscosity [153]. Clinical results of hemodilution in acute myocardial infarction have been inconclusive, but animal studies of hemodilution with oxygen-carrying fluids suggest that further studies would be worthwhile [136] (see Chapter 12).

Two recent studies have found that after recovery from myocardial infarction, coronary recurrence and death are related to the white cell count, but not to the hematocrit [154,155]. We have suggested that white cell capillary plugging may promote recurrent myocardial ischemia [155].

7.6. Thrombosis of arterial shunts and grafts

Relatively high hematocrits in patients with renal failure (greater than 30%) have been associated with occlusion of their arterial shunts [156]. Increased plasma fibrinogen levels have been associated with late occlusion of arterial grafts to the lower limb [55,157] and we have also associated increased hematocrit with late occlusion of lower limb grafts (J. Drury and G.D.O. Lowe, unpublished). These associations may reflect the rheological effects on platelets and thrombosis previously discussed in section 7.2. of this Chapter, and it would be interesting to know if similar associations apply in coronary arterial bypass grafts.

7.7. Microvascular thrombosis

7.7.1. Disseminated intravascular coagulation

Microvascular thrombosis (or disseminated intravascular coagulation, DIC) occurs in many forms of shock and in more chronic disorders such as malignant hypertension, hemolytic uremic syndrome and thrombotic thrombocytopenic purpura [158]. The etiology and pathogenesis are complex, but may include some rheological aspects. Fragmentation of red cells is commonly observed in blood films, and is thought to arise from damage by fibrin strands in the microcirculation. This microangiopathic hemolysis could activate platelets by release of ADP. DIC commonly arises in sick patients with high white cell counts and fibrinogen levels. Gurewich et al [159] showed a correlation between the extent of intravascular fibrin deposition induced by endotoxin in animals and the white cell count and fibrinogen level. These associations may partly reflect rheological influences of white cells and fibrinogen in the microcirculation of sick patients. For example, progressive white cell plugging of skeletal muscle capillaries occurs in shock [140], possibly promoting vascular injury and activation of coagulation.

7.7.2. Leukostasis

In hyperleukocytic leukemias, small blood vessels may be blocked by packed white cells, with or without fibrin. Leukostasis, or the "hyperleukocytic syndrome", is increasingly recognised as an important cause of morbidity and mortality in leukemia [160,161]. The clinical features appear to correlate with the rheology of different types of leukemic cells [161]. Harris [162] has drawn attention to the circulatory hazards of red cell transfusion, which may cause a further increase in viscosity, in such patients.

7.8. References

1. Hirsh J., Genton E., Hull R. 1981: Venous thromboembolism. New York: Grune and Stratton, 335 pp.
2. Sevitt S. 1984: Pathology and pathogenesis of deep vein thrombi. In: Tesi M., Dormandy J.A. (eds). Superficial and deep venous disorders of the lower limbs. Turin: Edizioni Panminerva Medici, pp. 45-58.
3. Mitchell J.R.A. 1976: Has our basic knowledge of cerebrovascular disease led to effective and rational treatment? In: Gillingham F.J., Mawdsley C., Williams A.E. (eds). Stroke. Edinburgh: Churchill Livingstone, pp. 301-316.
4. Dintenfass L. 1971: Blood microrheology-viscosity factors in blood flow, ischaemia and thrombosis. London: Butterworth, 445 pp.
5. Schmid-Schönbein H. 1983: Haemorheology and thrombosis. In: van de Loo J., Prentice C.R.M., Beller F.K. (eds): The thromboembolic disorders. Stuttgart: Schattauer, pp. 45-64.
6. Macfarlane R.G. 1977: Introduction. Br. Med. Bull. 33, 183-185.
7. Harker L.A., Slichter S.J. 1972: The bleeding time as a screening test for evaluation of platelet function. N. Engl. J. Med. 287, 155-159.
8. Sixma J.J. 1981: Role of blood vessel, platelet and coagulation interactions in haemostasis. In: Bloom A.L., Thomas D.P. (eds). Haemostasis and thrombosis. Edinburgh: Churchill Livingstone, pp. 252-267.
9. Tangelder G.J. 1982: Distribution and orientation of blood platelets flowing in small arterioles. Doctoral Thesis, Rijksuniversiteit Limburg, Maastricht.
10. Goldsmith H.L., Karino T. 1980: Physical and mathematical models of blood flow: experimental studies. In: Cokelet G.R., Meiselman H.J., Brooks D.E. (eds). Erythrocyte mechanics and blood flow. New York: Alan R. Liss, Inc., pp. 165-194.
11. Gaehtgens P., Brunner R., Pries A.R., Kanzow G. 1981: Physiological dilution of blood in the microvasculature. Bibl. Haematol. 47, 5-13.
12. Duke W.W. 1910: The relation of blood platelets to haemorrhagic disease. JAMA 60, 1185-1192.
13. Hellem A.J., Borchgrevink C.F., Ames S.B. 1961: The role of red cells in haemostasis: the relation between haematocrit, bleeding time and platelet adhesiveness. Br. J. Haematol. 7, 42-50.
14. Livio M., Gotti E., Marchesi D., Mecca G., Remuzzi K.G., de Gaetano G. 1982: Uraemic bleeding: role of anaemia and beneficial effect of red cell transfusions. Lancet 2, 1013-1015.
15. Small M., Lowe G.D.O., Cameron E., Forbes C.D. 1983: Contribution of the haematocrit to the bleeding time. Haemostasis 13, 379-384.
16. Jackson C.W., Smith P.J., Edwards C.C., Whidden M.A. 1979: Relationship between packed cell volume, platelets and platelet survival in red blood cell - hypertransfused mice. J. Lab. Clin. Med. 94, 505-509.
17. Challoner T., Bain B., Briggs C., Rampling M.W., Sirs J.A., Thomas D.J. 1981: Rheological, biochemical and haematological consequences of serial venesection. Abstracts of Second European Conference on Clinical Hemorheology, London, 1981, p. 40.
18. Turitto V.T., Baumgartner H.R. 1983: Platelet adhesion. In: Harker L.A., Zimmerman T.S. (eds). Measurements of platelet function. Edinburgh: Churchill Livingstone, pp. 46-63.

19. Ludlam C.A. 1981: Assessment of platelet function. In: Bloom A.L. and Thomas D.P. (eds). Haemostasis and thrombosis. Edinburgh: Churchill Livingstone pp. 775-795.
20. Turitto V.T., Weiss H.J. 1980: Red blood cells - their dual role in thrombus formation. Science 207, 541-543.
21. Aarts P.A.M.M., Bolhus P.A., Sakariassen K.S., Heethar R.M., Sixma J.J. 1983: Red blood cell size is important for adherence of blood platelets to artery subendothelium. Blood 62, 214-217.
22. Aarts P.A.M.M., Heethar R.M., Sixma J.J. 1984: Red blood cell deformability influences platelets - vessel wall interaction in flowing blood. Blood 64, 1228-1233.
23. Kinlough-Rathbone R.L., Packham M.A., Mustard J.F. 1983: Platelet aggregation. In: Harker L.A., Zimmerman T.S. (eds). Measurements of platelet function. Edinburgh: Churchill Livingstone, pp. 64-91.
24. Born G.V.R. 1962: Aggregation of blood platelets by adenosine diphosphate and its reversal. Nature 194, 927-929.
25. O'Brien J.R. 1962: Platelet aggregation. I. Some effects of the adenosine phosphates, thrombin and cocaine upon platelet adhesiveness. J. Clin. Pathol. 15, 446-452.
26. Frojmovic M.M. 1973: Quantitative parameterization of the light transmission properties of citrated, platelet-rich plasma as a function of platelet and adenosine diphosphate concentrations and temperature. J. Lab. Clin. Med. 82, 137-153.
27. Yu S.K., Latour J.G., Marchandise B., Bois M. 1978: Shear stress-induced changes in platelet reactivity. Thrombos. Haemostas. 40, 551-560.
28. Wurzinger L.J., Optiz R., Blasberg P., Eschweiler H., Schmid-Schönbein H. 1983: The role of hydrodynamic factors in platelet activation and thrombotic events: the effects of shear stress of short duration. In: Schettler G., Nerem R.M., Schmid-Schönbein H., Mörl H., Diehm C. (eds). Fluid dynamics as a localizing factor for atherosclerosis. Berlin: Springer Verlag pp. 91-102.
29. Anderson G.H., Hellums J.D., Moake J., Alfrey C.P. Jr. 1978: Platelet response to shear stress: changes in serotonin uptake, serotonin release, and ADP-induced aggregation. Thrombos. Res. 13, 1039-1047.
30. Stevens D.E., Joist J.H., Sutera S.P. 1980: Role of platelet-prostaglandin synthesis in shear-induced platelet alterations. Blood 56, 753-758.
31. Born G.V.R. 1977: Fluid-mechanical and biochemical interactions in haemostasis. Br. Med. Bull. 33, 193-197.
32. Zwaal R.F.A., Rosing J., Tans G., Bevers E.M., Hemker H.C. 1980: Topological and kinetic aspects of phospholipids in blood coagulation. In: Mann K.G., Taylor F.B. (eds): The regulation of coagulation. New York: Elsevier North Holland, pp. 95-112.
33. Yung W., Frojmovic M.M. 1982: Platelet aggregation in laminar flow - ADP concentration, time and shear rate dependence. Thrombos. Res. 28, 361-377.
34. Moritz M.W., Reimers R.C., Baker R.K., Sutera S.P., Joist J.H. 1983: Role of cytoplasmic and releasable ADP in platelet aggregation induced by laminar shear stress. J. Lab. Clin. Med. 101, 537-544.
35. Jen C.J., McIntire L.V. 1984: Characteristics of shear-induced aggregation in whole blood. J. Lab. Clin. Med. 103, 115-124.
36. Dewitz T.S., Martin R.R., Hung T.C., McIntire L.V. 1977: Mechanical trauma in leukocytes. J. Lab. Clin. Med. 90, 728-736.
37. Hellem A.J. 1960: The adhesiveness of human blood platelets in vitro. Scand. J. Clin. Lab. Invest. Supplement 51, 1-117.
38. Hellem A.J., Odegaard A.E., Skalhegg B.A. 1963: Investigations on adenosine diphosphate (ADP) induced platelet adhesiveness in vitro. I. The ADP-platelet reaction in various experimental conditions. Thrombos. Diath. Haemorrh. 10, 70-80.
39. Harrison M.J.G., Mitchell J.R.A. 1966: The influence of red blood-cells on platelet adhesiveness. Lancet ii, 1163-1164.
40. Schmid-Schönbein H., Born G.V.R., Richardson P.D., Cusack N., Rieger H., Forst R., Rohling-

Winkel I., Blasberg P., Wehmeyer A. 1981: Rheology of thrombotic processes in flow - the interaction of erythrocytes and thrombocytes subjected to high flow forces. Biorheology 18, 415-444.

41. Reimers R.C., Sutera S.P., Joist J.H. 1984: Potentiation by red blood cells of shear-induced platelet aggregation: relative importance of chemical and physical mechanisms. Blood 64, 1200-1206.
42. Born G.V.R., Bergqvist D., Arfors K.E. 1976: Evidence for inhibition of platelet activation in blood by a drug effect on erythrocytes. Nature 259, 233-235.
43. Bergqvist D., Arfors K.E. 1980: Haemostatic platelet plug formation in the isolated rabbit mesenteric preparation - an analysis of red blood cell participation. Thrombos. Haemostas. 44, 6-8.
44. Zawilska K.M., Born G.V.R., Begent N.A. 1982: Effect of ADP-utilising enzymes on the arterial bleeding time in rats and rabbits. Br. J. Haematol. 50, 317-325.
45. Born G.V.R., Wehmeyer A. 1979: Inhibition of platelet thrombus formation by chlorpromazine acting to diminish haemolysis. Nature 282, 212-213.
46. Zahavi J.: Personal communication.
47. Aursnes I., Gjesdal K., Abildgaard U. 1981: Platelet aggregation induced by ADP from unsheared erythrocytes at physiological Ca++ concentration. Br. J. Haematol. 47, 149-152.
48. Aursnes I., Vikholm V. 1984: On a possible interaction between ADP and mechanical stimulation in platelet activation. Thrombos. Haemostas. 51, 54-56.
49. Saniabadi A.R., Lowe G.D.O., Barbenel J.C., Forbes C.D. 1984: A comparison of spontaneous platelet aggregation in whole blood with platelet rich plasma: additional evidence for the role of ADP. Thrombos. Haemostas. 51, 115-118.
50. Saniabadi A.R., Lowe G.D.O., Barbenel J.C., Forbes C.D. 1984: Haematocrit, bleeding time, and platelet aggregation. Lancet i, 1409-1410.
51. Burgess-Wilson M.E., Green S., Heptinstall S., Mitchell J.R.A. 1984: Spontaneous platelet aggregation in whole blood: dependence on age and haematocrit. Lancet ii, 1213.
52. Turitto V.T., Baumgartner H.R. 1979: Platelet interaction with subendothelium in flowing rabbit blood: effects of blood shear rate. Microvasc. Res. 17, 38-54.
53. Juhan I., Buonocore M., Jouve R., Vague P., Moulin J.P., Vialettes B. 1982: Abnormalities of erythrocyte deformability and platelet aggregation in insulin-dependent diabetics corrected by insulin in vivo and in vitro. Lancet i, 535-537.
54. Lowe G.D.O. 1984: Defibrination, blood flow and blood rheology. Clin. Hemorheol. 4, 15-28.
55. Zucker M.B., Vroman I. 1969: Platelet adhesion induced by fibrinogen adsorbed onto glass. Proc. Soc. Exper. Biol. Med. 131, 318-320.
56. Hamer J.D., Ashton F., Meynell M.J. 1973: Factors affecting prognosis in the surgery of peripheral vascular disease: platelet adhesiveness, plasma fibrinogen and fibrinolysis. Br. J. Surg. 60, 386-389.
57. Lyman B., Rosenberg L., Karpatkin S. 1971: Biochemical and biophysical aspects of human platelet adhesion to collagen fibers. J. Clin. Invest. 50, 1854-1863.
58. Lowe G.D.O., Reavey M.M., Johnston R.V., Forbes C.D., Prentice C.R.M. 1979: Increased platelet aggregates in vascular and non-vascular illness - correlation with plasma fibrinogen and effect of ancrod. Thrombos. Res. 14, 377-386.
59. Meade T.W., Vickers M.V., Thompson S.G., Stirling Y., Haines A.P., Miller G.J. 1985: Epidemiological characteristics of platelet aggregability. Br. Med. J. 290, 428-432.
60. Egberg N., Johnsson H. 1972: Platelet aggregation induced by ADP and thrombin in reptilase defibrinated dogs. Thrombos. Res. 1, 95-112.
61. Turpie A.G.G., McNicol G.P., Douglas A.S. 1972: Platelet electrophoresis: effect of defibrination by ancrod (Arvin). Cardiovasc. Res. 6, 101-108.
62. Schultz J.S., Ciarkowski A.A., Lindenauer S.M., Penner J.A. 1978: Effects of hematological parameters on thrombus formation. Trans. Amer. Soc. Artif. Intern. organs. 24, 565-567.

63. Ernst E., Matrai A., Dormandy J.A. 1984: Shear dependence of blood coagulation. Clin. Hemorheol. 4, 395-399.
64. Ardlie N.G., Kinlough R.L., Schwartz C.J. 1966: In vitro thrombosis and platelet aggregation in myocardial infarction. Br. Med. J. i, 888-891.
65. Freidman A.H., Cliffton E.E. 1958: Effect of fibrinogen concentration on susceptibility of clots to in vitro lysis with plasmin. Thrombos. Diath. Haemorrh. 2, 269-278.
66. Brass E.P., Forman W.B., Edwards R.V., Lindan O. 1976: Fibrin formation: the role of the fibrinogen-fibrin monomer complex. Thrombos. Haemostas. 36, 37-48.
67. Copley A.L. (ed) 1983: The Endoendothelial Fibrin Lining. Oxford: Pergamon Press, 160 pp.
68. Copley A.L., King R.G. 1984: A survey of surface hemorheological experiments on the inhibition of fibrinogenin formation employing surface layers of fibrinogen systems with heparins and other substances. A contribution on antithrombogenic action. Thrombos. Res. 35, 237-256.
69. Karino T., Motomiya M. 1984: Flow through a venous valve and its implication for thrombus formation. Thrombos. Res. 36, 245-257.
70. Hamer J.D., Malone P.C., Silver I.A. 1981: The PO_2 in venous valve pockets: its possible bearing on thrombogenesis. Br. J. Surg. 68, 166-170.
71. Okoye G.C., Evans J.H., Beattie J., Lowe G.D.O., Lorimer A.R., Forbes C.D. 1984: Response of femoral venous oxygen tension to graduated pressure stockings - possible relationship to deep vein thrombosis. Thrombos. Haemostas. 51, 103-104.
72. Kakkar V.V. 1981: Prevention of venous thromboembolism. Clin. Haematol. 10, 543-582.
73. Chien S. 1975: Biophysical behavior of red cells in suspensions. In: Surgenor D.M. (ed). The Red Blood Cell. New York: Academic Press, pp. 1031-1133.
74. Wessler S. 1975: Factors in the initiation of deep venous thrombosis. In: Nicolaides A.N. (ed). Thromboembolism. Lancaster: Medical and Technical Publishing Co. pp. 9-28.
75. Lowe G.D.O. 1984: Blood rheology and venous thrombosis. Clin. Hemorheol. 4, 571-588.
76. Meyerowitz B.R., Nelson R. 1964: Measurement of the velocity of blood in lower limb veins with and without compression. Surgery 56, 481-486.
77. Wilkins R.W., Stanton J.R. 1953: Elastic stockings in the prevention of pulmonary embolism. N. Engl. J. Med. 248, 1087-1091.
78. Moyses C., Michel C.C. 1984: Fluid balance between blood and tissues in the feet. Int. J. Microcirc. Clin. Exper. 3, 354 (Abstract).
79. Pearson T.C., Wetherley-Mein G. 1978: Vascular occlusive episodes and venous haematocrit in primary proliferative polycythaemia. Lancet ii, 1219-1222.
80. Wasserman L.R., Gilbert H.S. 1963: Surgery in polycythaemia vera. N. Engl. J. Med. 269, 1226-1230.
81. Lawson D.H., Parker J.L.W. 1976: Deaths from severe megaloblastic anaemia in hospitalised patients. Scand. J. Haematol. 17, 347-352.
82. Mossey R.T., Kasabian A.A. Wilkes B.M., Mailloux L.U., Susin M., Bluestone P.A. 1982: Pulmonary embolism. Low incidence in chronic renal failure. Arch. Intern. Med. 142, 1646-1648.
83. Dormandy J.A. 1971: Influence of blood viscosity on blood flow and the effects of low molecular dextran. Br. Med. J. iv, 716-719.
84. Lowe G.D.O., Osborne D.H., McArdle B.M., Smith A., Carter D.C., Forbes C.D., McLaren D., Prentice C.R.M. 1982: Prediction and selective prophylaxis of venous thrombosis in elective gastrointestinal surgery. Lancet 1, 409-412.
85. Jones E.W., Mitchell J.R.A. 1983: Venous thrombosis in diabetes mellitus. Diabetologia 25, 502-505.
86. Lowe G.D.O., Campbell A.F., Meek D.R., Forbes C.D., Prentice C.R.M., Cummings S.W. 1978: Subcutaneous ancrod in prevention of deep-vein thrombosis after operation for fractured neck of femur. Lancet 2, 698-700.
87. Belch J.J.F., Meek D.R., Lowe G.D.O., Campbell A.F., Young A.B., Forbes C.D., Prentice

C.R.M. 1982: Subcutaneous ancrod in prevention of deep vein thrombosis after hip replacement surgery. Thrombos. Res. 25, 23-31.
88. Meissner A.G., O'Sullivan G., MacBeth R.A. 1976: The effect of defibrinogenation on pulmonary embolism in dogs. Thrombos. Diath. Haemorrh. 36, 140-145.
89. McGrath M.A., Wechsler F., Hunyor A.B.L., Penny R. 1978: Systemic factors contributing to retinal vein occlusion. Arch. Intern. Med. 138, 216-220.
90. Ring C.P., Pearson T.C., Sanders M.D., Wetherley-Mein G. 1976: Viscosity and retinal vein thrombosis. Br. J. Ophthalmol. 60, 397-410.
91. Trope G.E., Lowe G.D.O., McArdle B.M., Douglas J.T., Forbes C.D., Prentice C.R.M., Foulds W.S. 1983: Abnormal blood viscosity and haemostasis in long-standing retinal vein occlusion. Br. J. Ophthalmol. 67, 137-142.
92. Lowe G.D.O. 1984: Anticoagulants in cardiac thromboembolism, cardiac surgery, peripheral arterial disease and cerebrovascular disease. In: Meade T.W. (ed). Anticoagulants and Myocardial Infarction. A Reappraisal. Chichester: Wiley, pp. 203-221.
93. Asinger R.W., Mikell F.L., Elsperger J., Hodges M. 1981: Incidence of left ventricular thrombosis after acute transmural myocardial infarction: serial evaluation by two-dimenional echocardiography. N. Engl. J. Med. 305, 297-302.
94. Naumann A. 1979: Fluid dynamic aspects of mechanical haemolysis. In: Schmid-Schönbein H., Teitel P. (eds). Basic aspects of blood trauma. The Hague: Martinus Nijhoff, pp. 205-219.
95. Woolf N. 1982: Pathology of atherosclerosis. London: Butterworth Scientific, 322 pp.
96. Caro C.G. 1977: Mechanical factors in atherogenesis. In: Hwang W.H.C., Norman W.A. (eds). Cardiovascular flow dynamics and measurements. Baltimore: University Park Press, pp. 473-487.
97. Harker L.A., Schwartz S.M., Ross R. 1981: Endothelium and arteriosclerosis. Clin. Haematol. 10, 283-296.
98. Fox J.A., Hugh A.E. 1966: Localization of atheroma. A theory based on boundary layer separation. Br. Heart J. 28, 388-399.
99. Rowntree L.G., Shionaya T. 1927: Studies in experimental extracorporeal thrombus formation. Method for direct observation of extracorporeal thrombus formation. J. Exp. Med. 46, 7-18.
100. Mustard J.F., Murphy E.A., Rowsell H.C., Downie H.G. 1962: Factors influencing thrombus formation in vivo. Amer. J. Med. 33, 621-647.
101. Müller-Mohnssen H. 1976: Experimental results to the deposition hypothesis of atherosclerosis. Thrombos. Res. 8, 553-566.
102. Lowe G.D.O., Drummond M.M., Lorimer A.R., Hutton I., Forbes C.D., Prentice C.R.M., Barbenel J.C. 1980: Relationship between extent of coronary artery disease and blood viscosity. Br. Med. J. 1, 673-674.
103. Rhoads C.G., Blackwelder W.C., Stemmerman G.N., Hayashi T., Kagan A. 1978: Coronary risk factors and autopsy findings in Japanese-American men. Lab. Invest. 38, 304-311.
104. Tohgi H., Yamanouchi H., Murakami M., Kameyama M. 1978: Importance of haematocrit as a risk factor in cerebral infarction. Stroke 9, 369-374.
105. Harrison M.J.G., Pollock S., Kendall B.E., Marshall J. 1981: Effect of haematocrit on carotid stenosis and cerebral infarction. Lancet 2, 114-115.
106. Smith E.B., Alexander K.M., Massie I.B. 1976: Insoluble "fibrin" in human aortic intima. Quantitative studies on the relationship between insoluble "fibrin", soluble fibrinogen and low density lipoprotein. Atherosclerosis 23, 19-26.
107. Sadoshima S., Tanaka K. 1979: Fibrinogen and low density lipoprotein in the development of cerebral atherosclerosis. Atherosclerosis 34, 93-103.
108. Copley A.L. 1981: Hemorheological aspects of the endo-endothelial fibrin lining and of fibrinogen gel clotting. Their importance in physiology and pathological conditions. Clin. Hemorheol. 1, 9-72.
109. Kostis J.B., Turkerich D., Sharp J. 1984: Association between leukocyte count and the presence and extent of coronary atherosclerosis as determined by coronary arteriography. Amer. J. Cardiol. 53, 997-999.

110. De Wood M.A., Spores J., Notske R., Mouser L.T., Burroughs R., Golden M.S., Lang H.T. 1980: Prevalence of total coronary artery occlusion during the early hours of transmural myocardial infarction. N. Engl. J. Med. 303, 897-902.
111. Davies M.J., Thomas A. 1984: Thrombosis and acute coronary artery lesions in sudden cardiac ischaemic death. N. Engl. J. Med. 310, 1137-1140.
112. Capone G. J., Meyer B.B., Wolf N.M., Meister S.G. 1984: Incidence of intracoronary thrombi in patients with active unstable angina pectoris. Circulation 70, Supplement II, 415 (Abstract).
113. Meade T.W., Howarth D.J., Stirling Y., Welch T.P., Crompton M.R. 1984: Fibrinopeptide A and sudden coronary death. Lancet 2, 607-609.
114. Constantinides P. 1966: Plaque fissure in human coronary thrombosis. J. Atheroscler. Res. 6, 1-17.
115. Slaney G., Hamer J.D. 1973: Arterial embolism. In: Birnstingl M. (ed). Peripheral vascular surgery. London: Heinemann pp. 189-210.
116. Gautier J.C. 1979: Arterial pathology in cerebral ischaemia and infarction. In: Greenhalgh R.M., Rose F.C. (eds). Progress in Stroke Research I. Tunbridge Wells: Pitman Medical, pp. 28-39.
117. Harrison M.J.G. 1982: Pathogenesis. In: Warlow C., Morris P.J. (eds): Transient ischaemic attacks. New York: Marcel Dekker, pp. 21-46.
118. Haerem J.W. 1972: Platelet aggregates in intramyocardial vessels of patients dying suddenly and unexpectedly of coronary artery disease. Atherosclerosis 15, 199-213.
119. Elwood P.C., Benjamin I.T., Waters W.E., Sweetnam P.M. 1974: Mortality and anaemia in women. Lancet 1, 891-894.
120. Dawber T.R., Wolf P.A., Colton T., Nickerson R.J. 1977: Risk factors: comparison of the biological data in myocardial and brain infarctions. In: Zulch K.J., Kaufmann W., Hossman R.A., Hossman V. (eds). Brain and heart infarct. Berlin: Springer Verlag, pp. 226-252.
121. Böttiger L.E., Carlson L.A. 1980: Risk facors for ischaemic vascular death for men in the Stockholm Prospective Study. Atherosclerosis 36, 389-408.
122. Sorlie P.D., Garcia-Palmieri M.R., Costas R., Havlik R. 1981: Hematocrit and risk of coronary heart disease: the Puerto Rico Heart Health Program. Amer. Heart J. 101, 456-461.
123. Carter C., McGee D., Reed D., Yano K., Stemmermann G. 1983: Hematocrit and the risk of coronary heart disease: the Honolulu Heart Program. Amer. Heart J. 105, 674-679.
124. Friedman G.D., Klatsky A.L., Siegelaub A.B. 1974: The leukocyte count as a predictor of myocardial infarction. N. Engl. J. Med. 290, 1275-1278.
125. Zalokar J.B., Richard J.L., Claude J.R. 1981: Leukocyte count, smoking and myocardial infarction. N. Engl. J. Med. 304, 465-468.
126. Prentice R.L., Szatrowski T.P., Fujikura T., Kato H., Mason M.W., Hamilton H.H. 1982: Leukocyte counts and coronary heart disease in a Japanese cohort. Amer. J. Epidemiol. 116, 496-509.
127. Meade T.W., North W.R.S., Chakrabarti R., Stirling Y., Haines A.P., Thompson S.G., Brozovic M. 1980: Haemostatic function and cardiovascular death: early results of a prospective study. Lancet 1, 1050-1054.
128. Stone M.C., Thorp J.M. 1983: Plasma fibrinogen - a major coronary risk factor. In: Lenzi S., Descovitch G.C. (eds). Atherosclerosis and cardiovascular diseases. Bologna: Editrice Compositori, pp. 3-10.
129. Wilhelmsen L., Svardsudd K., Korsan-Bengtsen K., Larsson B., Welin L., Tibblin G. 1984: Fibrinogen as a risk factor for stroke and myocardial infarction. N. Engl. J. Med. 311, 501-505.
130. Heyman A., Karp H.R., Heyden S., Bartel A., Cassel J.C., Tyroler H.A., Hames C.G. 1971: Cerebrovascular disease in the biracial population of Evans County, Georgia. Arch. Intern. Med. 128, 949-955.
131. Kannel W.B., Gordon T., Wolf P.A., McNamara P. 1972: Hemoglobin and the risk of cerebral infarction: the Framingham Study. Stroke 3, 409-420.

132. Kagan A., Popper J.S., Rhoads G.G. 1980: Factors related to stroke incidence in Hawaii Japanese men: the Honolulu Heart Study. Stroke 11, 14-21.
133. Prentice R.L., Szatrowski T.P., Kato H., Mason M.W. 1982: Leukocyte counts and cerebrovascular disease. J. Chron. Dis. 35, 703-714.
134. Committee of Principal Investigators 1984: W.H.O. Co-operative trial on primary prevention of ischaemic heart disease with clofibrate to lower serum cholesterol: final mortality follow-up. Lancet ii, 600-604.
135. Garcia J.H., Conger K.A., Lossinsky A.S., Kauffmann F.C. 1979: Ultrastructural and biochemical evidence for reversibility of regional cerebral ischaemia. In: Zulch K.J., Kaufmann W., Hossmann K.-A., Hossmann V. (eds). Brain and heart infarct II. Berlin: Springer-Verlag, pp. 157-170.
136. Biro G.P. 1981: Effect of hemodilution with dextran, stroma-free hemoglobin solution and fluosol-DA on experimental myocardial ischemia in the dog. Bibl. Haematol. 47, 54-69.
137. Fischer E.G., Ames A. 1972: Studies on mechanisms of impairment of cerebral circulation following ischaemia: effect of hemodilution and perfusion pressure. Stroke 3, 538-542.
138. Kloner R.A., Ganote C.E., Jennings R.B. 1974: The "no-reflow" phenomenon after temporary coronary occlusion in the dog. J. Clin. Invest. 54, 1496-1508.
139. Dahlgren M.D., Peterson M.A., Engler R.L., Schmid-Schönbein G.W. 1984: Leukocyte rheology in cardiac ischemia. In: Meiselman H.J., Lichtman M.A., LaCelle P.L. (eds). White cell mechanics. Basic science and clinical aspects. New York: Alan R.Liss, Inc., pp. 271-283.
140. Bagge U. 1984: Leukocytes and capillary perfusion in shock. In: Meiselman H.J., Lichtman M.A., LaCelle P.L. (eds). White cell mechanics. Basic science and clinical aspects. New York: Alan R. Liss, Inc., pp. 285-294.
141. Lowe G.D.O., Jaap A.J., Forbes C.D. 1983: Relation of atrial fibrillation and high haematocrit to mortality in acute stroke. Lancet i, 784-786.
142. The National Institute of Neurological and Communicative Disorders and Stroke 1981: The national survey of stroke. Stroke 121, Supplement 23-24.
143. Fletcher A.P., Alkjaersig N., Davies A., Lewis M., Brooks J., Hardin W., Landau W., Raichle M. 1976: Blood coagulation and plasma fibrinolytic enzyme system pathophysiology in stroke. Stroke 7, 337-348.
144. Pollock S., Tsitsopoulos P., Harrison M.J.G. 1982: The effect of hematocrit on cerebral perfusion and clinical status following carotid occlusion in the gerbil. Stroke 13, 167-170.
145. Grotta J., Ackerman R., Correia J., Fallick G., Chang J. 1982: Whole blood viscosity parameters and cerebral blood flow. Stroke 13, 296-301.
146. Gottstein U. 1981: Normovolemic and hypervolemic hemodilution in cerebrovascular ischemia. Bibl. Haematol. 47, 127-138.
147. Hossmann V., Heiss W.D., Bewermeyer H., Wiedemann G. 1983: Controlled trial of ancrod in ischemic stroke. Arch. Neurol. 40, 803-808.
148. Yamakawa T. 1982: Dynamics of white blood cells and red blood cells in microcirculatory networks of the cat brain cortex during hemorrhagic shock: intravital microscopic study. Microvasc. Res. 24, 218.
149. Hartmann A. 1981: Effect of pentoxifylline on regional cerebral blood flow in patients with cerebrovascular disease. Pharmatherapeutica 2, 528-531.
150. Schmalzer E.A., Chien S. 1984: Filterability of subpopulations of leukocytes: effect of Pentoxifylline. Blood 64, 542-546.
151. Hershberg P.I., Wells R.E., McGandy R.B. 1972: Hematocrit and prognosis in patients with acute myocardial infarction. JAMA 219, 855-860.
152. Haines A.P., Howarth D., North W.R.S., Goldenberg E., Stirling Y., Meade T.W., Raftery E.B., Millar-Craig M.W. 1983: Haemostatic variables and the outcome of myocardial infarction. Thrombos. Hemostas. 50, 800-803.
153. European Collaborative Study Group (1979: Streptokinase in acute myocardial infarction. N. Engl. J. Med. 301, 797-802.

154. Schlant R.C., Forman S., Stamler J., Canner P.L. 1982: The natural history of coronary heart disease: prognostic factors after recovery from myocardial infarction in 2789 men. The 5-year findings of the Coronary Drug Project. Circulation 66, 401-414.
155. Lowe G.D.O., Machado S.G., Krol W.F., Forbes C.D. 1985: White cell count and recurrent coronary events after myocardial infarction - an effect of myocardial capillary plugging? Clin. Sci. 68, Suppl. 11, 32P (Abstract).
156. Remuzzi G., Livio M., Poletti E., Mecca G., de Gaetano G., Donati M.B. 1978: Factors influencing the occlusion of vascular access for regular haemodialysis. A retrospective analysis. In: Coccheri S. (ed). Proceedings of 5th International Congress on thromboembolism. Bologna: Quaderni della Coagulazione, p. 248.
157. Harris P.L., Harvey D.R., Bliss B.P. 1978: The importance of plasma lipids, glucose, insulin and fibrinogen in femoropopliteal surgery. Br. J. Surg. 65, 197-200.
158. Brozovic M. 1981: Acquired disorders of blood coagulation. In: Bloom A.L., Thomas D.P. (eds). Haemostasis and thrombosis. Edinburgh: Churchill Livingstone, pp. 411-438.
159. Gurewich V., Lipinski B., Hyde E. 1976: The effect of the fibrinogen concentration and the leukocyte count on intravascular fibrin deposition from soluble fibrin monomer complexes. Thrombos. Haemostas. 36, 605-614.
160. McKee L.C., Collins R.D. 1974: Intravascular leukocytic thrombi and aggregates as a cause of morbidity and mortality in leukaemias. Medicine 53, 463-478.
161. Lichtman M.A., Rowe J.M. 1982: Hyperleukocytic leukaemias: Rheological, clinical and therapeutic considerations. Blood 60, 279-283.
162. Harris A.L. 1978: Leukostasis associated with blood transfusion in acute myeloid leukaemia. Br. Med. J. ii, 1169-1171.

8
Hemorheology and blood diseases

Pierre F. Leblond
Associate Professor of Medicine (Hematology), Faculty of Medicine, Université Laval and Centre d'Hématologie et d'Immunologie clinique, Hôpital du Saint-Sacrement, 1050 Chemin Ste-Foy, Quebec, Canada, G1S 4L8

8.1. Introduction

In the midst of a recent flurry of enthusiasm towards hemorheology as a potentially exciting new field of clinical investigation, one still finds among blood diseases some of the best available models for the study of disorders affecting blood flow in man. Quantitative or qualitative modifications in the various constituents of blood, while providing excellent diagnostic clues, can also lead to rheological disturbances capable of causing specific symptoms of their own. The past fifteen years have been marked by considerable progress in our ability to understand the properties of blood not only as a tissue but also as a circulating fluid. In several well-known hematological diseases, such knowledge has led to a better understanding of the mechanisms underlying various symptoms and to the application of more rational and effective therapeutic strategies. It is probably fair to say that hematology in this regard has opened the way to the vast amount of research currently being conducted in various other fields of medicine on the role played by hemorheological disturbances.

In this chapter, I will first examine, how various hematological diseases can lead to alterations in the rheological properties of blood and how, in turn, such disturbances can produce symptoms. In so doing, an attempt will be made to reinforce the concept, already proposed by Wells [1], that hyperviscosity can no longer be restricted to a single clinical syndrome. Next, the various specific blood diseases will be discussed in greater detail according to the general mechanism by which their features can lead to disturbance of blood flow. An effort will be made in each case to indicate how rheological considerations relate to their diagnostic as well as therapeutic approach.

8.2. The pathophysiology of blood hyperviscosity

The clinical manifestations of hyperviscosity can best be understood by briefly reviewing the role played by the various factors that govern normal blood rheology. The reader is referred to the first few chapters of this book for a more comprehensive review and illustration of these basic concepts.

Human whole blood is an unusual fluid in that its apparent viscosity, when measured at 37°C under conditions of steady laminar flow, varies according to the speed at which it is set into motion. This is especially true at shear rates of 50 s^{-1} or less, where a steep rise in viscosity is typically observed. Such behavior is commonly referred to as the *non-Newtonian* character of whole blood viscosity. In contrast, plasma alone, when separated by centrifugation and examined under the same standard conditions, behaves as a rheologically simple (*Newtonian*) fluid, its viscosity remaining quite the same at all shear rates [2].

This fundamental observation already tells us about two important issues in clinical hemorheology. The first is that an in vitro measurement of the viscosity of serum or plasma alone never reflects the totality of events occurring in vivo in a patient's circulation. The second is that the cellular elements, by acting as particles in suspension, are primarily responsible for the above-described non-Newtonian behavior of blood. For these reasons, one should expect the occurrence of rheological abnormalities in diseases affecting the blood cells themselves rather than only, as tradition has it, in those characterized by abnormal plasma proteins.

Among circulating blood cells, erythrocytes interact most significantly with plasma, mainly as a function of the amount of space which they occupy within the suspension. This leads to the importance of the hematocrit, or true cell concentration, in determining the viscosity of whole blood in vivo [3,4]. Yet, as discussed in Chapters 2 and 3, erythrocytes are not ordinary particles, having physical properties of their own capable of directly influencing blood flow regardless of the hematocrit. Using the "rheoscope", which allows direct microscopic examination of the cells inside a viscometer, Schmid-Schönbein [5] has described the occurrence of two important erythrocyte properties that bear direct relationship to the non-Newtonian behavior of whole blood. The first is the spontaneous aggregation of red cells which occurs at rest and results in the formation of rouleaux. As movement is started and the shear rate steadily increased, the forces of attraction that hold the cells together are progressively overcome by the stress created in the suspension and these large flow-resistant aggregates begin to break-up into small pieces until they reach their point of complete dispersion at a shear rate of approximately 50 s^{-1}. Blood viscosity, meanwhile, decreases about fivefold from its original value. Rouleaux formation is probably the most significant determinant of the normal shear-dependent behavior of whole blood, and the degree to which this phenomenon occurs is intimately related to the same factors that directly influence the viscosity of plasma itself [6]. High-molecular-weight proteins such as fibrinogen and the various immunoglobulins, by being passively adsorbed onto the red cell membrane, contribute to the formation of macromolecular bridges between cells, with a strength that is directly proportional to their concentration in plasma [1,2]. Thus, when suspended in a protein-free solution, red cells do not form rouleaux and flow quite easily at low shear rates. In contrast, blood viscosity is almost invariably abnormal in patients with diseases characterized by excessive rouleaux formation.

The second rheologically important phenomenon concerns the morphology of individual red cells. As the rotational speed of the rheoscope or viscometer increases, the shape of red cells changes progressively from that of a biconcave disk, tumbling about in all directions, to that of a fluid droplet remaining well oriented in the axis of flow, thereby causing less viscous resistance [5]. Erythrocyte deformability thus represents another important determinant of blood viscosity because it can influence the effective amount of space occupied by each individual particle in relation to that into which the entire suspension is allowed to flow. This, as opposed to the hematocrit, has been designated by Chien as the effective cell concentration [2]. Factors such as a low shear rate (i.e. insufficient stress to produce optimal deformation) or cell crowding (i.e. insufficient space to reach optimal deformation) tend to maximize the influcence of this property on the viscosity of whole blood [7]. The rheological influence of cell deformability is perhaps even more crucial in the microcirculation where the diameter of capillaries is often smaller than that of the cells themselves [8]. Viscosity in these very small vessels would rise almost infinitely if the cells were unable to adapt their contours to the small diameter. In certain conditions, even a slight departure from the normal deformability of erythrocytes may lead to serious clinical consequences [9].

Table 8.1. Hyperviscosity syndromes in hematological diseases.

I. Syndrome of polycythemic hyperviscosity	Diseases characterized by an increase in the *concentration* of circulating blood cells	– Erythrocytosis – Hyperleukocytic leukemia
II. Syndrome of sclerocythemic hyperviscosity	Diseases characterized by a decrease in the *deformability* of erythrocytes	– Sickle cell disease – Hemolytic anemias
III. Syndrome of plasmatic hyperviscosity	Diseases characterized by increases in plasma viscosity and the *aggregation* of erythrocytes	– Paraprotein diseases – Hematological stress syndrome

Based on these simplified premises, the general concept of hyperviscosity in hematological diseases may be viewed as a grouping of three distinguishable syndromes (Table 8.1), each originating from a specific mechanism and giving rise to a pattern of symptoms accompanied by typical laboratory abnormalities. We will now review each of these syndromes and the various specific diseases which they encompass. The reader is also referred to Chapter 5 for discussions of the pathophysiological significance of the rheological changes.

8.3. The syndrome of polycythemic hyperviscosity

This syndrome is typically observed in association with a pathological increase in the number or volume concentration of circulating erythrocytes and leukocytes. In clinical practice, the problem most often originates from the red cell line which, under normal circumstances, already occupies more than 95% of the total cell volume in whole blood. Diseases characterized by an increased circulating platelet count, while frequently associated with thromboembolic complications, do not generally cause hyperviscosity in the sense described here. Their manifestations rather stem from the coexistence of acquired abnormalities in the hemostatic function of platelets [10], a subject which is beyond the scope of the present review. This section, therefore, will deal mostly with the generic condition known as ERYTHROCYTOSIS and with the rheological problems associated with HYPERLEUKOCYTIC LEUKEMIA.

8.3.1. Erythrocytosis

This condition is defined as an elevation in the packed red cell volume above the value which is usually considered normal in a given individual. In adults, at or near sea level, hematocrit values exceeding 0.52 in males and 0.48 in females usually warrant the diagnosis of erythrocytosis [11], but in newborn babies a hematocrit of up to 0.65 is still considered acceptable [12].

Erythrocytosis may be relative or absolute, depending on whether it is due to a decrease in the plasma volume (spurious polycythemia) or a true increase in the total circulating red cell mass [13]. In certain individuals, true erythrocytosis may develop as an adaptive response to a decreased capacity to saturate their arterial blood hemoglobin with oxygen. Through physiological feedback, this leads to an increased production of erythropoietin with consequent stimulation of committed stem cells in the bone marrow to produce more circulating erythrocytes [14]. Examples of such a mechanism are found in life at high altitude [15], severe lung or heart diseases (with right-to-left blood shunting) [16,17] or certain unusual hemoglobinopathies in which the mutant molecule has an abnormally high affinity for oxygen [18]. All of these conditions are typically associated with a decrease in the measured arterial blood oxygen saturation (SAO_2) and often lead to a significant so-called "secondary appropriate erythrocytosis" [19]. Secondary erythrocytosis may also be of the inappropriate type when observed despite a normal SAO_2; this occurs in individuals who are afflicted with certain erythropoietin-secreting tumors from the kidneys, liver, uterus or cerebellum [20]. Erythrocytosis may also occur as a primary event in the form of Polycythemia Rubra Vera, a well known hematological disease characterized by an uncontrolled proliferation of the bone marrow pluripotential stem cell [21]. Circulating erythropoietin levels are extremely low in these patients, and in vitro erythroid colony growth occurs even in the absence of the hormone, two observations that confirm the autonomous nature of this myeloproliferative disorder [22,23].

A major consequence of erythrocytosis is a rise in whole blood viscosity, a phenomenon responsible for many of the symptoms experienced by patients afflicted with this condition [24]. The relationship between hematocrit and blood viscosity is not a linear one. As shown in Fig. 8.1, changes in hematocrit within the physiological range have a much lesser impact on viscosity than those which occur at higher, pathological values. This is due to the progressive inability of the more tightly packed erythrocytes to reach optimal deformation for streamlining, even at high shear rates, thus causing greater resistance to flow [25]. This phenomenon becomes even more pronounced at lower shear rates, when the stress necessary to produce deformation is reduced.

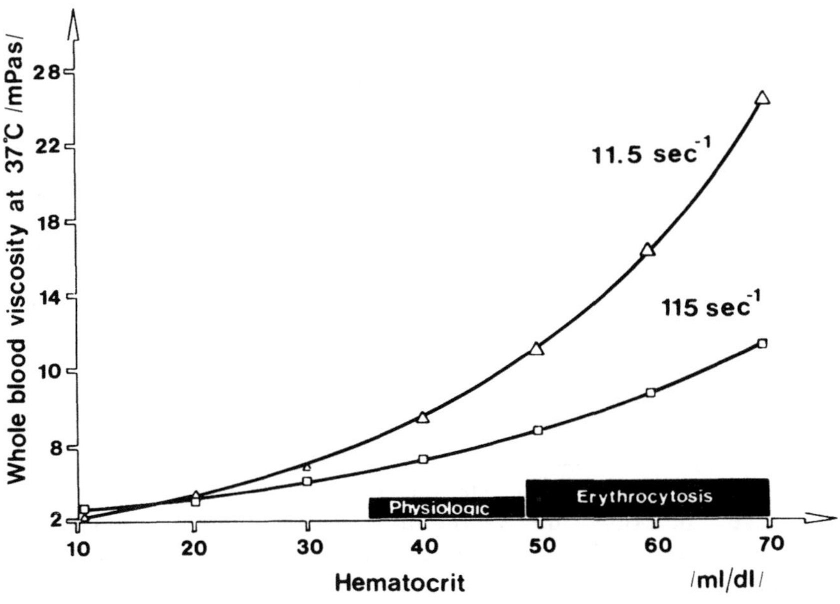

Figure 8.1. Relationship between whole blood viscosity and hematocrit. The non-linearity results in a greater rheological impact of small variations in hematocrit in individuals with erythrocytosis, especially at lower shear rates.

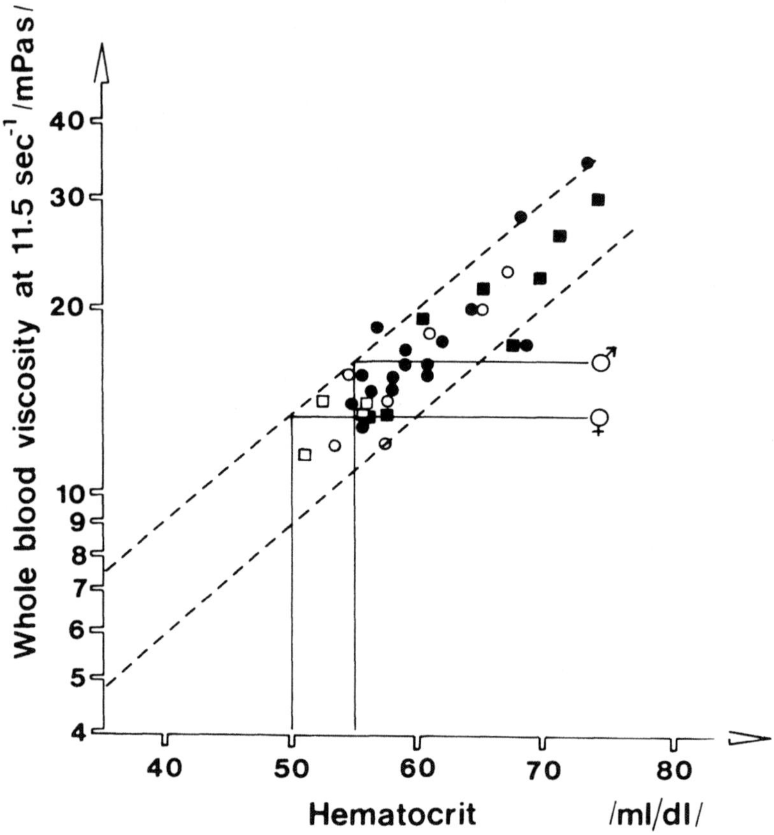

Figure 8.2. Whole blood viscosity in 22 individuals with relative or secondary erythrocytosis (circles) and 13 individuals with Polycythemia Vera (squares). Closed and open symbols represent males and females respectively. The dashed lines indicate the 95% confidence limits of the regression line of log viscosity vs. hematocrit established in 10 normal subjects at hematocrit values of 0.20 to 0.70. The solid lines indicate the upper limits of normal viscosity for a hematocrit of 0.50 in females and 0.55 in males.

Our experience with the measurement of whole blood viscosity in patients with erythrocytosis is depicted in Fig. 8.2. Viscosity is plotted here on a logarithmic scale, which results in a near-linear relationship with the hematocrit over the entire study range. The dotted lines represent the 95% confidence limits of the mean regression line established after testing blood samples from ten healthy volunteers (5 males and 5 females) at hematocrit values adjusted in the laboratory between 0.20 and 0.70. The mean (± 2 SD) value obtained for whole blood viscosity at 11.5 s^{-1} was 17.24 ± 5.13 mPas in 22 patients with relative or secondary erythrocytosis and 18.09 ± 5.06 mPas in 13 patients with Polycythemia

Vera, as compared to 7.88 ± 0.79 mPas in the normal controls. The average hematocrit in each group was 0.602, 0.616 and 0.428, respectively. Using the cut-off points indicated in the figure as the upper limits of normal for males and females, the existence of an absolute hyperviscosity was relatively more frequent in Polycythemia Vera patients [10/13 = 77%) than in those with other types of erythrocytosis [11/22 = 50%). A possible explanation for this phenomenon may relate to the more frequent occurrence of microcytosis due to iron deficiency in individuals with treated Polycythemia Vera [26], although such a contention has been recently disputed [27].

Most published series have confirmed the fact that patients with erythrocytosis, whatever the mechanism of their disease, experience thromboembolic complications with a frequency that exceeds that observed in a control age- and sex-matched population. Commonly cited figures indicate that 40% to 60% of these patients will develop vascular occlusive events of one type or another during the course of their disease corresponding to 7.5 episodes/10 patient-years, as opposed to an expected rate of 0.2/10 patient-years in the normal population [28]. Venous and arterial thromboses seem to occur with approximately the same frequency.

The cerebral circulation in these patients is significantly affected by the increase in blood viscosity, as demonstrated by the existence of an inverse relationship between cerebral blood flow and venous hematocrit [29]. A specific role of hyperviscosity is suggested by the fact that the improvement in blood flow observed after phlebotomy cannot be explained only by a change in the oxygen-carrying capacity of their circulating blood [28-30]. Complaints such as lightheadedness, vertigo, tinnitus and blurry vision are frequent in the early stages of the disease and may progress to typical cerebrovascular accidents, ranging from mild attacks of aphasia to the classical picture of a major stroke. Death due to cerebral thrombosis has been reported to occur up to five times more frequently in this disease than in a comparable population with a normal hematocrit [31]. Coronary artery disease, although to a lesser degree, is also a frequent complication when compared to its natural incidence, especially in females. Patients with Polycythemia Vera are also prone to develop peripheral microvascular complications, such as transient amaurosis or numbness in their fingers, sometimes evolving to pre-gangrenous lesions. Such events, however, are more likely to result from the coexistence of an increased platelet reactivity than from hyperviscosity itself, as judged by the beneficial effect obtained from the administration of low doses of aspirin [32].

Venous thrombosis most often affects the lower limbs, with or without pulmonary embolization. Although less frequent, thrombosis of the deep abdominal veins (portal, hepatic) has also been reported [13]. There is no doubt that the combination of an elevated hematocrit with the low shear rate that normally characterizes venous blood flow must act as a major determinant of hyperviscosity and blood stasis in these patients.

Erythrocyte aggregation, plasma viscosity or red cell deformability are otherwise usually normal in erythrocytosis [27]. Hence, in a given case, the approximate degree of hyperviscosity can be estimated from the level of the hematocrit by use of a mathematical formula that expresses the near exponential relationship between the two variables at a given shear rate. Data obtained in our laboratory using a Wells-Brookfield cone-in-plate viscometer have led us to use the following:

$$\text{at } 11.5\ s^{-1}: \ln(\text{viscosity}) = 0.0401 \times \text{Hct} + 0.3893 \quad (1)$$

$$\text{at } 115.0\ s^{-1}: \ln(\text{viscosity}) = 0.0255 \times \text{Hct} + 0.6333 \quad (2)$$

The relationship between blood viscosity and hematocrit is treated in more detail in Chapter 2.

Therapeutic measures should aim primarily at reducing the hematocrit. For this reason, phlebotomy remains the single most immediately effective remedy in these patients. Besides removal of the underlying cause when possible, long-term management of the disease should include the establishment of a chronic blood-letting program in order to prevent thromboembolic complications. Current evidence suggests that maintenance of the hematocrit towards the lower end of the normal range during treatment offers greater protection against vaso-occlusive episodes (0.20 vs 0.92 per 10 patients-years) than at the higher end [33]. This in itself raises interesting questions as to the existence of a possible relationship between the hematocrit and the incidence of vascular complications in the normal, non-erythrocytotic population, especially when other risk factors are present.

8.3.2. Hyperleukocytic leukemias

Approximately 5% of all patients with leukemia present with an extremely high leukocyte count accompanied by symptoms that strongly suggest the existence of underlying vascular occlusions in the lung, brain, retina and sometimes other organs [34]. Hyperviscosity due to the increased number of circulating white blood cells has frequently been advocated to explain the clinical manifestations that characterize this "hyperleukocytic syndrome".

It has been shown by Lichtman [35] that white blood cells can influence the bulk viscosity of whole blood in the same manner as erythrocytes, depending on the relative volume which they occupy within the suspension. Being less deformable, their comparative effect on viscosity is more pronounced than that of red cells and becomes apparent as soon as their concentration exceeds 0.15 (Fig. 8.3). Depending on the volume of individual leukemic cells, "leukocrits" of such magnitude may require circulating cell counts as high as 300,000/μl in acute or chronic myeloid leukemia and 800,000/μl in chronic lymphocytic leukemia [36]. Not only are such events quite rare, but consideration must also be given to the fact that hyperleukocytic leukemias are invariably accompanied by anemia in

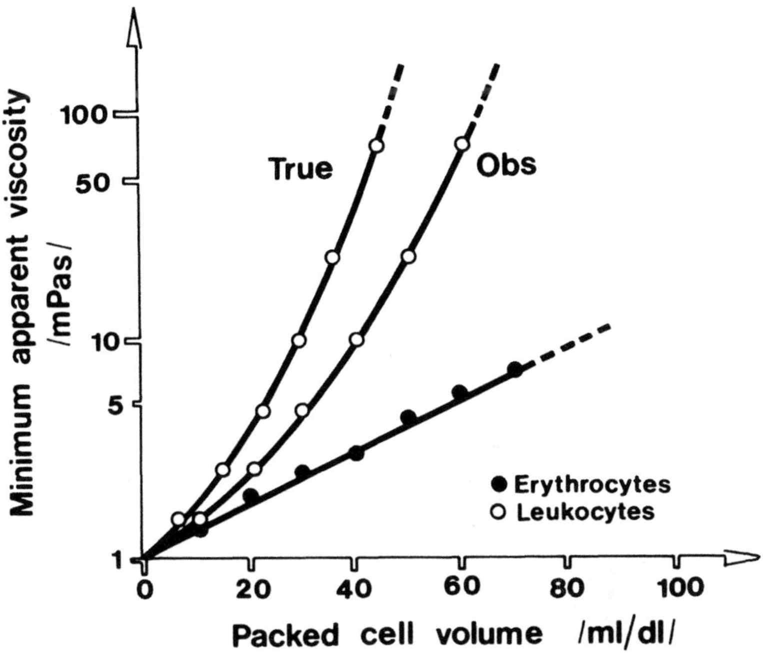

Figure 8.3. Comparative viscosity of suspensions of human erythrocytes and leukocytes in plasma following adjustment to specific packed cell volumes. The true leukocrit (True) was corrected for trapped plasma after multiplying the observed leukocrit (Obs) by the packing factor of 0.7. Minimum apparent viscosity is a value derived from the Casson equation fitted to the data for shear rates between 2 and 200 s^{-1}. Reproduced from (34) with permission of Dr. Lichtman and of Grune & Stratton.

which a fall in the erythrocrit usually exceeds the rise in leukocrit. The net result is that a measurable increase in the bulk viscosity of circulating whole blood is extremely rare in leukemia (Fig. 8.4) and remains virtually confined to a few cases of chronic myelogenous leukemia, especially when the disease occurs in younger patients [37].

Histopathological studies have shown that leukemic cell thrombi often seem to occlude small vessels in the lung or brain of hyperleukocytic patients [38], suggesting that blood stasis in the microcirculation plays an important role in the development of the syndrome. As already mentioned, cell deformability acts as a prime determinant of flow at the microcirculatory level, and the increased resistance of leukemic leukocytes, as opposed to normal mature cells, to traverse small porous membranes [39,40] or micropipette tips [41] in vitro suggests that their presence in large numbers in a patient's circulation could lead to the occlusion of vessels whose caliber is 75% or less that of the leukemic cell diameter [36]. This probably explains why the hyperleukocytic syndrome is often observed

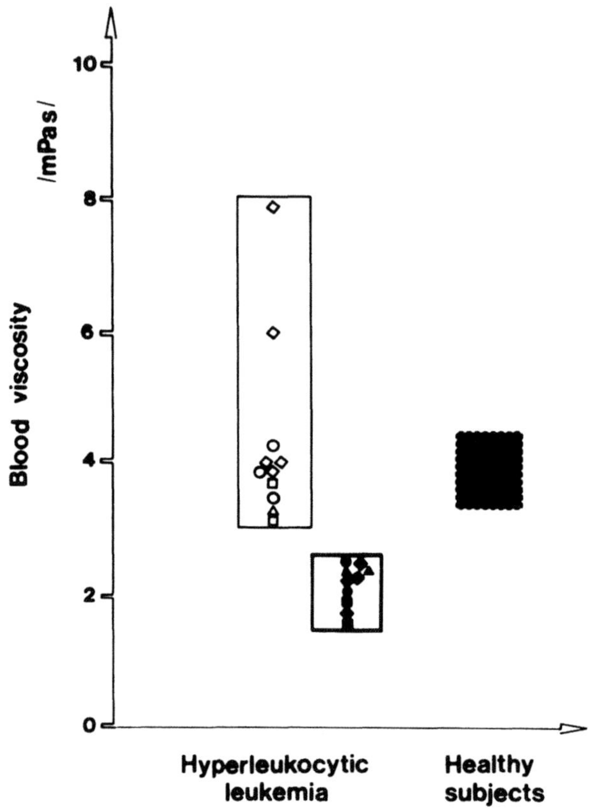

Figure 8.4. Blood viscosity in 11 subjects with hyperleukocytic leukemia compared to that of healthy controls. Open diamonds represent patients with chronic myeloid leukemia with leukocyte counts of 210,000 to 620,000/μl. Open circles are from three patients with acute myeloblastic leukemia with leucocyte counts of 160,000 to 230,000/μl. Open squares represent patients with acute lymphoblastic leukemia with leukocyte counts of 350,000 to 750,000/μl. The single open triangle is from a subject with chronic lymphocytic leukemia with a white cell count of 890,000/μl. The closed symbols represent the blood of these leukemic patients at the same erythrocrit but following removal of the original leukocytes. Reproduced from (34) with permission of Dr. Lichtman and of Grune & Stratton.

in patients whose blood viscosity, measured by standard techniques, is normal despite a very high circulating leukocyte count. The latter alone, from the clinician's viewpoint, certainly justifies the undertaking of specific measures to prevent irreversible tissue damage resulting from such a mechanism.

Most hematologists will consider that patients with acute leukemia presenting with a leukocyte count of 100,000/μl or more are at serious risk of developing leukostatic complications to the central nervous system [42] or the lungs [43], if they have not already done so. The preventive application of therapeutic measures starting at cell counts of 50,000/μl has also been advocated [37]. In chronic myeloid leukemia, the threshold appears to lie somewhat higher, i.e. in the vicinity of 250,000 to 300,000 cell/μl, whereas the risk seems practically non-existent in patients with chronic lymphocytic leukemia, despite leukocyte counts sometimes as high as 800,000/μl at the time of presentation.

Leukapheresis and the use of cytotoxic drugs are the two most effective measures which are applicable to alleviate the risk of hemorheological complications in patients with hyperleukocytic leukemias [44,45]. Since these procedures will not reverse the damage already caused by prior thrombotic events, it is highly important that their use be considered as soon as possible after initial evaluation of the patient. A single apheresis procedure using any one of the currently available cell separators may decrease the circulating leukocyte count by 20% to 60% in a few hours, depending on the total blood volume processed. Filtration leukapheresis should not be employed since most immature white blood cells will not adhere to glass or nylon wool as normal granulocytes do. In our experience, a rise in leukocytosis to pre-treatment levels almost inevitably occurs within 12 to 24 hours of the procedure if leukapheresis is utilized alone; hence it is important to institute concomitant treatment with one or more cytotoxic drugs, while continuing the use of apheresis until safe numbers are reached.

In hospitals where a cell separator is not available, the rapid institution of chemotherapy alone is the best way to obtain a rapid reduction in the leukocyte count. Fast-acting drugs such as hydroxyurea in sufficient doses are usually recommended for this purpose [45]. Appropriate care must be applied, in such circumstances, to minimize the extent of cytolysis-induced metabolic complications such as hyperuricemia and hyperkalemia, using proper adjunctive therapeutic and supportive measures.

8.4. The syndrome of sclerocythemic hyperviscosity

The common rheological denominator of this second syndrome is a decrease in the normal deformability of red blood cells. As mentioned previously, this property is of major importance in the microcirculation where the diameter of capillaries is often smaller than that of the cells themselves. Congenital or acquired disorders affecting the cell membrane, the hemoglobin molecule or the internal metabolic machinery of erythocytes are most often responsible for a decrease in erythrocyte deformability [46]. The consequences of such a situation depend in large part on the degree of resulting cell rigidity in relation to the specific requirements of the various portions of the microcirculation. Severe abnormalities such as those associated with SICKLE CELL DISEASE usually result in loss of tissue perfusion with acute and dramatic clinical consequences. In contrast, more subtle changes such as those associated with a variety of other

HEMOLYTIC ANEMIAS occur mostly at the expense of the red cells themselves, with little if any direct consequence to the body tissues.

Only the rheological aspects pertaining to this group of hematological diseases will be discussed here, as excellent reviews dealing with their clinical and biological characterization can be found elsewhere [47,48].

8.4.1. *Sickle cell disease*

Despite the progress accomplished in the past few decades concerning the origin, nature and pathophysiology of this devastating disease, little if any change has occurred in the ability of modern medicine to deal effectively with the painful crises experienced by patients afflicted with sickle-cell anemia, let alone to prevent their recurrence and the ensuing tissue damage which leads to premature death [49].

There is no doubt that the best available solution would be to prevent the sickling phenomenon, or the intense rigidification of hemoglobin S-containing erythrocytes that occurs at low oxygen tension, since there lies the essence of the problem. Unfortunately, the attempts that have been so far made at improving the solubility of deoxygenated hemoglobin S molecule using various pharmacological agents have been either unsuccessful or simply inapplicable [50]. While it appears that research along these same lines (i.e. anti-sickling agents) should remain an important priority, others feel that a careful examination of the rheological events that characterize the various clinical phases of sickle-cell disease represent another possible avenue for the development of useful therapeutic strategies [51].

In the asymptomatic steady state of sickle-cell anemia, whole blood viscosity, when adjusted to a standard hematocrit, is higher than that of normal control blood [52]. This is largely due to the presence of irreversibly sickled cells (ISC) in proportions that range between 1% and 40% depending on individuals, but that usually remain stable in any given patient throughout his lifetime [53]. While representing the morphological hallmark of the disease, ISC are also the erythrocytes that have the shortest in vivo survival in sickle-cell patients. It is believed that their formation results from the repetitive alternate exposure to oxygenated and deoxygenated atmospheres in the circulation, leading to irreversible membrane damage with losses of potassium and cell water and an intracytoplasmic accumulation of calcium [54,55]. These cells have been shown by a variety of techniques to be the densest and the least deformable erythrocytes in the blood of sickle-cell patients [56-60]. However, despite such striking abnormalities, there seems to be little if any correlation between the percentage of circulating ISC and the clinical severity of the disease in general [51].

Measurement of the bulk viscosity of sickle-cell blood following removal of ISC by centrifugation reveals the persistence of abnormally high values, even when the cells are resuspended in Ringer's solution to exclude the possible effects of fibrinogen and immunoglobulins on erythrocyte aggregation [61]. This strongly suggests that other non-ISC erythrocytes also have a reduced deformability. Recent studies on fully oxygenated red blood cells from homozygous sickle-cell patients have confirmed the existence of an abnormally high cytoplasmic viscosity and membrane visco-elasticity in a small but significant proportion of morphologically normal cells, corresponding with a higher-than-normal density and with an increased intracellular concentration of hemoglobin S [59]. When exposed in vitro to progressively decreasing oxygen tensions, red cell suspensions from asymptomatic patients, as one might expect, become progressively less deformable, a phenomenon which is less pronounced in heterozygous individuals and absent in normal controls [51]. Thus it appears that the reduction in red cell deformability in this disease is by no means confined to the ISC population. Although only a small fraction of these patients' erythrocytes are abnormally rigid at arterial oxygen saturation, their effect on the microcirculation may become magnified by a slower transit time. At the capillary level, where oxygen tension normally falls to much lower values, stasis caused by these flow-resistant cells may provide the necessary trigger to a chain of events ending in vascular obstruction with downstream tissue infarction.

Rheological studies performed during sickle cell crisis have shown an increase in whole blood viscosity when compared to baseline values obtained in the steady state. This may partly be explained by a parallel increase in the concentration of plasma fibrinogen during the first few days of the crisis, in association with the acute inflammatory response to tissue injury. Serial measurements, however, indicate that viscosity increases very early on during the crisis, even before the observed rise in fibrinogen, suggesting that red cell deformability may have a role in initiating the vasco-occlusive event [51]. In a careful study by Kenny et al [62], it was found that a significant reduction in erythrocyte filterability, as compared to steady-state values, occurred on day 1 and preceded by 4 to 5 days any significant rise in plasma viscosity. These authors have also found that ISC counts tend to remain stable or even to decrease slightly during crisis, and, therefore, that they cannot be responsible for this early fall in the deformability of the patient's erythrocytes. Further work will be required to clarify the exact nature of the rheological changes that occur at the very beginning of a sickle-cell crisis.

Animal models transfused with human sickle erythrocytes have been useful in confirming the ability of hemoglobin S-containing cells to retard capillary flow in vivo [63-66]. In these experiments, vascular obstruction was most often followed by a compensatory phase of "bolus flow" in response to an increase in the perfusion pressure to values exceeding those normally observed in arteriolar capillaries. Recently, Rodgers and coworkers, using a laser-Doppler velocimetry technique to study skin blood flow in six asymptomatic patients with sickle-cell disease, have demonstrated the existence of unique periodic oscillations in capillary flow [67]. Such broad oscillations were found neither in normal subjects nor in comparably anemic patients with beta-thalassemia, and they disappeared in one of their test-patients after the proportion of hemoglobin S-containing erythrocytes had been decreased to less than 40% by exchange transfusion with normal donor red cells. These results suggest that a significant reduction of flow in vivo may be caused by a small sub-population of rigid erythrocytes in asymptomatic patients with sickle-cell disease and that a synchronized vasomotor response operating at the arteriolar level probably acts as a compensatory mechanism [68]. Further use of this technology to document the dynamic state of the microcirculation during sickle-cell crisis in vivo will certainly be watched with considerable interest in the near future. However, at the present time, the nature of the rheological events that might possibly occur to the development of the painful crises of sickle-cell disease remain poorly understood.

8.4.2. Hemolytic anemias

Normal human erythrocytes survive on average 120 days in the circulation. From their initial migration across the bone marrow sinus walls [69] to their eventual removal from the vascular compartment, their survival is intimately related to their capacity to deform through the countless meanders of the microcirculation [70]. The hemolytic anemias are a group of hematological diseases characterized by a shortened survival of red blood cells in vivo. Their origin may be congenital or acquired, and usually relates to a defect in either the membrane, shape, metabolism or cytoplasmic content of the cell. Whatever the exact cause, a reduced deformability of erythrocytes stands out as the common denominator underlying the accelerated rate of cell destruction in most cases. The spleen by virtue of its unique microvasculature, plays an important role in this process [71].

The composite scanning electronmicrographs in Fig. 8.5 show the outside and inside surfaces of a sinusoid capillary from the red pulp of a human spleen. Blood cells entering the organ and progressing through the cords of Billroth must deform through the tiny slit-like apertures between endothelial cells in order to reach the sinus lumen and, eventually, the splenic vein [72]. This obstacle is probably the severest rheological test imposed upon individual red blood cells in vivo, and it is believed that the spleen, under normal circumstances, uses this mechanism to filter out naturally defective or senescent erythrocytes. In the hemolytic anemias, clinical and ultrastructural evidence (Fig. 8.6) suggests that this function becomes overtly exaggerated [73,74].

Membrane filtration and micropipette aspiration have been two of the most widely used techniques to study the deformability of circulating erythrocytes in patients with hemolytic anemias [75,70]. Fig. 8.7 shows the "filtration resistance index" measured in our laboratory with a Nuclepore membrane method in 40 patients with hemolytic anemias of various etiologies, compared to that obtained

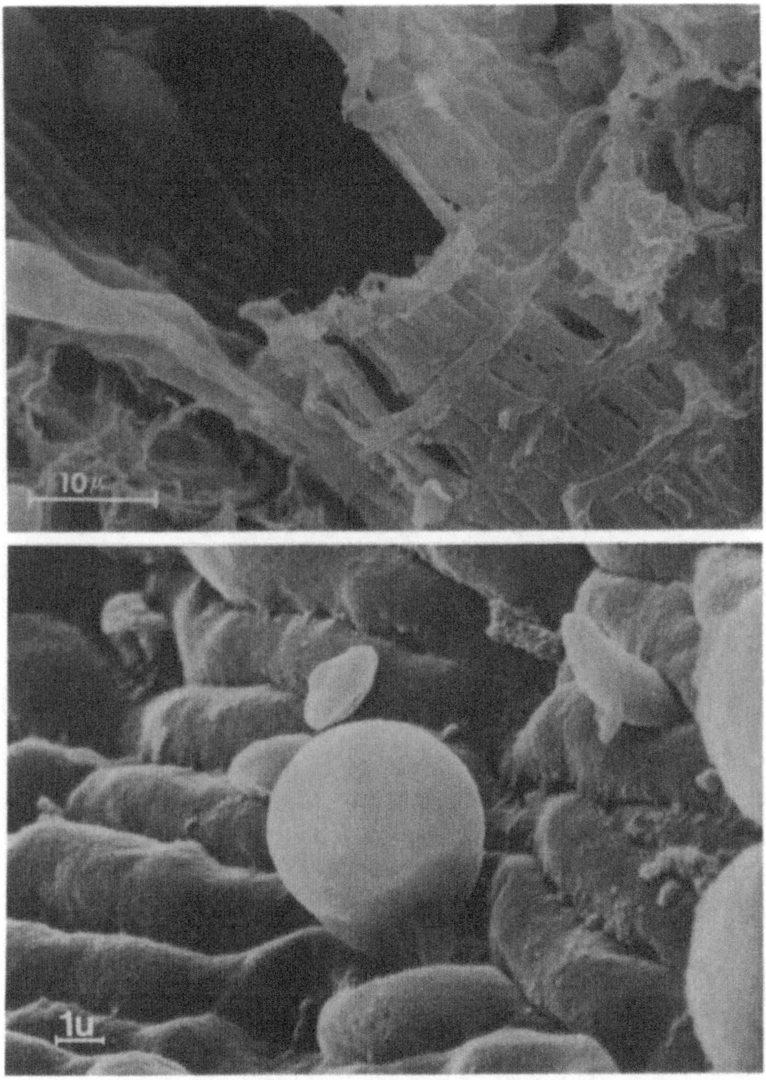

Figure 8.5. Scanning electron micrographs of post-surgical human spleen, rinsed and fixed by perfusion. Top: outer surface of a large sinusoid capillary showing parallel alignment of endothelial cells surrounded by "staves" of basement membrane material. Blood cells coming from the cords of Billroth must enter the lumen of the sinus by squeezing through tiny inter-endothelial slits. Bottom: inner surface of sinusoid with portion of a deformed red cell emerging from inter-endothelial space, presumably on its way from the cord.

in normal and splenectomized controls. Combined studies, using a single cell elastimetry (micropipette aspiration) technique, have shown that the presence of immature or "shift" reticulocytes in the blood of many of these patients also

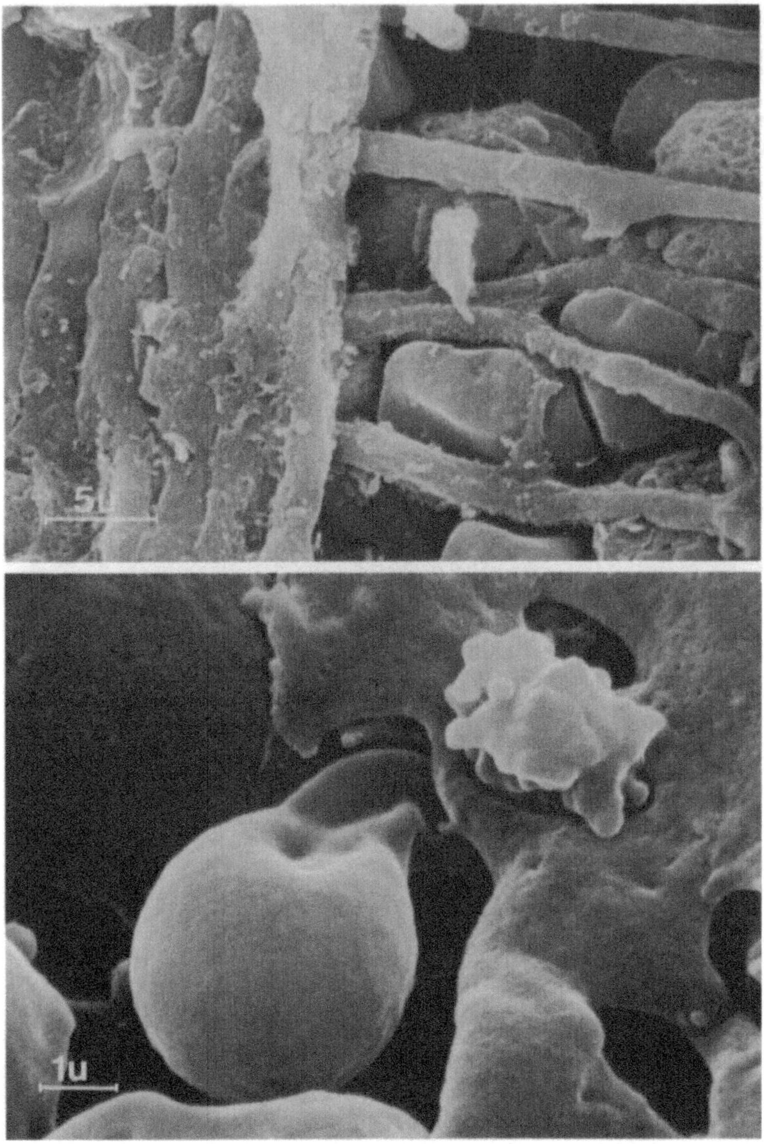

Figure 8.6. Top: human spleen from a patient with spherocytic, auto-immune, hemolytic anemia. Disruption of sinus endothelial wall shows the adjacent packing of spherocytes sequestered in the cord of Billroth due to their inability to deform. Bottom: rat spleen following phenylhydrazine-induced, hemolytic anemia. Several erythrocytes, such as the one shown here, remained attached to the sinus wall by their rigid Heinz-body containing portion.

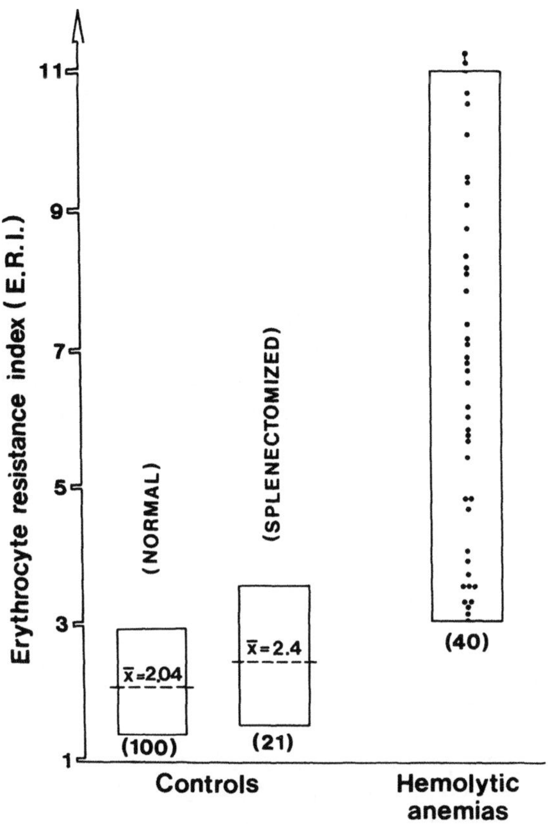

Figure 8.7. Erythrocyte resistance index (derived from ratio of final over initial pressures) to filtration across Nuclepore membrane with 3μm-diameter pores in patients with hemolytic anemias of various etiologies, as compared to normal and splenectomized controls. Numbers between parentheses indicate number of subjects in each group.

contributes to the observed decrease in the average deformability of their circulating erythrocytes [76]. Teitel, using a slightly different filtration technique, has obtained similar results, with a good correlation between the filtration index and the measured red cell survival time in over 200 patients [77]. Little doubt remains that most if not all hemolytic anemias in man arise from the rheological incompetence of pathologically altered red blood cells to meet the unique requirements of the splenic microcirculation. This forms the basis for the classical role of splenectomy in the treatment of these disorders [78].

One might speculate that the spleen plays a protective role in these diseases by preventing the most rigid red cells from remaining in the peripheral circulation where they would impede blood flow to more vital organs. If this were the case, splenectomy might result in unwanted vascular complications. Except in the case of sickle-cell anemia, clinical observation does not support such a concept, since the frequency of microcirculatory disturbances following splenectomy in patients with other hemolytic anemias does not appear to increase significantly. One must therefore conclude that the rheological defect documented in these patients with the use of currently available methods is not of sufficient magnitude to cause vascular occlusion elsewhere than in the spleen. By the same token, this leaves a number of unresolved questions with regards to the exact significance of similar in vitro observations purporting to the existence of a decreased erythrocyte deformability in patients with peripheral microvascular diseases such as diabetes [79], intermittent claudication [80], or coronary insufficiency [81], which are discussed in Chapters 6 and 10. As will be discussed in the following section, the influence of rheological factors extrinsic to the erythrocytes, rather than the erythrocytes themselves, may have led to the observed results in these studies.

8.5. The syndrome of plasmatic hyperviscosity

The term *hyperviscosity syndrome* was first coined in the literature by Fahey and coworkers [82], establishing the relationship between a group of symptoms previously described in certain individuals [83] and the existence in their plasma or serum of large concentrations of abnormal proteins capable of influencing viscosity [84,85]. As we now know, this syndrome represents only one of several ways in which the viscosity of whole blood may be altered in hematological diseases. In this section, the rheological problems associated with a group of disorders commonly known as the PARAPROTEIN DISEASES will first be examined. This will be followed by a short discussion of a more recently defined condition, the HEMATOLOGICAL STRESS SYNDROME, with regards to its effects on rheological measurements in patients with vascular diseases.

8.5.1. Paraprotein diseases

A group of malignant blood diseases, including multiple myeloma, Waldenström's macroglobulinemia and occasional cases of lymphoproliferative disorders such as chronic lymphocytic leukemia and non-Hodgkin's lymphoma, is characterized by the presence, in plasma, of abnormal immunoglobulin molecules known as paraproteins. Being the secretion products of uncontrolled malignant B-lymphocytic cell clones, these proteins, in contrast to normal immunoglobulins, are usually present in high concentrations and bear only one of the two usual light chain types (kappa or labda), hence their alternative designation as monoclonal immunoglobulins. Such proteins, depending on their concentration, size and shape, have a tendency to form intermolecular bridges, with a resulting fluid structure capable of influencing the viscosity of plasma (1). In whole blood, their adsorbtion on the surface of erythrocytes further causes the formation of a cell-protein-cell lattice which results in a synergistic increase in the viscosity of the entire suspension, especially at low shear rates (3). Two well-known hematological clues reflecting the latter phenomenon in the blood of individuals with these diseases are the observation of an extremely elevated erythrocyte sedimentation rate and that of an increased formation of rouleaux on the stained peripheral blood smear.The viscosity of serum or plasma, as measured by different methods, has been found elevated in the majority of patients with paraproteinemia (86,87). Values up to eight times those observed in normal controls have been reported in certain patients with macroglobulinemia. This increase in viscosity reflects both the concentration and the intrinsic properties of the abnormal protein. As with the hematocrit in whole blood, plasma viscosity varies as an approximately exponential function of the paraprotein concentration, hence the risk created in these patients by even a moderate degree of dehydration such as that incurred in the preparation for an intravenous pyelogram. At a given shear rate, the slope of the *plasma viscosity - protein concentration* relationship is further influenced by the molecular weight of the paraprotein (IgM, IgA or IgG), as well as by its natural tendency to form complexes of high intrinsic viscosity, such as in the case of certain IgA or IgG_3 molecules, which may elevate the viscosity of plasma even at relatively low concentrations (88). Except in rare cases, the measurement of plasma or serum viscosity alone is of limited value in predicting clinical symptoms of hyperviscosity; other factors, such as the hematocrit and the state of the microvasculature, also play an important role in determining the clinical picture (86,87,89). Measuring the viscosity of whole blood has proved more informative for assessing the state of the circulation in these patients. Fig. 8.8 shows the values obtained in our laboratory in 26 individuals with paraproteinemia whose blood viscosity was measured at 11.5 s^{-1}, which is about the lowest shear rate at which reliable measurements can be obtained with the Wells-Brookfield viscometer.

When the low hematocrit values in these patients are ignored, the blood viscosity values were most often within the range observed at the same shear rate in 10 healthy control individuals (6.3 to 9.4 mPas). An "absolute hyperviscosity" was therefore documented in three patients only. When comparison is made on the basis of the viscosity-hematocrit relationship, in 21 cases blood viscosity was higher than that predicted for the patient's hematocrit. Such results are comparable to those previously reported by Somer using a similar viscometer (86). McGrath and Penny, using a coaxial-cylinder instrument, were able to measure blood viscosity at a shear rate of 0.18 s^{-1} in 65 individuals with various paraproteins (87). With this method, they found an absolute hyperviscosity in over 50% of their patients despite the coexistence of a reduced hematocrit in most cases. The apparent advantage of measuring whole blood viscosity at the lowest possible shear rate stems from the fact that cell-protein interactions become

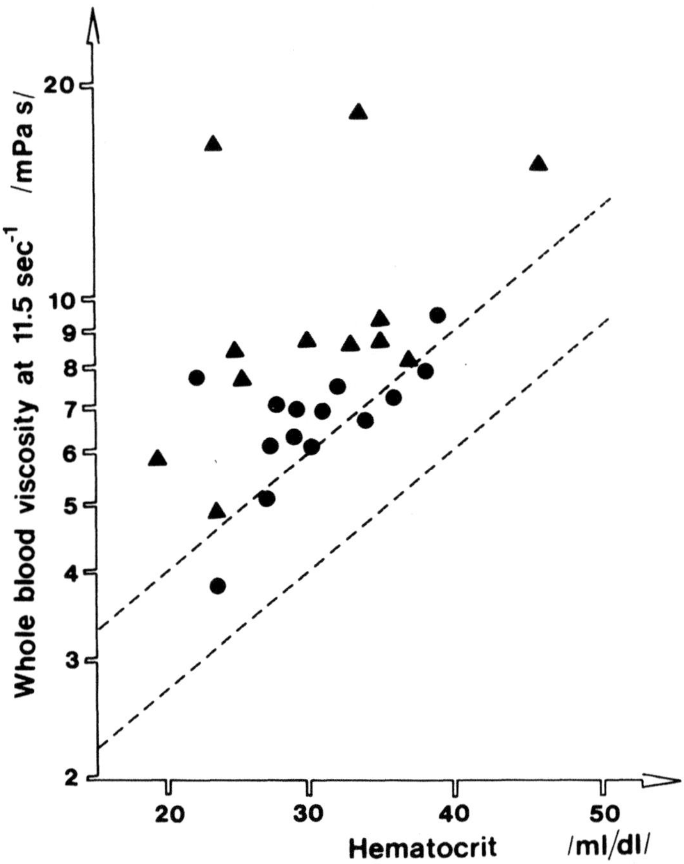

Figure 8.8. Whole blood viscosity in 26 individuals with paraproteinemia. Patients with IgM paraproteins are represented by triangles, while those with either IgG or IgA are represented by circles. The diagonal dashed lines represent the 95% confidence limits of the regression line of the log viscosity - hematocrit relationship established in ten control individuals.

increasingly more important as one approaches creep-flow values similar to those encountered in vivo during the low amplitude phase of pulsatile flow. Nonetheless, the reduction in hematocrit which almost always accompanies the disease probably serves as a protective mechanism against absolute hyperviscosity in many of these patients and provides the best possible compromise for optimizing oxygen transport in the presence of high plasma viscosity (Chapter 5). For this reason, several authors have cautioned against the risk of transfusing them with concentrated erythrocytes for fear of augmenting their symptoms (4,87-89).The most frequently reported clinical features of the plasma hyperviscosity syndrome are those involving the retinal circulation, the central nervous system, the cardiac function and the peripheral vascular system (87,90). The finding of typical funduscopic abnormalities, such as tortuous retinal veins or the presence of exudates and hemorrhages has been considered essential by some to sustain a clinical diagnosis of plasma hyperviscosity (90). Complaints relating to ischemia in the central nervous system may resemble those observed in severe erythrocytosis, although somnolence or coma are more frequent presenting features than typical stroke. Peripheral vascular or neurological manifestations are less frequent, and this probably reflects the tendency of the paraprotein to cryoprecipitate in certain individuals. Heart failure due to a combination of anemia, hypervolemia and a generalized increase in peripheral resistance is also frequently observed (91). Excessive bleeding due to interactions between the paraprotein and either the platelets or fibrinogen is another common problem in patients with severe plasma hyperviscosity (92). As already mentioned, attempts to correlate the clinical abnormalities with the serum or plasma viscosity alone in paraproteinemic patients have gained limited success because such measurements largely disregard the important rheological contributions of both the hematocrit and cell-protein interactions. Correlation of clinical abnormalities with whole blood viscosity measured at low shear rate appears to be much better, although some degree of variability must be expected to account for differences, among patients, in other important factors such as pre-existing vascular disease, heart condition or special temperature-related manifestations (87).Plasmapheresis is the most effective therapeutic method to obtain a rapid reduction in whole blood viscosity in patients with symptomatic paraproteinemia (93). The removal of large quantities of noxious immunoglobulins with this technique usually results in a rapid and dramatic reversal of the clinical syndrome (94). Plasma viscosity and whole blood viscosity decrease exponentially as the concentration of the paraprotein is reduced. In patients with IgM macroglobulins, which are largely distributed within the vascular compartment, a single exchange of 2.5 to 3.0 liters of plasma with an equivalent volume of a 5% human albumin-NaCl solution usually results in the removal of 60-65% of the circulating paraprotein (95). In contrast, sufficient clearance of the smaller IgG or IgA molecules may require several exchange procedures, because each step induces the recruitment of these proteins from the extravascular fluid space, where up to 60% of the original paraprotein load is normaly distributed. A further benefit of plasmapheresis is to correct the hypervolemia and to provide the necessary "rheological space" for the safe transfusion of packed erythrocytes when clinically needed. Once these immediate goals have been satisfactorily achieved, other therapeutic approaches, such as chemotherapy, should normally be instituted to control the proliferative nature of the underlying disease.

8.5.2. Hematological stress syndrome

Several diseases may be accompanied by a non-specific response to tissue injury manifested by an increased hepatic synthesis of various proteins as well as an increased production of granulocytes and platelets by the bone marrow. Such changes are best known to occur in acute situations such as trauma, infections, or myocardial infarction and are usually referred to as the acute-phase response of inflammatory disorders. Patients in the steady state of certain chronic disorders may show similar biological changes in their blood. These changes, which include anemia, leukocytosis, thrombocytosis and hyperfibrinogenemia associated with an accelerated rate of erythrocyte sedimentation and the presence of rouleaux on the peripheral blood smear, have been collectively described by Reizenstein as the *hematological stress syndrome* (96). Many of these non-specific hematological manifestations resemble those described in the paraprotein disorders in that there is an increase in plasma concentrations of high-molecular-weight, asymmetrical proteins, namely fibrinogen and the alpha-2 macroglobulins, which have similar effects on plasma and whole blood viscosity. Interleukin-1, a substance derived from activated monocytes and macrophages, has been proposed as a possible mediator of the acute-phase response, on account of its ability to stimulate both the synthesis of fibrinogen from hepatic cells (97) and the release of granulocytes from the bone marrow (98). Rheological studies in patients with vascular diseases have often shown an increase in blood viscosity and a decreased erythrocyte deformability as measured by standard filtration techniques (79-81). Whether such abnormalities reflect the cause or the consequence of the disease remains at present an area of debate (see Chapter 6). Characteristic manifestations of acute and chronic phase responses have also been documented in the same disorders (99), which suggests that the apparent reduction in erythrocyte deformability might be due to other factors, such as plasma proteins and leukocytes. Pursuing this hypothesis several investigators have emphasized the need for being extremely careful in removing leukocytes and plasma while preparing erythrocyte suspensions for filtration (100-102). Using a method of whole blood pre-filtration through cotton wool columns followed by washing in buffer, Kenny et al (103) and Winkenwender et al (105) have shown that after elimination of these extrinsic variables, the filterability of erythrocytes from diabetic and atherosclerotic patients with peripheral vascular disease was not significantly different from that of control erythrocytes (104). Such improvements in methodology are important to prevent further spurious hemorheological findings in vascular diseases and should allow us to concentrate on other abnormalities that are perhaps more relevant to the effective clinical management of these patients. The clinical importance of the hematological stress syndrome in producing specific symptoms in patients with chronic vascular disease has yet to be determined. Therapeutic measures such as hemodilution (106), plasmapheresis (107) or Arvin defibrinogenation (108), which have all been attempted in acute diseases to decrease the viscosity of whole blood, would require application for long periods of time and therefore do not seem very practical. Drugs taken orally and capable of causing a long-term reduction in the level of circulating fibrinogen by inhibition of interleukin-1 or other appropriate mediators of the inflammatory response would appear more promising and should be the object of further research (see Chapter 12).

8.6. Summary and conclusions

Blood diseases may cause hemorheological disturbances by three major mechanisms linked respectively with the concentration of circulating blood cells, the deformability of erythrocytes and the intrinsic viscosity of plasma. Corresponding *hyperviscosity syndromes* are described in which the demonstration of specific rheological abnormalities in vitro provides a rational explanation for the various clinical manifestations encountered in diseases such as erythrocytosis, leukemia, sickle-cell disease, hemolysis, paraproteinemias and the more recently described hematological stress syndrome which accompanies several chronic disorders. Useful concepts on patient management have emerged from these studies, especially with regards to the appropriate use and monitoring of blood transfusions and plasmapheresis in certain cases. Over the years, improvements in methodology have contributed significantly to provide new and more relevant information on the rheological implications of blood disease. Measuring the viscosity of whole blood over a wide range of shear rates as opposed to that of plasma or serum alone in simple capillary tubes represents one of the best examples of the progress accomplished during the past few decades. Yet, as we have seen with the recent wide-spread application of erythrocyte filtration tests, new techniques may sometimes lead to erroneous interpretations regarding a specific parameter such as red cell deformability until further refinements are introduced to sort out or eliminate other variables. Hence it is of importance in hemorheological research to maintain a close and constant relationship between the clinician and his laboratory colleagues. Blood rheology in vivo is a far more complex entity than the rather simple conditions prevailing in most labortatory tests. While the development of methods to quantify blood flow in various parts of the human body are still in their infancy, the emergence of new technologies such as laser-Doppler velocimetry seems very promising as judged by the results already obtained in a few patients with sickle-cell disease. The further applications of this and other similar methods should aim at enhancing our ability to detect microcirculatory disturbances in patients before the development of clinical manifestations. Future research on the rheological aspects of blood disorders will hopefully bring us a step forward towards prevention rather than the simple treatment of diseases.

References

1. Wells R. 1970: Syndromes of hyperviscosity. N. Engl. J. Med. 283, 183-186.
2. Chien S. 1975: Biophysical behavior of red cells in suspension. In: The Red Blood Cell (Vol. II), Surgenor D.M. (ed), Academic Press, New York: 1031-1133.

3. Chien S., Usami S., Taylor H.M. 1964: Effects of hematocrit and plasma proteins on flow properties of erythrocyte suspensions. Amer. J. Physiol. 207, 1035-1040.
4. Leblond P.F. Lacasse M., Morillon M., Huot-Petitclerc M.C. 1983: Le rôle de l'hématocrite sur la viscosité sanguine. Union. Med. Can. 112, 22-25.
5. Schmid-Schönbein H., Wells R., Schildkraut R. 1969: Microscopy and viscometry of blood flowing under uniform shear rate. J. App. Physiol. 26, 674-678.
6. Chien S., Usami S., Dellenback R.J., Gregersen M.I., Nanninga L.B., Guest M.M. 1967: Blood viscosity: influence of erythrocyte aggregation. Science 157, 829-831.
7. Chien S., Usami S., Dellenback R.J., Gregersen M.I. 1967: Blood viscosity: influence of erythrocyte deformation. Science 157, 827-829.
8. Driessen G.K., Fischer T.M., Haest C.W.M., Inhoffen W., Schmid-Schönbein H. 1984: Flow behaviour of rigid red cells in the microcirculation. Int. J. Microcirc. Clin. Exp. 3, 197-210.
9. Leblond P.F. 1976: L'importance rhéologique de la déformabilité érythrocytaire. Un. Med. Can. 105, 177-185.
10. Schafer A.I. 1984: Bleeding and thrombosis in the myeloproliferative disorders. Blood 64, 1-12.
11. Cohen J., Lichtman M.A. 1978: Polycythemia. In: Hematology for practitioners. Lichtman M.A. (ed). Little Brown, Boston 87-103.
12. Nathan D.G., Oski F. 1981: Hematology of infancy and childhood. (2nd ed). W.B. Saunders, Phildelphia 1507.
13. Berlin N.I. 1973: Diagnosis and classification of the polycythemias. Semin. Hematol. 12, 605-608.
14. Halvorsen S. 1984: Regulation of erythropoiesis. In. J. Microcirc. Clin. Exp. 3, 109-114.
15. Lenfant C., Sullivan K. 1971: Adaptation to high altitude. N. Eng. J. Med. 284, 1298-1309.
16. Cocking J.B., Darke C.S. 1972: Blood volume studies in chronic obstructive non-specific lung disease. Thorax 27, 44-51.
17. Rosenthal A., Button L.N., Nathan D.G. 1972: Blood volume changes in cyanotic congenital heart disease. Am. J. Cardiol. 29, 162-167.
18. Nagel R.L., Bookchin R.M. 1974: Human hemoglobin mutants with abnormal oxygen binding. Semin. Hematol. 11, 385-403.
19. Balcerzak S.P., Bromberg P.A. 1975: Secondary polycythemia. Semin. Hematol. 12, 353-382.
20. Hammond D., Winnick S. 1974: Paraneoplastic erythrocytosis and ectopic erythropoietin. Ann. N.Y. Acad. Sci. 230, 219-227.
21. Gilbert H.S. 1975: Definition, clinical features and diagnosis of polycythemia vera. Clin. Hematol. 4, 263-290.
22. Stohlman F. 1966: Pathogenesis of erythrocytosis. Semin. Hematol. 3, 181-192.
23. Eaves C.J., Eaves A.C. 1978: Erythropoietin dose-response curves for three classes of erythroid progenitors in normal human marrow and in patients with polycythemia vera. Blood 52, 1196-1210.
24. Leblond P.F., Weed R.I. 1975: The peripheral blood in polycythemia vera and myelofibrosis. Clin. Haematol. 4, 353-371.
25. LaCelle P.L., Weed R.I. 1979: The contribution of normal and pathologic erythrocytes to blood rheology. Progress in Hematology 7, 1-31.
26. Hutton R.D. 1979: The effects of iron deficiency on whole blood viscosity in polycythemia patients. Brit. J. Haematol. 43, 191-199.
27. Kenny M.W., Gyde O.H.B., Stuart J. 1984: Influence of cell size on erythrocyte deformability in treated polycythemia vera. Clin. Hemorheol. 4, 381-386.
28. Pearson T.C., Humphrey P.R.D., Thomas D.J., Wetherley-Mein G. 1981: Hematocrit, blood viscosity, cerebral blood flow and vascular occlusion. In: Clinical aspects of blood viscosity and cell deformability. Lowe G.D.O., Barbenel J.C., Forbes C.D. (eds), Springer-Verlag, Berlin and New York 97-107.
29. Thomas D.J., du Boulay G.H., Marshall J., Pearson T.C., Ross Russell R.W., Symon L., Wetherley-Mein G., Zilkha E. 1977: Cerebral blood flow in polycythemia. Lancet 2, 161-163.

30. Humphrey P.R.D., du Boulay G.H., Marshall J., Pearson T.C., Ross Russel R.W., Symon L., Wetherley-Mein G., Zilkha E. 1979: Cerebral blood flow and viscosity in relative polycythaemia. Lancet 2, 873-878.
31. Chievitz E., Thiede T. 1962: Complications and causes of death in polycythemia. Acta Med. Scand. 172, 513-523.
32. Mundall J., Quintero P., von Kaulla K.N., Harmon R., Ansoin J. 1972: Transient monocular blindness and increased platelet aggregability treated with aspirin. Neurol. 22, 280-295.
33. Pearson T.C., Wetherley-Mein G. 1978: Vascular occlusive episodes and venous haematocrit in primary proliferative polycythaemia. Lancet 2, 1219-1222.
34. Lichtman M.A., Rowe J.M 1982: Hyperleukocytic leukemias: rheological, clinical and therapeutic considerations. Blood 60, 279-283.
35. Lichtman M.A. 1973: Rheology of leukocytes, leukocyte suspensions and blood in leukemia. Possible relationship to clinical manifestations. J. Clin. Invest. 52, 350-358.
36. Lichtman M.A. 1984: The relationship of excessive white cell accumulation to vascular insufficiency in patients with leukemia. In: White cell mechanics: Basic science and clinical aspects. Alan R. Liss, New York. KROC Found. Sci. 295-306.
37. Rowe J.M., Lichtman M.A. 1984: Hyperleukocytosis and leukostasis: common features of childhood chronic myelogenous leukemia. Blood 63, 1230-1234.
38. McKee L.C. Jr., Collins R.D. 1974: Intravascular leukocyte thrombi and aggregates as a cause of morbidity and mortality in leukemias. Medicine 53, 463-478.
39. Lichtman M.A., Kearny E.A. 1976: The filterability of normal and leukemic leukocytes. Blood Cells 2, 491-506.
40. Albanese B., Morini R., Pasquini G., Manescalchi P.G., Guidi S., Bartholi V. 1984: The hemorheological findings in leukemia. Clin. Hemorheol. 4, 505-512.
41. Lichtman M.A. 1970: Cellular deformability during maturation of the myeloblast. Possible role in marrow egress. N. Engl. J. Med. 283, 943-948.
42. Preston F.E., Sokol R.J., Lilleyman J.S., Winfield D.A., Blackburn E.K. 1978: Cellular hyperviscosity as a cause of neurological symptoms in leukemia. Br. Med. J. 1, 476-478.
43. Vernant J.P., Brun B., Mannoni P., Dreyfus B. 1979: Respiratory distress of hyperleukocytic granulocytic leukemias. Cancer 44, 264-268.
44. Lane T.A. 1980: Continuous flow leukapheresis for rapid cytoreduction in leukemia. Transfusion 20, 455-457.
45. Murinson D.S. 1981: Clinical pharmacology of anti-neoplastic agents. In: Practical cancer chemotherapy. Rosenthal S.N., Bennet J.M. (eds), Medical Examination Publishing, Garden City (NY), 55-56.
46. Mohandas N., Clark M.R., Jacobs M.S., Shohet S.V. 1980: Analysis of factors regulating erythrocyte deformability. J. Clin. Invest. 66, 563-573.
47. Serjeant G.R. 1974: The clinical features of sickle-cell disease. American Elsevier, 208-219.
48. Prankerd T.A.J., Bellingham A.J. (eds) 1975: Hemolytic anemias. Clin. Hemorheol. (Vol. 4). W.B. Saunders, London.
49. Dean J., Schechter A.N. 1978: Sickle cell anemia: molecular and cellular bases of therapeutic approach (parts I and II). N. Eng. J. Med. 299, 752-763, 804-811.
50. Dean J., Schechter A.N. 1978: Sickle cell anemia: molecular and cellular bases of therapeutic approach (part III). N. Eng. J. Med. 299, 863-870.
51. Stuart J. 1984: Sickle cell disease and vascular occlusion - rheological aspects. Clin. Hemorheol. 4, 193-207.
52. Chien S., Usami S., Jan K.M., Smith J.A., Bertles J.F. 1976: Blood rheology in sickle cell disease. In: Proceedings of the symposium on molecular and cellular aspects of sickle cell disease. Hercules J.I., Cottam G.L., Waterman M.R., Schechter A.N. (eds). US Department of Health, Education and Welfare, Bethesda, Publication No. (NIH) 76-1007, 277-303.
53. Serjeant G.R., Serjeant B.E., Milner P.F. 1969: The irreversibly sickled cell: a determinant of haemolysis in sickle cell anemia. Br. J. Haematol. 17, 527-533.

54. Glader B.E., Nathan D.G. 1978: Cation permeability alterations during sickling: relationship to cation composition and cellular dehydration of irreversibly sickled cells. Blood 51, 983-989.
55. Eaton J.W., Skelton T.D., Swofford H.S., Koplin C.E., Jacob H.S. 1973: Elevated erythrocyte calcium in sickle cell disease. Nature (Lond.) 246, 105-106.
56. Schmid-Schönbein H. 1982: Continuous viscous deformation of red blood cells in flow and their disturbance in sickle cell disease. Blood Cells 8, 29-51.
57. Smith C.M., Kuettner J.F., Tukey D.P., Burris S.M., White J.G. 1981: Variable deformability of irreversibly sickled erythrocytes. Blood 58, 71-77.
58. Clark M.R., Mohandas N., Shohet S.B. 1980: Deformability of oxygenated irreversibly sickled cells. J. Clin. Invest. 65, 189-196.
59. Evans E., Mohandas N., Leung A. 1984: Static and dynamic rigidities of normal and sickle erythrocytes. Major influence of cell hemoglobin concentration. J. Clin. Invest. 73, 477-488.
60. Nash G.B., Johnson C.S., Meiselman H.J. 1984: Mechanical properties of oxygenated red cells in sickle cell (HbSS) disease. Blood 63, 73-82.
61. Chien S., Usami S., Bertles J.F. 1970: Abnormal rheology of oxygenated blood in sickle cell anemia. J. Clin. Invest. 49, 623-634.
62. Kenny M.W., Meakin M., Worthington D.J., Stuart J. 1981: Erythrocyte deformability in sickle cell crisis. Brit. J. Haematol. 49, 103-109.
63. LaCelle P.L. 1977: Oxygen delivery to muscle cells during capillary vascular occlusion by sickled erythrocytes. Blood Cells 3, 273-281.
64. Klug P.P., Lessin L.S. 1977: Microvascular blood flow of sickled erythrocytes: a dynamic morphological study. Blood Cells 3, 263-272.
65. Kaul D.K., Fabry M.E., Windisch P., Baez S., Nagel R.L. 1983: Erythrocytes in sickle cell anemia are heterogeneous in their rheological and hemodynamic characteristics. J. Clin. Invest. 72 (1), 22-31.
66. Lipowsky H.H., Usami S., Chien S. 1982: Human SS red cell rheological behavior in the microcirculation of cremaster muscle. Blood Cells 8, 113-126.
67. Rodgers G.P., Schechter A.N., Noguchi C.T., Klein H.G., Nienhius A.W., Bonner R.F. 1984: Periodic microcirculatory flow in patients with sickle cell disease. N. Eng. J. Med. 311, 1534-1538.
68. Chien S. 1984: Rheology of sickle cells and the microcirculation (Editorial). N.Eng. J. Med. 311, 1567-1569.
69. Leblond P.F., Lacelle P.L., Weed R.I. 1971: Cellular deformability: a possible determinant of the normal release of maturing erythrocytes from the bone marrow. Blood 37, 40-46.
70. LaCelle P.L. 1969: Alteration of the deformability of the erythrocyte membrane in stored blood. Transfusion 9, 238-245.
71. Weiss L. 1974: A scanning electron microscopic study of the spleen. Blood 43, 665-691.
72. Chen L.T., Weiss L. 1973: The role of the sinus wall in the passage of erythrocytes through the spleen. Blood 41, 529-537.
73. Bowdler A.J. 1975: The spleen and haemolytic disorders. Clin. Haematol. 4, 231-246.
74. Leblond P.F. 1973: Etude au microscope electronique à balayage de la migration des cellules sanguines à travers les parois des sinusoïdes spléniques et médullaires chez le rat. Nouv. Rev. Fr. Hématol. 13, 771-788.
75. Leblond P.F., Coulombe L. 1979: The measurement of erythrocyte deformability using micropore membranes: a sensitive technique with clinical applications. J. Lab. Clin. Med. 94, 133-143.
76. Leblond P.F., Coulombe L., Lyonnais J. 1978: Erythrocyte populations in pyruvate kinase deficiency anemia following splenectomy: II. Cell deformability. Brit. J. Haematol. 39, 63-70.
77. Teitel P. 1967: Le test de la filtrabilité érythrocytaire. Nouv. Rev. Fr. Hematol. 7, 195-214.
78. Tillmann W., Schröter W. 1983: Deformability of red cells and splenectomy in hemolytic anemias. Clin. Hemorheol. 3, 409-428.
79. Hanss M., Attali J.R., Helou C., LeMarie J.C. 1983: Erythrocytes, deformability and diabetes. Clin. Hemorheol. 3, 383-391.

80. Reid H.L., Dormandy J.A., Barnes A.J., Lock P.J., Dormandy T.L. 1976: Impaired red cell deformability in peripheral vascular disease. Lancet 1, 666-668.
81. Dintenfass L. 1981: Blood viscosity, red cell rigidity and arterial blood pressure in patients with severe coronary occlusions or chest pains. Effect of submaximal exercise test. Clin. Hemorheol. 1, 121-134.
82. Fahey J.L., Barth W.F., Solomon A. 1965: Serum hyperviscosity syndrome. JAMA 192, 464-467.
83. Waldenström J. 1944: Incipient myelomatosis or essential hyperglobulinemia with fibrinogenopenia - a new syndrome? Acta Med. Scand. 117, 216-247.
84. Wintrobe M.M., Buell M.V. 1933: Hyperproteinemia associated with multiple myeloma. Bull. Johns. Hopk. Hosp. 52, 156-165.
85. Albers D. 1937: Multiple Myelome und Viskosität. Z. Klin. Med. 132, 807-811.
86. Somer T. 1966: The viscosity of blood, plasma and serum in dys- and para-proteinemias. Acta Med. Scand. (Suppl) 456, 1-97.
87. McGrath M., Penny R. 1976: Paraproteinemia. Blood hyperviscosity and clinical manifestations. J. Clin. Invest. 58, 1155-1162.
88. Preston F.E., Cooke K.B., Foster M.E., Winfield D.A., Lee D. 1978: Myelomatosis and the hyperviscosity syndrome. Br. J. Haematol. 38, 517-530.
89. Mannik M 1974: Blood viscosity in Waldenström's macroglobulinemia. Blood 44, 87-98.
90. Preston F.E. 1981: Circulatory complications of leukaemia and paraproteinaemia. In: Clinical aspects of blood viscosity and cell deformability. Lowe G.D.O., Barbenel J.C., Forbes C.D. (eds), Springer Verlag, Berlin and New York 123-132.
91. Russel J.A., Powles R.L. 1978: The relationship between serum viscosity, hypervolemia and clinical manifestations associated with circulating paraprotein. Brit. J. Haematol. 39, 163-175.
92. Lackner H., Hunt V., Zucker M.B., Pearson J. 1970: Abnormal fibrin ultrastructure polymerization and clot retraction in multiple myeloma. Brit. J. Haematol. 18, 625-636.
93. Powles R., Smith C., Kohn J., Hamilton Fairley G. 1971: Method of removing abnormal protein rapidly from patients with malignant paraproteinemias. Br. Med. J. 3, 664-667.
94. Shumak K.H., Rock G.A. 1984: Therapeutic plasma exchange. N. Eng. J. Med. 310, 762-771.
95. Buskard N.A., Galton D.A.G., Goldman J.M., Kohner E.M., Grindle C.F., Newman D.L., Twinn K.W., Lowenthal R.M. 1977: Plasma exchange in the long term management of Waldenström's macroglobulinemia. Can. Med. Assn. J. 117, 135-137.
96. Reizenstein P. 1979: The haematological stress syndrome. Brit. J. Haematol. 43: 329-334.
97. Kampschmidt R.F., Upchurch H.F., Pulliam L.A. 1982: Characterization of a leukocyte-derived endogenous mediator responsible for increased plasma fibrinogen. Ann. N.Y. Acad. Sci. 389, 338-353.
98. Bornstein D.L. 1982: Leukocytic pyrogen: a major mediator of the acute-phase reaction. Ann. N.Y. Acad. Sci. 389, 323-337.
99. Stuart J., George A.J., Davies A.J., Auckland A., Hurlow R.A. 1981: Haematological stress syndrome in atherosclerosis. J. Clin. Pathol. 34, 464-467.
100. Alderman M.J., Ridge A., Morley A.A., Ryall R.G., Walsh J.A. 1981: Effect of total leucocyte count on whole blood filterability in patients with peripheral vascular disease. J. Clin. Pathol. 34, 163-166.
101. Chien S., Schmalzer E.A., Lee M.M., Impelluso T., Skalak R. 1983: Role of white blood cells in filtration of blood cell suspensions. Biorheology 20 (1), 11-27.
102. Stuart J. 1984: The acute-phase reaction and haematological stress syndrome in vascular disease. Int. J. Microcirc. Clin. Exp. 3, 115-129.
103. Kenny M.W., Meakin M., Stuart J. 1983: Methods for removal of leucocytes and platelets prior to study of erythrocyte deformability. Clin. Hemorheol. 3 (2), 191-200.
104. Stuart J., Kenny M.W., Aukland A., George A.J., Neumann V., Shapiro L.M., Cove D.H. 1983: Filtration of washed erythrocytes in atherosclerosis and diabetes mellitus. Clin. Hemorheol. 3 (1), 23-30.

105. Winkenwerder W., Adams K., Lineberger T., Johnson G. 1982: Blood filtration in patients with peripheral vascular disease. Clin. Hemorheol. 2, 201-207.
106. Messmer K., Schmid-Schönbein H. (eds) 1972: Hemodilution, theoretical basis and clinical application. Karger, Basel.
107. Dodds A.J., O'Reilly M.J.G., Yates C.J.P., Cotton L.T., Flute P.T., Dormandy J.A. 1979: Haemorheological response to plasma exchange in Raynaud's syndrome. Br. Med. J. 2, 1186-1187.
108. Dormandy J.A., Reid H.L. 1978: Controlled defibrination in the treatment of peripheral vascular disease. Angiology 29, 80-88.

9
Obstetrics, neonatology and gynaecology

Peter C. Buchan
Department of Obstetrics and Gynaecology, St. James's University Hospital, Leeds LS9 7TF United Kingdom

9.1. Why rheology in obstetrics, gynaecology and neonatology?

> *"It is the heart by whose virtue and pulse the blood is moved, perfected and made apt to nourish, and is preserved from corruption and coagulation."*
>
> William Harvey (1628) [1]

The quotation from Harvey's classic work contains the essence of rheology in obstetrics, gynecology and neonatology. The adequacy of placental blood flow, on both maternal and fetal sides of the placenta, is critical for fetal growth and development, and abnormal rheology has been reported as a final common pathway for fetal intrauterine growth retardation in many different pregnancy pathologies. Hemorheological therapy in obstetrics is well established and being rapidly developed. In gynecology the importance of venous thrombo-embolism is as great as in any surgical speciality, and the role of hormones, which are used in pregnancy, contraception and replacement therapy, in producing rheological changes that predispose to thrombosis has been well defined. The neonate has a particularly vulnerable microcirculation, and there are clearly defined hyper-viscosity syndromes for which appropriate hemorheological therapy holds an established place in neonatological practice. This chapter reviews the current state of knowledge of hemorheology in three important clinical disciplines.

9.2. Maternal rheology in normal pregnancy

Pregnancy presents a unique challenge to maternal cardiovascular physiology, and the changes that take place during pregnancy are among the most extreme alterations occurring in non-pathological states. Not only is blood flow to many, if not all, maternal organs increased, but a virtually new vascular bed is also developed which demands, over an extended period, up to 15 per cent of the cardiac output. In the non-pregnant state the uterine blood flow is on the order of 20 ml per minute, whereas at term the pregnant uterus has a blood flow of between 500 and 750 ml per minute. To cope with the increased demands of pregnancy, the cardiac output rises from the non-pregnant level of around five litres per minute to between 6.1 and 6.8 litres per minute by 12 weeks, this level being maintained until term, the blood volume also increases by 30 per cent above non-pregnant levels. The rise in cardiac output might be expected to lead to an increase in mean arterial pressure, but in fact the mean arterial pressure falls in the first trimester of pregnancy, remaining low until the third trimester, when it rises. This fall in mean arterial pressure in the face of increased cardiac output indicates a significant fall in the total peripheral resistance. Bader et al [2] showed, in cardiac catheterisation studies, that the total peripheral resistance was 1,250 dyne · sec · cm^{-5} in the non-pregnant state; this fell to 986 dyne · sec · cm^{-5} by 14 to 24 weeks of pregnancy, and then rose slowly towards the normal non-pregnant figure of 1,250 dyne · sec · cm^{-5} at term. These changes in peripheral resistance are effected in two ways; firstly, there is clear evidence of vascular dilatation in arterioles and capillaries and in the venous side of the circulation. These changes are present by 12 weeks and are maintained until term, returning quickly to non-pregnant levels in the puerperium. Secondly, peripheral resistance may be lowered by reduction in whole blood viscosity [3]. In a state of vascular dilatation, such as exists in pregnancy, hemorheological factors become of primary importance in the regulation of the peripheral circulation, and abnormal maternal blood rheology has been shown to be associated with increased perinatal mortality and morbidity in both mother and child.

Before considering the changes in maternal and fetal hemorheology found in pathological pregnancy, it is important to have a good understanding of the maternal and fetal hemorheological profiles throughout healthy normal pregnancy. Whole blood viscosity throughout normal pregnancy and its major determinants, i.e. hematocrit, erythrocyte deformability, plasma viscosity, plasma fibrinogen concentration and total serum protein concentration, are graphically displayed in Figs. 9.1 and 9.2 [4]. The literature with regard to whole blood viscosity requires careful attention to the methods of measurement and the calculations by which viscosity is derived. By and large, the British and American workers have reported straight forward whole blood viscosity measurements, as shown in Figs. 9.1 and 9.2, whereas German investigators have reported either "relative viscosity", i.e. the ratio of whole blood to plasma viscosity, or whole blood viscosity corrected to standard hematocrit. Pillisiers [5], using a Hess capillary viscometer, showed that whole blood viscosity was lowered by the later months of pregnancy and Esiaschwili [6] by an undisclosed technique, found a fall in whole blood viscosity during normal pregnancy. The two most comprehensive studies throughout pregnancy are those of Cohen and Thomson [7], who derived whole blood viscosity by a calculation based on the hematocrit, and

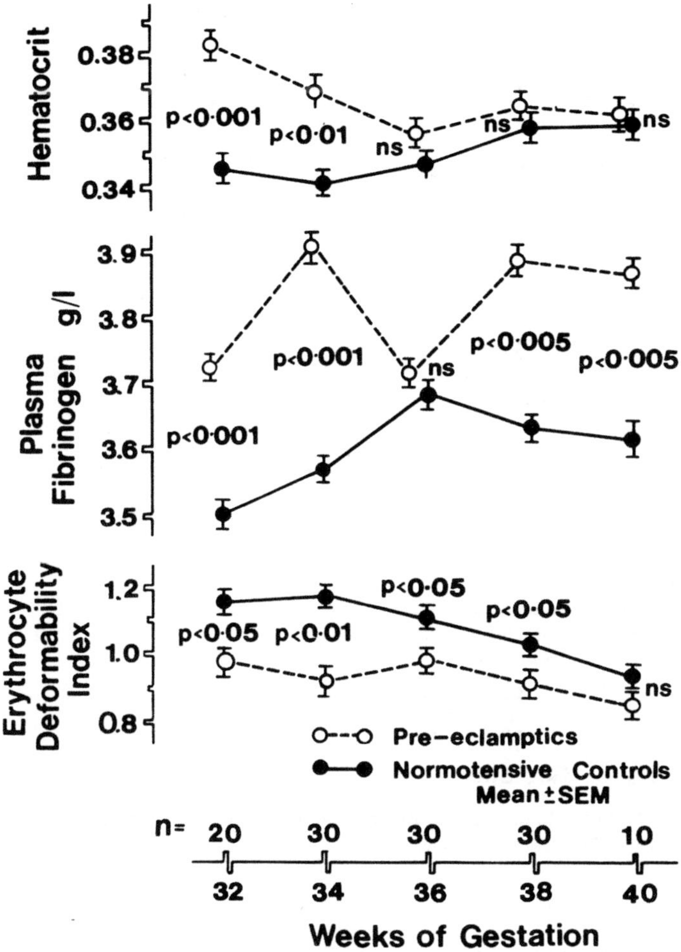

Figure 9.1. Hematocrit plasma fibrinogen and erythrocyte deformability in serial study through normal pregnancy [4].. Data given refers to red cell filtration through 5 μm Nuclepore filters.

Hamilton [8], who used an Ostwald viscometer. Their results show similar changes to those shown in Figs. 9.1 and 9.2, with a gradual fall in whole blood viscosity to a nadir between 30 and 34 weeks, followed by a rise towards term. Leonhardt et al [9] using a Wells-Brookfield viscometer and correcting the whole blood viscosity to a standard hematocrit, reported a significantly raised "corrected whole blood viscosity" in pregnancy, but in fact this merely reflects the raised plasma concentrations of fibrinogen and its effect on plasma viscosity and erythrocyte aggregation. Schmid-Schönbein et al [10] reported the results from 11 pregnant women whom they investigated for various hemorheological parame-

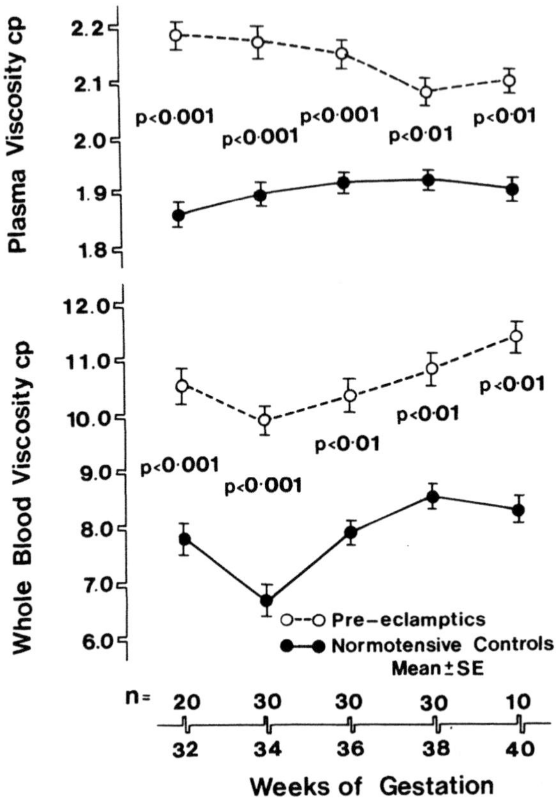

Figure 9.2. Plasma viscosity, and whole blood viscosity in serial study throughout normal pregnancy [4]. (viscometry with the Deer variable stress rheometer)

ters, using a modified Wells-Brookfield viscometer. They found a rise in "relative viscosity" of blood and increased erythrocyte aggregation.

Whole blood viscosity is a complex parameter which is influenced by many other hemorheological factors (see Chapter 2). Pregnancy presents us with a hemorheological workshop where the cellular and plasma constituents of blood are physiologically varied, so their interaction may be studied.

The changes in hematocrit in Fig. 9.1 confirm the findings of other studies. The whole blood viscosity profile throughout pregnancy follows that of hematocrit most closely, but in the first half of pregnancy the fall in whole blood viscosity is attenuated by the rapidly rising fibrinogen concentrations (Fig. 9.1). The literature is confused as regards in effect of pregnancy on erythrocyte deformability (Fig. 9.1). There are reports of a decrease [11], no change [12], and an increase [13]. In all these investigations microfiltration techniques were used for deformability measurement, but the first two studies [11,12] were made on washed red cells suspended in artificial media, whereas the third [13] used red cells suspended in their native plasma. Erythrocyte aggregation is a physiological property of human blood whereby erythrocytes form rouleaux, and this has a significant effect on blood viscosity at low shear rates [14] and has been shown to vary in pregnancy [15] with elevation of aggregation proportional to the increased plasma fibrinogen concentrations in pregnancy. Three studies of plasma viscosity throughout pregnancy have been published, presenting conflicting data. Hamilton [8] using an Ostwald viscometer, found plasma viscosity to be consistently reduced during pregnancy, whereas Eastham [16] and Buchan [4] showed an increase in plasma viscosity throughout pregnancy, mirroring the rise in plasma fibrinogen concentration. The plasma viscosity changes represent a balance between the rising fibrinogen and falling total serum protein concentrations shown in Fig. 9.2.

The hemorheological changes in the maternal blood are of obvious advantage in the hyperdynamic circulation of pregnancy described in the introduction to this chapter, and help to explain the changes in peripheral resistance that have been described in pregnancy [2]. The reduction in peripheral resistance shown in early pregnancy and the rise towards term mirror the described changes in whole blood viscosity and reciprocate the changes in erythrocyte deformability (Fig. 9.1). The part played by hemorheological factors in the peripheral resistance in pregnancy may be considerable, with the degree of arterio-venous dilatation and arteriolar insensitivity to pressor stimuli that are present. Modification of the hemorheological changes of pregnancy could affect blood flow in the sensitive placental circulation, the hemorheological profiles of pathological pregnancy are reviewed later in this Chapter (section 9.4.).

9.3. Normal fetal hemorheology

The delivery of oxygen and nutrients and the removal of waste products and hormones to and from the feto-placental unit may be affected by alterations in the blood flow on either the maternal or fetal side of the placenta. The fetal placental circulation is particularly vulnerable to hemorheological alterations, with the extensive microcirculation of the villi being susceptible to changes in erythrocyte deformability, plasma, and whole blood viscosity. The hemorheological profile of the normal fetus has been studied by several workers [4,13,17,18].

Comparison of neonatal with term-pregnant and non-pregnant adult female hemorheology (Table 9.1) [13] clearly shows that the fetus is poorly situated to cope with an increase in any of his hemorheological parameters. With an elevated hematocrit [13,17] and reduced erythrocyte deformability [13,18] combining to give an elevated whole blood viscosity, however, when measured at standard hematocrit, the fetal blood has a lower viscosity because of the reduced fibrino-

Table 9.1. Hemorheological measurements in adult females, pregnant women and full term fetuses.

	Pregnant women n = 20 (SD)	Full term infants n = 20 (SD)	Adult women n = 20 (SD)
Mean whole blood viscosity (centipoise)	9.8 (2.8) **	16.8 (2.4) **	12.7 (3.1)
Mean plasma viscosity (centipoise)	2.25 (0.46) **	1.46 (0.33) *	1.75 (0.40)
Mean hematocrit	0.373 (0.028) **	0.492 (0.037) *	0.447 (0.033)
Mean erythrocyte deformability index	1.13 (0.14) **	0.72 (0.10) *	0.81 (0.11)
Mean plasma fibrinogen (g/l)	4.32 (0.81) **	1.76 (0.73) *	2.80 (0.69)

Comparison of measurements with those from adult women using Student's t-test.
* $p < 0.05$; ** $p < 0.001$.

gen concentrations [13,19] and the lower erythrocyte aggregation [19]. The changes in hemorheology with advancing gestational age are shown in Table 9.2 [4]. With increasing gestation several workers have found a rising hematocrit [4,20] and rising concentrations in plasma fibrinogen and proteins [16]. It has been suggested [21] that during intrauterine life there are two separate mechanisms at work in the development of the blood picture seen in the fetus at birth. Firstly, there is an increase in hemoglobin and erythrocytes as part of the normal growth and maturation of the fetus. Secondly, an increased production of hemoglobin and erythrocytes may be forced at any stage of the pregnancy by a fall in the oxygen supply to the placenta, and the effect of this abnormal stimulation may be superimposed on the normal growth pattern (Fig. 9.3) [22].

A similar situation may well pertain with the whole range of hemorheological parameters. Hepatic and immunological maturation results in gradually rising concentrations of plasma fibrinogen, albumin, and globulins; maturation of the hemopoietic system results in a rising hematocrit. Consequent upon these changes, the plasma viscosity and whole blood viscosity rise. Stress situations may cause an acceleration in production of plasma proteins and erythrocytes; then a vicious

Table 9.2. Variations in the fetal hemorheological profile with gestational age–cross-sectional study.

Gestational age in weeks		34–35	36–37	38–39	40–41	42+
Number of subjects		15	25	45	75	30
Hematocrit	Mean	0.421	0.459 *	0.488 *	0.512 *	0.564 ***
	SD	0.032	0.031	0.033	0.032	0.037
Plasma viscosity (centipoise)	Mean	1.24	1.38 n.s.	1.43 n.s.	1.46 n.s.	1.69 *
	SD	0.25	0.29	0.26	0.33	0.35
Whole blood viscosity (centipoise)	Mean	12.5	14.6 *	15.5 n.s.	16.8 n.s.	19.7 *
	SD	1.8	2.1	2.3	2.3	3.5
Erythrocyte deformability	Mean	0.65	0.69 n.s.	0.72 n.s.	0.72 n.s.	0.64 **
	SD	0.11	0.08	0.09	0.09	0.11

Statistical significance of difference between result marked and preceding result using Student's t-test.
n.s. $p > 0.05$; * $p < 0.05$; ** $p < 0.01$; *** $p < 0.001$.

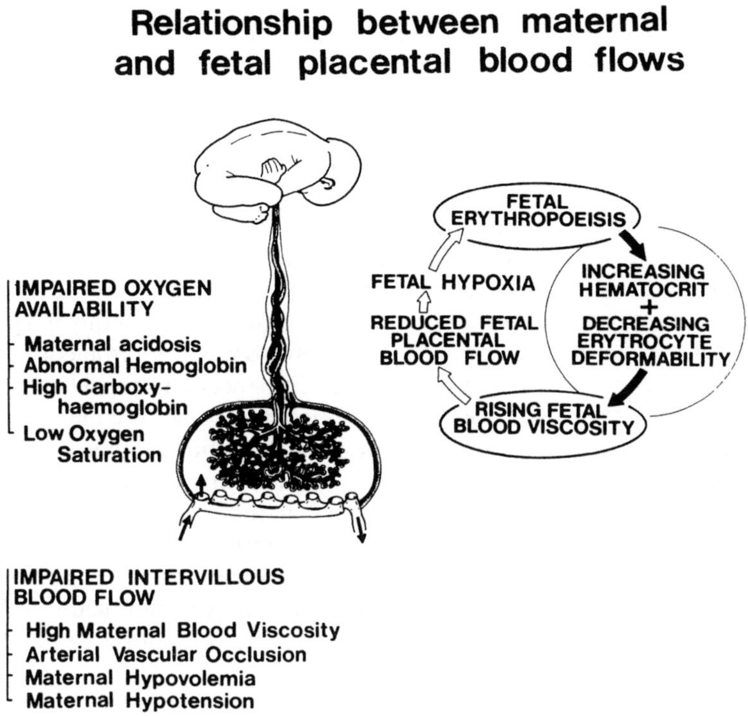

Figure 9.3. Diagramatic representation of fetal and maternal placental circulations [22].

circle is set up, with hyperviscosity leading to impaired placental perfusion, and further hypoxia adding renewed stimulus to erythropoiesis. It is known that post-maturity of the fetus is associated with an increased risk of fetal distress in labour and with an increased perinatal mortality and morbidity. The cumulative effect of these changes in fetal blood rheology would be a significant reduction in villous perfusion on the fetal side of the placenta, as well as an increased strain on the fetal heart because of the increase in peripheral resistance. Once again, the situation is open for a vicious circle of hypoxia and hyperviscosity, leading to impaired perfusion and further hypoxia. This situation could well make a significant contribution to the etiology of fetal distress in labour in post-mature fetuses, where any intrapartum anoxia would further exacerbate the already compromised hemorheological state of the placental blood flow.

9.4. Pathological pregnancy

Fetal intrauterine growth retardation is associated, except in the cases of congenital infection and developmental anomalies, with fetal hypoxia. The three most commonly identifiable causes of fetal hypoxia are: maternal cigarette smoking, pre-eclampsia, and maternal diabetes mellitus. The maternal and fetal hemorheology of these three conditions are described in this section.

9.4.1. Maternal smoking in pregnancy

A large volume of evidence has accumulated implicating cigarette smoking in low birth weight, preterm delivery, increased fetal wastage, and long term impairment of mental and physical growth. Smokers also show an increased incidence of abruptio placente, placenta previa, and other causes of ante-partum hemorrhage and premature rupture of the membranes [23].The chemistry and pharmacology of tobacco is complex and not fully understood. The mechanisms whereby cirgarette smoking affects fetal growth are not clear. Nicotine crosses the placenta, and in animal experiments injection of nicotine into the pregnant mother results in reduction of fetal birthweight. Suzuki et al [24] concluded that nicotine caused vasoconstriction of uterine vessels, with consequent reduction in intervillous blood flow and hence fetal asphyxia. Carbon monoxide appears in much higher levels in the blood of smokers and crosses the placental barrier. Astrup et al [25] exposed pregnant rabbits to different levels of ambient carbon monoxide and found a pronounced effect on average litter weight, fetal development and neonatal death rates.

The effect of cigarette smoking on hemorheological parameters has been studied in non-pregnant subjects. Chmiel et al [26] observed an increase in blood viscosity in smokers, this increase being much more marked immediately after smoking. Dintenfass [27] carried out a comparison of male smokers and matched controls. He reported that smokers had an increase in hematocrit, plasma fibrinogen, plasma and whole blood viscosity, and erythrocyte aggregation. All these findings have been confirmed in a study by Leonhardt et al [28]. It is probable that cigarette smoking affects fetal growth by several routes. Nicotine causes a reduction in intervillous blood flow, carbon monoxid decreases oxygen availability for the fetus, and there is clear evidence, at least in the fetus, of a hemorheological effect (Table 9.3) [29] that would further reduce placental perfusion and exacerbate fetal hypoxia.

The only clear difference in the maternal hemorheology of pregnancy, between smokers and non-smokers, was the reduced erythrocyte deformability index throughout pregnancy in smokers [29]. This is probably due to carboxyhemoglobin, which alters the internal viscosity of the erythrocyte and affects the oxygen availability for the cell's metabolism, thus reducing deformability. Clear differences existed in all parameters, except for plasma viscosity, when measurement were made at the postnatal visit [28]. These findings are in keeping with the published effects of smoking in non-pregnant subjects [26,27]. The alteration in hemorheology produced by smoking was much more pronounced in the fetus.

Table 9.3. Hemorheological profile of infants born to cigarette smoking and non-smoking mothers.

	Non-smokers	Smokers	Statistical comparison
Number of subjects	40	40	
Gestational age (weeks)			
Mean + SD	39.4 + 0.6	38.7 + 0.8	n.s.
Birth weight (g)			
Mean + SD	3215 +210	2897 +252	$p < 0.01$
Hematocrit			
Mean + SD	0.496 + 0.031	0.558 + 0.041	$p < 0.001$
Plasma viscosity (centipoise)			
Mean + SD	1.47 + 0.34	1.49 + 0.35	n.s.
Whole blood viscosity (centipoise)			
Mean + SD	16.3 + 2.2	18.7 +2.8	$p < 0.02$
Erthrocyte deformability index			
Mean + SD	0.79 + 0.10	0.65 + 0.11	$p < 0.02$

Statistical comparison using Student's t-test.

The whole blood viscosity was elevated because of the raised hematocrit and reduced erythrocyte deformability. Chronic fetal hypoxia has been suggested as a stimulus for erythrocyte production [20]; as with postmature infants, a vicious circle could be set up with carbon monoxide causing fetal hypoxia, leading to stimulation of erythropoiesis, elevation of hematocrit and blood viscosity, reduction of placental perfusion, and hence further fetal hypoxia. In support of this hypothesis, elevated levels of erythropoietin and hematocrit have been reported in cord blood from babies whose mothers smoked during pregnancy [30] and the increased whole blood viscosity and decreased erythrocyte deformability found in the present study complete the circle.

9.4.2. Pre-eclampsia

The clinical association between pre-eclampsia and increased perinatal morbidity and mortality is well documented, but the exact etiology of pre-eclampsia is complex, with several different pathological processes interacting and combining to produce the widespread changes seen in the mother, placenta, and fetus. Abnormalities of the immunological relationship between the maternal host and the feto-placental graft have been described, as have breakdown of the normal hemostatic mechanisms, abnormalities of the renin-angiotensin system, and morphological changes in the utero-placental vasculature. Although the order and importance of these abnormalities in the pathogenesis of pre-eclampsia is not clear, the end result, from the fetal point of view, is seen in the blood supply to the microvasculature of the placenta.

The association between pre-eclampsia and reduced intervillous blood flow is well established by clinical studies. McClure et al [31] demonstrated a 33 per cent reduction in intervillous blood flow in patients with toxemia. Morris et al [32] and others [33] indicated that the severity of pre-eclampsia was proportional to the degree of reduction in blood flow. It is not clear from these studies if the pre-eclampsia or the reduced placental blood flow comes first.

Animal experiments have shown that artificial uterine ischemia, induced by partial occlusion of the uterine artery in pregnant animals, produces a situation with maternal and fetal effects almost identical to pre-eclampsia. Utero-placental ischemia, as a basic etiological factor in the development of pre-eclampsia, has been postulated for many years, but it is only recently that attention has been focussed on the rheology of pre-eclampsia. Fahraeus [34] described eclampsia as "a disease of the checked microcirculation". Certainly the results of a cross-sectional study of blood rheology in patients with pre-eclampsia (Figs. 9.4 and 9.5) [35] would indicate that, in pre-eclampsia, hemorheological factors are altered in such a way as to increase peripheral resistance, elevate blood pressure, and reduce blood flow in the microcirculation. Independent of any vascular constriction, the increased whole blood and plasma viscosity and reduced erythrocyte deformability seen in maternal blood in pre-eclampsia would reduce intervillous blood flow. A 10 per cent increase in whole blood viscosity is associated with a 20 per cent reduction in peripheral blood flow. Several studies have shown similar findings [35-39]. The elevation in maternal hematocrit in pre-eclampsia has been previously reported, as have the elevations in fibrinogen and plasma viscosity. Heilmann et al [36] investigated the hemorheology of 27 women with pre-eclampsia and found an increase in relative blood viscosity and a reduction in erythrocyte deformability.

The cause of the observed phenomena is not clear. Certainly an increase in hematocrit may be due to the reduction in plasma volume seen in patients with pre-eclampsia. Increased plasma viscosity is related to raised fibrinogen levels and also to an increase in immunoglobulins which occurs in pre-eclampsia. Loss of water from the intravascular compartment due to abnormal capillary permeability may explain the alterations in all hemorheological parameters in pre-eclampsia without implicating an increased production of any factor. The protein concentration does not rise significantly because the albumin leaves the capillary with the water, leaving behind only the higher molecular weight globulins.

The relationship between hyperviscosity and disseminated intravascular coagulation is in speculation at present. Slowing of the microcirculation due to hyperviscosity, by leading to further hypoxia and hyperviscosity, will predispose to the formation of thrombi in the microvasculature. This process will operate not only in the placenta, but also in maternal organs such as the liver, kidneys and brain, which are all affected by microvascular coagulation in eclampsia.

The only consistent effect of pre-eclampsia on fetal hemorheology was an increase in the whole blood viscosity due to elevated hematocrit (Table 9.4) [34].

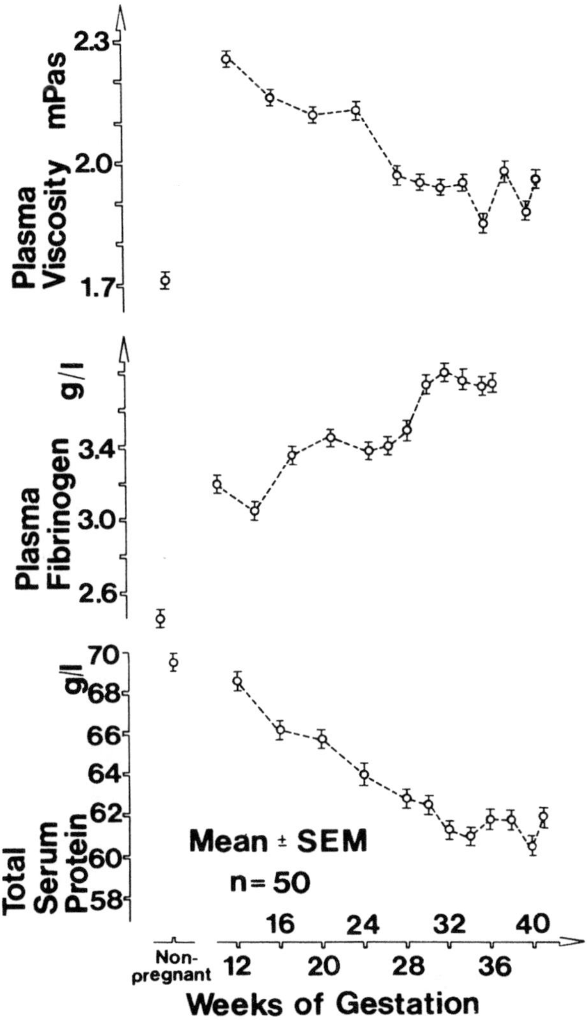

Figure 9.4. Plasma viscosity, fibrinogen and total serum protein in cross-sectional study of patients with pre-eclampsia [35].

Walker and Turnbull [20] proposed that fetal hypoxia, due to placental insufficiency from whatever cause, resulted in a secondary polycythemia, and this may be the main hemorheological consequence of maternal pre-eclampsia. If, however, fetal hypoxia became more pronounced, due to either a worsening maternal pre-eclampsia or the onset of labour, then a deteriorating hemorheological situation could develop, with decreased erythrocyte deformability, hypercoagulability, and elevated whole blood viscosity. The situation would then be ripe for

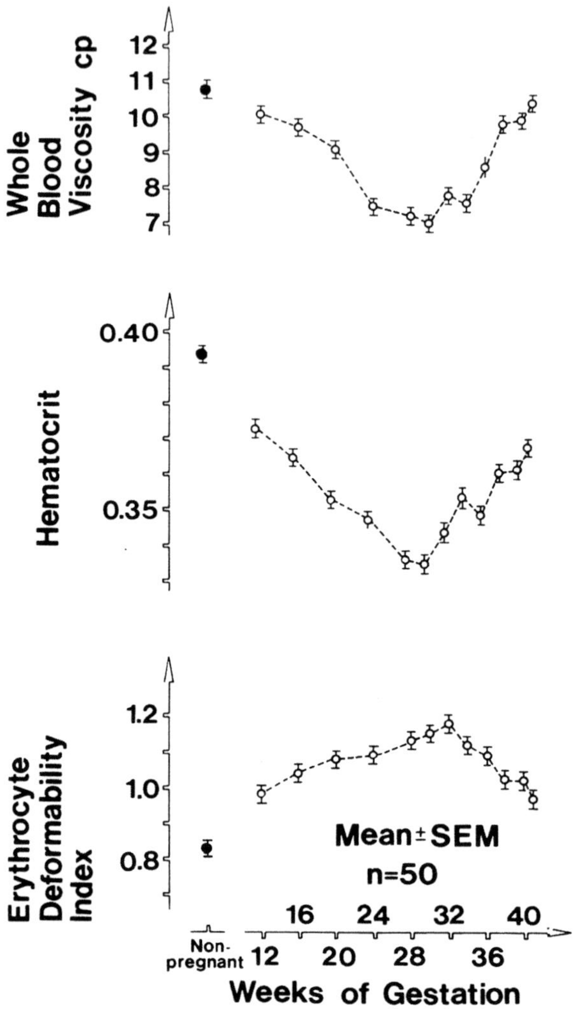

Figure 9.5. Whole blood viscosity hematocrit, and erythrocyte deformability index in cross-sectional study of patients with pre-eclampsia [35].

acute fetal distress and for thrombosis and hemorrhage at vulnerable areas of the fetal circulation.

9.4.3. Hemorheological therapy in pre-eclampsia

It is interesting to note that some commonly used treatment regimes in the management of pre-eclampsia have a hemorheological basis to their actions. The

Table 9.4. Hemorheological profile of infants born to mothers with pre-eclamptic toxaemia and normotensive controls–cross-sectional study.

	Normotensive controls	Pre-eclamptic patients	Statistical compa-comparison
Number of subjects	30	30	
Gestational age (weeks)			
Mean + SD	38.6 + 0.6	36.3 + 0.7	n.s.
Birth weight (g)			
Mean + SD	3175 + 209	2885 + 215	$p < 0.05$
Hematocrit			
Mean + SD	0.477 + 0.024	0.537 + 0.037	$p < 0.01$
Plasma viscosity (centipoise)			
Mean + SD	1.42 + 0.30	1.55 + 0.34	n.s.
Whole blood viscosity (centipoise)			
Mean + SD	15.8 + 1.9	17.9 + 2.1	$p < 0.01$
Erythrocyte deformability index			
Mean + SD	0.72 + 0.10	0.67 + 0.11	n.s.

Statistical comparison using Student's t-test.

restoration of normal plasma volume with salt-poor albumin [40,41,42] or low molecular weight dextran [43,44], has been shown to improve fetal outcome and maternal renal function in pre-eclampsia, by increasing peripheral blood flow due to reduction in hematocrit and whole blood viscosity. In order to avoid overloading of the circulation while giving plasma volume expanders, central venous pressure monitoring is essential [41,43]. Another common treatment of pre-eclampsia is to give thiazide diuretics. These will further reduce plasma volume and increase hematocrit, plasma viscosity and whole blood viscosity, and on the basis of these changes would be expected to reduce placental blood flow. Indeed, an increasing number of clinical studies have shown that diuretic therapy is not only unhelpful in the treatment of pre-eclampsia but may, in fact, be detrimental, and there is certainly a good hemorheological basis to support this view.

9.4.4. Diabetes mellitus in pregnancy

Abnormal hemorheology in non-pregnant diabetics has been extensively reported [45] and is discussed in Chapter 10. The main components of diabetic hyperviscosity are reduced erythrocyte deformability and elevated plasma fibrinogen levels. Poorly controlled diabetes is associated with a considerable morbidity and mortality for the fetus and neonate, but little has been done to investigate the hemorheology of either mother or fetus in pregnancy. Foley et al [46] showed a significantly elevated blood viscosity in the newborn and this has been shown to be due to both polycythemia and increased plasma viscosity. The blood viscosity of infants born to diabetic mothers is also elevated because of reduced erythrocyte deformability (P.C. Buchan, unpublished). These infants not infrequently show signs and symptoms of the hyperviscosity syndrome and can be greatly helped by isovolemic hemodilution.

9.5. Rheology in the neonate

Microcirculatory disorders in the neonate have been recognised for many years. Neonatal hyperviscosity syndrome occurs in three to six per cent of all newborns and is associated with cardiorespiratory failure, hyperbilirubinemia, convulsion, and neurological damage [47]. Long-term follow-up of infants with polycythemic hyperviscosity has shown a 50% incidence of neurological abnormality [48]. In a large series of 1,830 neonates, Oats et al [49] found an incidence of 6.6% of infants with hyperviscosity. They defined hyperviscosity as greater than two standard deviations above the mean for normal infants. They found that 34 per cent of the hyperviscous infants were polycythemic (two standard deviations above the mean hematocrit). They found a significant relation between birth weight and blood viscosity, with 15.2 per cent of growth-retarded infants exhibiting hyperviscosity. However, they point out that 70 per cent of the hyperviscous infants had birth weights appropriate for gestational age. The etiological factors responsible for neonatal hyperviscosity are extensive and include pre-term delivery, small for gestational age, intrapartum asphyxia, pre-eclampsia, diabetes mellitus, late cord clamping, and twin-twin transfusion.

9.6. Treatment of neonatal hyperviscosity

Infants with a hematocrit above 0.65 who exhibit symptoms of hyperviscosity (plethora, cyanosis, respiratory distress, cardiomegaly and central nervous system signs) should have treatment. The cerebral, pulmonary and renal disorders can be alleviated rapidly by partial exchange hemodilution. There is some doubt as to whether correction of hyperviscosity will prevent the long-term neurological sequelae - it must be remembered that fetal hyperviscosity of many months' duration may precede birth. The target hematocrit in hemodilution therapy is around 0.50, and great care must be taken not to reduce the oxygen-carrying capacity of the blood too far. Infants with hyperviscosity and without polycythemia require plasma exchange therapy if they have symptoms, however, little has been done in this area as yet.

9.7. Rheological sequelae of oral contraception

A vast amount of epidemiological, clinical and laboratory evidence has linked the use of combined oral contraceptives with certain types of cardiovascular disease, especially venous thromboembolism, hypertension, thrombotic stroke and myocardial infarction [50]. The introduction of low-estrogen oral contraceptives resulted in a dramatic reduction in venous thromboembolism, but the frequency of arterial complications remained unchanged, and several studies have implicated the progestogen in the combined oral contraceptive in the etiology of these arterial problems [51]. Raised blood viscosity has been reported in women taking combined oral contraceptives [52,53] and hyperviscosity is known to be associated with increased risk of venous thromboembolism, occlusive arterial disease and hypertension [54]. Estrogen and progestogens singly or in combination cause a rise in blood viscosity. These two hormones, however, affect the determinants of blood viscosity differently and this may account for the differing cardiovascular pathologies associated with oestrogen and progestogen therapy (Table 9.5) [55].

Classically, the high estrogen content of oral contraceptives is associated with venous thromboembolism. The predominant effect of estrogen on the hemorheological profile of blood is to raise plasma fibrinogen and hematocrit. These two parameters are raised in pregnancy [4] and post-surgery conditions also associated with increased risk of venous thromboembolism. Estrogen, either alone or in combination, has a direct effect on vascular smooth muscle, with increase in both arterial dilatation and venous compliance, predisposing to venous stasis and with an elevated fibrinogen to venous thrombosis. Reduction of the estrogen dose in the combined oral contraceptive has drastically decreased the risk of associated venous thromboembolism.

Progestogens, conversely, have no direct effect on vascular smooth muscle. With blood viscosity being elevated by a raised hematocrit and reduced erythrocyte deformability, there is an increase in peripheral resistance with reduced peripheral perfusion and increased blood pressure. Reduced erythrocyte deformability and raised hematocrit are also features of intermittant claudication [56], ischemic heart disease [54] and hypertension [57]. The common hemorheological profile of progestogen therapy and occlusive arterial disease is suggestive that this may be one of the links in the association between progestogens and occlusive vascular disease. The balance between the amount of estrogen and progestogen seems to be important. The relatively high progestogen level necessary for cycle control with very low estrogen dosage has potentially serious implications for arterial occlusive disease; evaluation of the new generation of triphasic and sequential combined oral contraceptives must be made to determine whether they have a more balanced effect on the hemorheological, hemostatic and biochemical profiles of blood related to cardiovascular disease.

Table 9.5. Effects of estrogen and progestogen alone and in combination on blood viscosity and its major determinant; mean (SEM).

	Ethinylestradiol		Norethisterone		Combined ethinylestradiol and norethisterone	
	Pre-treatment	Post-treatment	Pre-treatment	Post-treatment	Pre-treatment	Post-treatment
Number	20	20	20	20	20	20
Hematocrit	0.348 (0.006)	0.382 (0.007) **	0.342 (0.005)	0.390 (0.007) *	0.373 (0.009)	0.417 (0.008) *
Plasma fibrinogen g/l	2.400 (0.090)	3.100 (0.120) *	2.430 (0.100)	2.410 (0.090) n.s.	2.420 (0.100)	2.830 (0.170) *
Erythrocyte deformability index	0.810 (0.030)	0.970 (0.050) **	0.780 (0.030)	0.610 (0.020) *	0.830 (0.060)	0.770 (0.090) **
Blood viscosity mPa s	10.200 (0.800)	12.200 (1.200) *	10.400 (0.800)	13.100 (1.400) *	9.700 (1.200)	11.900 (1.300) *

Statistical comparison using Student's paired t-test.
* $p < 0.01$; ** $p < 0.05$; n.s. $p > 0.05$.

9.8. References

1. Harvey W. 1628: Exercitatio Anatomica de Moty Cordis et Sanguinis in Animalibus. Translated by K.J. Franklin [1957]. Oxford: Blackwell.
2. Bader R.A., Bader M.E., Rose D.J., Braunwald E. 1955: Haemodynamics at rest and during exercise in normal pregnancy as studied by cardiac catheterisation. J. Clin. Invest. 34, 1524-1536.
3. Hales S. 1753: Statistical Essays. Vol. 2. London, Imrys and Mauby.
4. Buchan P.C. 1984: Maternal and fetal blood viscosity throughout normal pregnancy. J. Obst. and Gyn. 4, 343-350.
5. Pellisier M.P. 1912: La viscosité du sang total chez la femme enceinte et accouchée et ses rapports avec la tension arterielle. Arch. Obstét. 11, 306-320.
6. Esiashwili I. 1933: Blutgerinnung und Viskosität in der Schwangerschafts- und Nachgeburtsperiode. Zentralblatt für Gynäkologie 57, 2712-2728.
7. Cohen M.E., Thomson K.J. 1936: Studies on the circulation in pregnancy. The velocity of blood flow and related aspects of the circulation in normal pregnant women. J. Clin. Invest. 15, 607-625.
8. Hamilton H.F.H. 1950: Blood viscosity in pregnancy. J. Obstet. Gynecol. (Brit. Comwth.) 57, 530-538.
9. Leonhardt H., Uthoff A., Stelter I. 1975: Veränderungen der Blut- und Plasmaviskosität bei Patienten mit Risikofaktoren. Medizinische Klinik 70, 1997-2005.
10. Schmid-Schönbein H., von Hugo R., Rieger H. 1976: In: Die Beckenvenen. Ed. Ludwig H., Karz E. p. 87.
11. Durocher J.R., Weir M.S., Lundblad E.G., Patow W.E., Conrad M.E. 1975: Effecta of oral contraceptives and pregnancy on erythrocyte deformability and surface charge. Proc. Soc. Exp. Biol. Med. 150, 368-370.
12. Murphy J.R. 1968: Haemoglobin CC disease - Rheological properties of erythrocytes and abnormalities in cell water. J. Clin. Invest. 47, 1483-1495.
13. Buchan P.C. 1980: Evaluation and modification of whole blood filtration in the measurement of erythrocyte deformability in pregnancy and the newborn. Br. J. Haematol. 45, 97-105.
14. Chien S. 1975: Biophysical behaviour of red cells in suspensions. In: Surgenor D. Mc. Ed: The Red Blood Cell, New York. Vol. 2, Academic Press, Inmc., 1031-1133.
15. Ozanne P., Linderkamp O., Miller F.C., Meiselman H.J. 1983: Erythrocyte aggregation during normal pregnancy. Am. J. Obstet. and Gyn. 147, 576-583.
16. Eastham R.D. 1964: Plasma viscosity in the improved haematological screening of antenatal patients. J. Obstet. Gynaecol. Brit. Comwth. 71, 763-764.
17. Foley M.E., Isherwood D.M., McNicol G.P. 1978: Viscosity, haematocrit, fibrinogen and plasma proteins in maternal and cord blood. Br. J. Obstet. Gyn. 85, 500-504.
18. Linderkamp O., Sengespeik H.C., Vermold H.T., Bethke K. 1983: Hemorheology in preterm and full-term neonates (Abstract). European Journal of Paediatrics 140, 81.
19. Foley M.E., Collins R., MacDonald D. 1984: Whole blood viscosity in umbilical cord blood, adult pregnant and non-adult pregnant blood: The influence of plasma factors. In: Heilmann L., Buchan P.C. Ed. Hemorheological disorders in Obstetrics and Neonatology. Schattauer, Stuttgart, pp. 92-97.
20. Linderkamp O., Sengespeik H.C., McKay C.B., Meiselman H.J. 1984: Rheological properties of blood in preterm and full-term neonates. In: Heilmann L., Buchan P.C. Ed: Hemorheological disorders in Obstetrics and Neonatology. Schattauer. Stuttgart, pp. 83-91.
21. Walker J., Turnbull E.P.N. 1953: Haemoglobin and red cells in the fetus and their relation to the oxygen content of the blood in the vessels of the umbilical cord. Lancet 2, 312-318.
22. Buchan P.C. 1984: Impaired erythrocyte deformability and raised blood viscosity and perinatal hypoxic brain damage - an in vitro and in vivo study. In: Heilmann L., Buchan P.C. Ed. Hemorheological disorders in Obstetrics and Neonatology. Schattauer. Stuttgart, pp. 98-103.
23. Pirani B.B.K. 1978: Smoking in pregnancy. Obstet. Gynaecol. Surv. 33, 1-13.

24. Suzuki K., Horiguchi T., Comas-Urrutia A.C., Müller-Heuback E., Morishima H.O., Adamson K. 1971: Pharmacological effects of nicotine upon the fetus and mother in the rhesus monkey. Am. J. Obstet. Gynecol. III, 1092.
25. Astrup P., Trolle D., Olsen H.M., Kjieldsen K. 1972: Effect of moderate carbon monoxide exposure on fetal development. Lancet 2, 1220-1223.
26. Chmiel H., Effert S., Mathey D. 1973: Rheologische Veränderungen des Blutes beim akuten Herzinfarkt und dessen Risikofaktoren. Dtsch. Med. Wochenschr. 98, 1641-1649.
27. Dintenfass L. 1975: Elevation of blood viscosity, aggregation of red cells, haematocrit values and fibrinogen levels in cigarette smokers. Med. J. Aust. 1, 617-620.
28. Leonhardt H., Grigoleit H.G., Reinhardt I. 1978: Auswirkungen von Zigarettenrauch und oralen Kontrazeptiva auf die Plasma- und Vollblutviskosität. Med. Welt 29, 880-886.
29. Buchan P.C. 1981: Effect of cigarette smoking on maternal and fetal blood viscosity in pregnancy. Clin. Haemorheol. 1, 459.
30. Finne P. 1968: Erythropoietin production in fetal hypoxia and in anaemic uraemic patients. Annals of the New York Academy of Science 149, 497.
31. McClure Browne J.C., Veal N. 1953: The maternal placental blood flow in normotensive and hypertensive women. J. Obstet. Gynaecol. Brit. Comwth. 60, 141-148.
32. Morris M., Osborn S.D., Wright H.P. 1955: Effective circulation of the uterine wall in late pregnancy measured with ^{24}NaCl. Lancet 1, 323-324.
33. Pritchard J.A. 1965: Changes in the blood volume during pregnancy and delivery. Anaesthesiology, 26, 393.
34. Fahraeus P. 1962: Eclampsia - a disease of the checked microcirculation. Acta Obstet. Gynaecol. Scand. 41, 101-110.
35. Buchan P.C. 1982: Pre-eclampsia - a hyperviscosity syndrome. American J. Obstet. Gynaecol. 142, 111-112.
36. Heilmann L., Mattheck C., Kurz E. 1977: Rheologische Veränderungen des Blutes in der normalen und pathologischen Schwangerschaft und deren Einfluß auf die Sauerstoffsdiffusion. Arch. Gynäkol. 223, 283-298.
37. Kaibara M., Marumoto Y., Taniguchi I., Kobayahi T. 1982: Blood viscosity at low shear rate in normal and abnormal pregnancies. Clin. Hemorheol. 2, 209-217.
38. Hobbs J.B., Oats J.N., Palmer A.A., Long P.A., Mitchell G.M., Lou A., McIver M.A. 1982: Whole blood viscosity in pre-eclampsia. Am. J. Obstet. Gynecol. 142, 288-292.
39. Thorburn J., Drummond M.M., Whigham K.A., Lowe G.D.O., Dorbes C.O., Prentice C.R., Whitfield C.R. 1982: Blood viscosity and haemostatic facors in late pregnancy, pre-eclampsia and fetal growth retardation. Br. J. Obstet. Gynaecol. 89, 117-122.
40. Buchan P.C. 1983: Fetal and maternal response to haemodilution in gestosis in "Dilemmas in Gestosis". Janisch H., Reinold E. Ed. Thieme, New York, pp. 157-158.
41. Maclean A.B., Doig J.R., Aickin D.R. 1978: Hypovolaemia, pre-eclampsia and diuretics. Br. J. Obstet. Gynaecol. 85, 597-603.
42. Schroeck R. 1984: Hemodilution in Obstetrics: Significance and monitoring of hypertonic dilution procedures with 20% human serum albumin. In: Heilmann L, Buchan P.C. Ed. Haemorheological disorders in Obstetrics and Neonatology. Schattauer. Stuttgart, pp. 54-62.
43. McGrath M.A., Penny R. 1976: Paraproteinaemia: hyperviscosity and clinical manifestation. J. Clin. Invest. 58, 1155-1162.
44. Heilmann L., Sieckmann U., Fischer W.M. 1981: Therapy of disturbed microcirculation on toxaemia of pregnancy. J. Fetal Med. 1, 39-43.
45. Barnes A.J. 1981: Blood viscosity in Diabetes Mellitus. In: Editors Lowe G.D.O., Barbenel J.C. and Forbes C.D. Clinical Aspects of Blood Viscosity and Cell Deformability. Springer Verlag. Berlin, pp. 151-162.
46. Foley M.E., Collins R., Stronge J.M., Drury M.I., MacDonald D. 1981: Blood viscosity in umbilical cord blood from babies of diabetic mothers. J. Obstet. Gynaecol. 2, 93-96.

47. Mentzer W.C. 1978: Polycythaemia and the hyperviscosity syndrome in newborn infants. Clin. Haematol. 7, 63-74.
48. Goldberg K.E., Lubchenco L.O., Guggenheim M.A. 1975: Sequelae of neonatal hyperviscosity. Paediatric Research 9, 488.
49. Oats J.N., Drew J.H., Hobbs J.B., Palmer A.A., Mitchell G.M., McIver M.A. 1984: Neonatal hyperviscosity. In: Editors Heilmann L., Buchan P.C. Haemorheological disorders in obstetrics and neonatology. Schattauer, Stuttgart, pp. 110-115.
50. Vessey M.P. 1980: Female hormones and vascular disease - an epidemiological overview. British Journal of Farm Planning 6, Suppl. 1-12.
51. Meade T.W., Chakrabarti R., Haines A.P., Howarth A.P., North W.R.S., Stirling Y. 1977: Haematocrit, lipid and blood pressure profiles of women or oral contraceptives containing 50 or 30 ug oestrogen. Lancet 11, 948-951.
52. Buchan P.C., MacDonald H.N. 1980: Altered haemorheology in oral contraceptive users. Br. Med. J. 280, 978-979.
53. Lowe G.D.O., Drummond M.M., Forbes C.D., Barbenel J.C. 1980: Increased blood viscosity in young women using oral contraceptives. Am. J. Obstet. Gynecol. 137, 840-842.
54. Dormandy J.A. 1975: Blood: its viscosity and circulation. In: Harcus A.W., Adamson L. Ed: Arteries and Veins, New York, Churchill Livingstone, p. 99-135.
55. Buchan P.C. 1982: Haemorheological consequences of oestrogen and progestogen therapy. International Journal of Microcirculation Clinical and Experimental 1, 262.
56. Dormandy J.A., Hoare E., Colley J., Arrowsmith D.E., Dormandy R.L. 1973: Clinical, haemodynamic, rheological and biochemical findings in 126 patients with intermittent claudication. Br. Med. J. 4, 576-581.
57. Tibblin G., Bergentz S.E., Bjure J., Wilhelmsen L. 1966: Haematocrit, plasma proteins, plasma volume and viscosity in early hypertensive disease. Am. Heart J. 72, 165-176.

10
Diabetes

Adrian Barnes and Elizabeth Willars
Barnet General Hospital, Wellhouse Lane, Barnet, Herts. United Kingdom

10.1. Introduction

Diabetes is a disease of major social and economic importance. In Western Europe it is estimated that approximately 2% of the population suffer from the condition. Not only is diabetes the most common cause of blindness between the ages of 20 and 60 years, but it is also one of the leading causes of renal failure and a powerful risk factor for coronary, cerebral and peripheral circulatory disease. Many diabetics also have abnormalities in peripheral and autonomic neural functions that lead to distressing and often debilitating symptoms. Before reviewing and discussing the literature on diabetes and hemorheology it would be helpful to outline the nature of diabetes and to examine the pathophysiology of some of these diabetic complications, so that rheological changes can be seen in the context of the overall pathology that they are reported to induce. At the end of the chapter rheological abnormalities in diabetes will be discussed in relation to other factors that diabetologists think might be of importance in the etiology and progression of these lesions.

10.2. Diabetes and its complications

Although controversy continues as to the exact definition of diabetes the condition is generally held to be a syndrome resulting from a relative or absolute deficiency of insulin. Type 1, or juvenile, diabetes is characterised by extensive or total insulin deficiency; patients usually develop the disorder under the age of 40 and require daily injections of insulin to survive. Type 2 or maturity onset, diabetes occurs in middle or latter life. It is the most common type of diabetes and patients are treated with diet alone or diet and tablets. Here insulin secretion is delayed; there is variable peripheral insulin resistance, and islet cell damage is much less extensive. Both types of diabetes are associated with micro- and macrocirculatory disease. The microangiopathy is specific to diabetes itself, whereas large vessel disease in diabetes is histologically indistinguishable from that of non-diabetics. The pathophysiological features of the microcirculatory disturbance of diabetes are best considered in relation to the target organs involved. A more detailed account of diabetic complications may be read elsewhere [1].

In the eye, thickening of the basement membrane of capillaries occurs as an early change [2]. The chemical composition of the membrane has been shown to be altered, and it becomes more permeable to a variety of substances [3]. The capillary endothelial cells themselves behave abnormally by several different criteria, and loss of pericytes is a readily observed microscopic feature [4]. The key pathophysiological event in the eye in diabetes, however, is capillary non-perfusion [5]. This may be seen on fluorescein angiography and is presumed to be due to occlusion of capillaries. Over a sustained time period the increasing number of occluded capillaries lead to foci of retinal hypoxia. It is postulated that the damaged retina produces an as yet unidentified factor that stimulates new vessel formation within the eye; presumably in an attempt to revascularize the areas of ischaemia. Initially the new vessels lie flat on the posterior aspect of the vitreous, but as associated fibrous tissue contracts, retinal detachment and hemorrhage may occur - both of which may result in impairment or loss of vision. This chain of events is not a feature specific to diabetes, and many conditions in which retinal hypoxia occurs have been observed to be associated with neovascularization (Table 10.1) [2,6]. Interestingly, although this failure of capillary flow is clinically the central pathological event in diabetic retinopathy, one of the earliest changes observeable in diabetes is capillary and venous dilatation, and retinal blood flow appears to be actually increased before extensive retinopathy develops [2]. The cause of this hemodynamic change is unknown but raised blood flow to several organs has been reported in diabetes [7-9], and cardiac output [10] is increased. The basal metabolic rate (BMR) has recently been shown to be high in diabetics [11], and it is possible that the hemodynamic changes represent adaptation to the abnormally high metabolic demands of diabetic tissue. When strict glycaemic control is restored to diabetic patients, the BMR, cardiac output and organ blood flow revert to near normal levels.

In the kidney, as in the eye, there is thickening of the capillary basement membrane. The turnover of the latter is retarded and its chemical composition abnormal [12]. Basement membrane-like material accumulates in the mesangial zone which may be related in part to trapping of fibrinogen and other macromolecules. Light microscopy of renal tissue shows nodular, diffuse and exudative changes in the glomeruli, with a common end point of hyalinization - diabetic glomerulosclerosis. Arteriosclerosis is common, with both efferent and afferent vessel walls showing hyaline and fatty degeneration. Although atheroma is said to be more common in diabetes there is no accurate documentation of any increases in its incidence in large renal vessels. On the other hand, diffuse intimal fibrosis in these vessels is more common and more extensive than in non-diabetics [13]. Glomerular filtration rate is increased in most patients, but reports on renal

Table 10.1. Conditions in which new blood vessels may be seen in the retina.

Disease	Hemorheological deficit
Diabetes mellitus	+
Eales vasculopathy	0
Sickle cell disease	+
Thalassaemia	+
Dysproteinaemia	+
Von Willebrands disease	−
Chronic myeloid leukaemia	+
Polycythaemia	+
Sarcoidosis	0
Branch vein occlusion	+
Hypertension (with vein occlusion)	+
Takayasu's disease	0
Carotid-cavernous fistula	0
Carotid insufficiency	0
Radiation retinopathy	0
Retrolental fibroplasia	0
Coate's disease	0
Intraocular foreign body	0

+ present; − absent; 0 not investigated.

plasma flow have given variable results. Proteinuria (predominantly albuminuria) occurs partially as a result of basement membrane abnormalities, but it is also related to hemodynamic and other factors.

Diabetic neuropathy is a complex and varied clinical entity [14]. Symmetrical sensory and autonomic neuropathies are characterised histologically by segmental demyelination and axonal degeneration and are considered to have a metabolic etiology. Mononeuropathies, however, may have a vascular basis. Here isolated or multiple involvment of cranial or peripheral nerves occurs, palsies of the 3rd and 6th cranial nerves and lesions of ulnar, radial, median, femoral and peroneal nerves being the most common. Onset may be abrupt or insidious, and damage may be sensory, motor or mixed. Occlusion of intraneural blood vessels with fibrin and cellular material has been described in association with these lesions, implicating the possible etiological importance of hemodynamic factors.

There is an increased frequency of peripheral, coronary and cerebral circulatory disease in diabetes [15-17]. In the periphery, atherosclerosis frequently involves the arteries below the knee. Indeed, gangrene of the lower limb is estimated to be forty times more common in diabetics than in non diabetics [18]. Claudication is also significantly increased. Although reduced blood flow to the leg may be clinically inferred in many individuals, other diabetics have warm feet with pounding foot pulses, and increased leg blood flow has been amply demonstrated in these subjects. Such changes may well be due to arteriovenous shunting (possibly related to neuropathy) and distal nutrient flow may still be impaired [19]. Besides ischemia, both neuropathy and infection can contribute to the diabetic foot which is often an entity of complex pathology.

Clinical cardiac disease and cardiac mortality are more frequent in diabetes. These findings are not entirely explained by coronary artery disease, and other known risk factors and a specific diabetic cardiomyopathy has been postulated [20]. This may in part be related to microangiopathy, but metabolic and other factors may also be important. Like coronary artery disease, disability and death from cerebrovascular disease appear to be more common in diabetics. For example, in Japan cerebral arterial disease is the most frequent single cause of death amongst diabetics, with brain infarction, rather than hemorrhage as the principal factor. Resting cerebral blood flow has been found to be similar in diabetics and non-diabetics; in both groups flow declining with increasing age. Unlike controls, however, many diabetics are unable to increase cerebral blood flow in response to hypercapnia, and these individuals seem to have diminished ciculatory reserves [21].

10.3. Relevance of blood rheology in diabetes

The retinal manifestations of diabetes provided the stimulus for early workers to examine blood rheology in this condition [22,23]. Distended veins, micro-aneurysms, hemorrhages and neovascularization occur not only in diabetes, but also in other conditions which are associated with an increased viscosity of blood, macroglobulinemia, leukemia and sickle cell disease being notable examples. Furthermore, some of these retinal changes have been induced in experimental animals after increasing their blood viscosity with infusions of high molecular weight dextran [24]. An additional piece of evidence implicating hemorheology in microcirculatory disease was a study showing that patients with retinal branch vein thrombosis, who had developed capillary occlusion had higher levels of blood viscosity than patients with a vasodilatory response [25].

Of the three primary determinants of blood flow, vessel radius (vascular morphology) has received by far the most attention in diabetes. A reduction in vessel radius or alterations in vascular geometry are actually more common in diabetics than in non-diabetics and are certain to play an important role in the circulatory disease of many patients. Impaired circulation due to altered perfusion pressure in diabetes is more difficult to define. Many vessels are subjected to increased flow (rather than reduced flow) with higher pulse pressures for reasons already discussed. The implications of sustained elevations of shear stress on large and small vessel walls in diabetes must remain speculative but they may have a damaging influence on these structures. Reduced perfusion pressure seems unlikely to be of significance in diabetic complications, since hypertension rather than hypotension tends to occur in diabetes [26] and even in capillaries pressure does not seem to be reduced. Interestingly the reduction in perfusion pressure and volume flow in the retina, which follows improvement in metabolic control, has been recently put forward to explain the initial deterioration of retinopathy observed after one year of initiating continuous subcutaneous insulin infusion (CSII) therapy [27]. It is presumed that such hemodynamic changes promote the occlusion of capillaries. The physical properties of blood, the other primary determinant of flow, may well have importance in both large and small vessels in diabetes, particularly when these are diseased and are no longer able to respond to changes in tissue demands by alterations of internal radius. The possibility that impaired metabolic control may adversely affect blood rheology and at the same time increase tissue demands for blood flow requires further careful evaluation.

10.4. Macrorheology of blood in diabetes

10.4.1. Whole blood viscosity

The bulk viscosity of blood has been shown to be a determinant of flow in vessels of greater than capillary size, and measurement of this variable is therefore of great interest in patients with diabetic macroangiopathy, in particular ischemia of the lower limb. In addition to expressing viscosity in this way many workers have also expressed their data after correcting blood viscosity to a standard hematocrit (usually 0.40-0.45). The reasons for doing this are that hematocrit varies both between and within patients, and in particular it may be readily influenced by the circumstances of venepuncture. This may be of greater relevance in diabetes, as it has been shown that changes in hematocrit in response to exercise are more striking in diabetics with complications than in non-diabetics, probably due to greater fluid loss from the intravascular compartment [28]. This was thought to be related to structural and chemical changes in the walls of small vessels. Excursions of blood sugar have also been shown to influence hematocrit both in diabetics and non diabetics [29]. Thus, diabetics are susceptible to greater than normal variations of red cell concentration, and notice should be taken of both the hematocrit corrected and uncorrected whole blood viscosity values.

Although Swank [30] reported an elevation of whole blood viscosity in five diabetics as part of a larger study of patients with general vascular disease in 1959, the first full survey of this variable in diabetes was that of Skovborg et al in 1966 [23]. Using a Wells-Brookfield viscometer at shear rates between 1.15 and 230 s^{-1}, he and his group found a 20% increase in whole blood viscosity when compared to non-diabetic controls. A number of patients investigated had complications, but the authors did not comment on differences between individuals with and without microangiopathy. However, in his doctorate thesis [31], Skovborg subsequently examined a much larger number of diabetics ($n = 143$) and commented that there was no statistically significant correlation between the presence of retinopathy and elevated blood viscosity. Interestingly within the group of patients with retinopathy a statistically significant correlation was found between the presence of proliferative retinopathy and elevated blood viscosity. In a group of 10 diabetic patients, blood viscosity was highest in the day and lowest at night, with meals usually being followed by a reduction of this variable (the results in this way were similar to a group of non-diabetic control subjects). The variation in blood viscosity was best correlated statistically with the change in hematocrit and to a lesser extent the concentration of albumin, fibrinogen and beta globulin or alpha-2-globulin, while blood glucose concentrations did not have any significant correlation.

In 1967 Rees et al [32], using the more sophisticated GDM rotational viscometer, made rheological measurements on suspensions of diabetic erythrocytes in native plasma at a standard hematocrit of 0.40. Extrapolated yield shear stress values in diabetics in the early stages of retinopathy were no different from normal. By contrast, patients with progressive hemorrhagic proliferative retinopathy complicating uncontrolled diabetes, infection and the nephrotic stages of diabetic nephropathy were consistently associated with an increase in plasma fibrinogen and macroglobulin. The authors concluded that multiple non-specific factors can increase the yield shear stress of blood in diabetics, which may in turn contribute to the fulminating progression of established microangiopathy. Pursuing this approach Ditzel [33] examined whole blood viscosity with a Wells-Brookfield viscometer in 35 diabetics without retinopathy and found no differences compared with non-diabetics. He reasoned that if one accepted that the development of retinopathy was a slow chain of events starting from the earliest evidence of diabetes, then an inability to find an elevation in viscosity in the initial stages of diabetes did not support the view that blood viscosity was etiologically important in the very early retinal lesions. Like Rees et al [32], he felt that the increased viscosity present in long standing cases of diabetes might contribute to the progression of an already established retinopathy. Interestingly, plasma fibrinogen was increased in the complication-free diabetics of Ditzel's study, suggesting a possible increase in low shear viscosity which remained undetectable using the relatively insensitive Wells Brookfield viscometer. Zingg et al [34] have subsequently reported an increase in hematocrit corrected whole blood viscosity in diabetic children (compared with adult controls) prior to the development of clinically manifest complications.

Since these initial publications of whole blood viscosity in diabetes, a number of groups have worked in this area investigating different types of diabetes and using varying instrumentation. Many of these are shown in Table 10.2. Most reports have indicated an increase in whole blood viscosity in ambulant diabetics which tended to be more marked when corrected to a standard hematocrit. Differences in viscosity were larger at lower shear rates which are best evaluated by viscometers more sensitive than the Wells Brookfield microviscometer used by most authors. This suggests that factors promoting red cell aggregation have a major role in the hyperviscosity of diabetes. The majority of studies found an increase in plasma fibrinogen and where measured, globulins, especially alpha-2-macroglobulin, in their patients and these proteins usually correlated well with hematocrit corrected whole blood viscosity. The reasons for the raised circulating proteins in diabetics were not explored in any of the publications.

Examining their data for evidence of a relationship between blood rheology and metabolic control, several authors found no correlation between blood viscosity and either the prevailing blood sugar or HbA_1c [31,41,44,50,51]. This is perhaps not surprizing in the case of the former as glucose varies rapidly and extensively throughout the day in diabetes. Others, however, found increases in viscosity to be higher in patients with higher fasting blood glucose values [34,36]. One group reported that red cell aggregation correlated with blood glucose [43]. In two studies diabetics were examined before and after periods of improved metabolic control, showing decreases of whole blood viscosity, hematocrit corrected whole blood viscosity and plasma viscosity respectively [47,51]. The highest levels of blood viscosity in diabetes probably occur during ketoacidotic coma or precoma. As long ago as 1953, calculated blood viscosity during diabetic coma in 9 patients (using Lamport's formulae which utilize hematocrit and plasma protein concentrations) was found to be nearly twice as high compared with post-treatment values [55]. These results were later confirmed by actual measurements of blood viscosity in ketoacidotic patients [47,56,57]. The high levels of viscosity were related to hemoconcentration, hyperproteinemia and possibly to impaired red cell deformability [40].

Other factors which have interested workers as possible determinants of blood hyperviscosity in diabetes have been the duration of the condition and the type of anti-diabetic therapy used. Two authors [37,49] reported that higher blood viscosity levels were present with increased duration of diabetes, whereas others failed to confirm this. Whole blood viscosity and plasma fibrinogen may in fact increase with age; as diabetics with long standing disease are usually older than their newly diagnosed counterparts it is difficult to implicate the duration of their diabetes "per se" as a major contributor to their abnormal rheological state.

No systematic comparison of the effect of different treatment regimes in diabetes has been published, but no differences between the effects of insulin, sulphonylureas, biguanides or diet alone on several rheological variables have been reported [39,58]. Sulphonylurea-treated patients have been shown to have higher plasma fibrinogen concentrations than diabetics on insulin or biguanides [59]. Others found plasma viscosity to be similar in 314 insulin treated and 134 tablet-treated individuals [49].

The relationship between the presence of different diabetic circulatory, microcirculatory and other complications and the abnormalities in blood viscosity has intrigued some workers but failed to interest others. Indeed in many of the studies patient selection does not enable comparisons of patients with and without complications to be made. Increases in measured or hematocrit corrected

Table 10.2. Summary of whole blood and plasma viscosity studies in diabetes mellitus.

Author	Viscometer shear rates in brackets	Diabetics (patients, treatment, severity, complications)	Controls	Native viscosity	Hematocrit corrected viscosity	Plasma viscosity	Plasma/ serum Proteins	Correlation with blood glucose	Other comments
Swank 1959 (30)	Screen filtration ?	5 Rx (not stated)	37	–	–	–	–	–	No direct comparison made between diabs. & controls
Skovborg et al. 1966 (23)	Wells Brookfield (1.15–230 s-1)	16 (Rx not stated No retinop. 2 mild retinop. 5 severe retinop. 9)	16	↑	↑	No difference	Fibrinogen ↑ alpha 2 globulin ↑ Albumin ↓	–	Viscosity correlated with alpha 2 & beta globulins.
Rees et al. 1967 (32)	GDM	(not stated)	–	–	–	–	alpha 2 Macroglob. ↑ Fibrinogen ↑	–	Yield stress at HCT 40% only increased when diab. had nephropathy, ketoacidosis or infection.
Ditzel 1968 (33)	Wells Brookfield (2.3–230 s-1)	35 (Rx mainly insulin. No comps.)	90	–	No difference	No difference	Fibrinogen ↑	–	–
Bollinger et al. 1969 (35)	Wells Brookfield (11.5–46s-1)	53	60	No difference	No difference	–	Fibrinogen ↑	–	–
Isogai et al. 1971, 1976 (36)(37)	Wells Brookfield (23–230s-1)	127 (Rx mainly tabs/diet)	56	No difference	↑	↑	Fibrinogen ↑	yes	Diabs. with higher fasting glucose & longer duration had increased viscosity.
Labib et al. 1971 (38)	Capillary	73 (Rx not stated Retinop. 62 Non retinop. 11)	13	↑	–	–	–	–	Viscosity highest in non retinopathy.

Langer et al. 1971 (28)	Brookfield Synchro-electric (23–230s-1)	15 Rx insulin No retinop 9 Retinop 6 Nephrop 1	10	No difference	–	No difference	Fibrinogen ↑	–	Hematocrit after exercise increased more in diabs.
Zingg et al. 1971 (34)	Wells Brookfield (11.5–230s-1)	76 children	46	–	↑	–	–	Yes	Visc. increase more marked in diabs. with higher fasting glucose.
Skovborg 1974 (31)	Wells Brookfield (2.3–230 s-1)	143 Rx diet 3 tabs 8 insulin 132 with or without complications	71	↑	–	No difference	Fibrinogen ↑ Globulins ↑ Albumin ↓	No	Presc. of retinop not assoc. with raised visc. but proliferative patients had higher visc. No correlation with duration disease.
Hoare et al. 1975 (39)	Wells Brookfield (23–230 s-1) Contraves LS (0.77s-1)	100 35 Rx mixed with or without complications	100 36	No difference	↑ ↑	– –	Fibrinogen ↑ Fibrinogen ↑	–	Visc. higher in patients with retinopathy. Type of treatment had no effect.
Schmid-Schönbein & Volger 1976 (40)	Wells Brookfield (8–160s-1)	46 Rx not stated	43	–	↑	↑	–	Yes	Rheological variables related to metabolic control. No diffs. in pats. ± profil. retinop.
Barnes et al. 1977 (41)	Contraves LS 100 (0.77–2.62s-1)	64 Rx insulin 53 tablets 11 with and without complications	61	↑	↑	–	Fibrinogen ↑ Globulins ↑ Albumin ↓	No	Hematocrit corrected visc. related to extent of diab. comps. Type of Rx no effect.

Table 10.2 (continued)

Author	Viscometer shear rates in brackets	Diabetics (patients, treatment, severity, complications)	Controls	Native viscosity	Hematocrit corrected viscosity	Plasma viscosity	Plasma/ serum Proteins	Correlation with blood glucose	Other comments
Dintenfass 1977 (42)	Dintenfass Rhombosphe-roid (180s-1)	12 Rx not stated Retinop	19 Non diabs. with retinop	–	–	No difference	Fibrinogen ↑ both gps	–	Both gps had pats with various rheological abnorms. Blood visc ↑ in non diab retinops. Interrelation of variables examined in detail.
Dintenfass & Davis 1977 (43)	Dintenfass Rhombosphe-roid (180s-1)	14 Ashkenazi Jews comp. with 45 Sephardi Jews. No control group		–	–	–	–	RBC aggrega-tion corre-lated with glucose	Diffs in rheolog. variables found bet-ween gps, influenced by sex. social class & ABO blood groups.
Lowe et al. 1980 (44)	Dintenfass cone in cone (100s-1) Contraves LS (0.94s-1)	38 Rx insulin No retinop. 20 Retinopathy 18 Young males	38	↑	↑	↑	Fibrinogen ↑	None	Measured & corrected visc. raised in all diab. measured visc. higher in retinops. & correlated with duration of diab.
McMillan et al. 1980 (45)	Contraves LS	20 Rx not stated No adv. retinop or nephropathy	20	–	↑	–	–	–	Slight visc elevation in diabs at high shear, low shear sig. inc. in diabs.
Paisey et al. 1980 (46)	Contraves LS Capillary	12 + 10 mainly insulin mixed comps.	none	with ↑ poor control	–	with ↑ poor control			Visc and fibrinogen independent of diabet complications but higher in poor metabolic control

Barnes 1981 (47)	Contraves LS (0.77–2.62s-1)	32 Rx newly diagnosed maturity onset	61	↑	↑	–	Fibrinogen ↑	Yes	Fall in native visc in response to improve cont. with either diet tabs or insulin.
Rand et al. 1981 (48)	Wells Brookfield (21–212s-1)	42 Rx insulin 16 tabs 26 Mixed comps	36	–	↑	No difference	–	None	Results similar in patients with and without complications.
Stoltz et al. 1981 (49)	Not stated (0.23–1.16s-1)	448 Rx not stated Mixed comps	Not stated	↑	–	↑	–	–	High visc in patients with more extensive comps. ↑ duration of diab. enhanced this relationship.
Hill et al. 1982 (50)	concentric cylinder (0.1–100s-1)	26 children	Not stated	↑	–	–	Fibrinogen ↑ alpha2-macroglob. ↑	None with glucose or HbA1c	No correlation of ↑ blood visc with microalbuminuria.
Poon et al. 1982 (51)	Contraves LS (0.7–94s-1)	32 Rx insulin no retinop. 12 mild retinop. 10 prolif. retinop. 10	10	↑	No change	↑	–	None with glucose or HbA1c	36 additional patients with improved HbA1c and glucose over 1 year had a fall in corrected and plasma visc.
Leiper et al. 1983 (52)	Contraves LS (0.94–94s-1) & Harkness	22 Rx insulin Mainly comp free	22	↑	↑	n ↑	–	Yes	Poor control ass. with worse rheology. Diff types of insulin–no effect on rheology.
Stuart et al. 1983 (53)	Contraves LS (128s-1)	55 Rx insulin 38 tabs 17 Mixed comps	37	–	No difference	No difference	–	–	–

↑ = elevated
↓ = decreased
Other papers of interest include: Rouselle et al. 1980 (54) and Grigoleit et al. 1973 (128).

blood viscosity in patients with proliferative retinopathy compared to diabetics with mild/background or no retinopathy were found in some studies [31,39,41,44,51]. Others found no significant changes in patients with retinopathy alone (severity not documented), but a hyperviscosity state was present when retinopathic patients had other vascular and microvascular complications in addition [32,49]. Finally, lower blood viscosity values in patients with severe diabetic retinopathy than in those with mild or absent retinopathy were reported to two groups [37,38]. A major problem with attempting to analyze relationships between specific rheological variables and individual diabetic complications is that several microvascular or vascular sequelae often occur simultaneously in the same patient. Furthermore, even in the absence of a clinically manifest complications, a significant degree of subclinical pathology may be present. Attempts have been made to minimize this problem by examining only diabetics with normal creatinine and urea levels [44]. Different groups were carefully matched for cigarette consumption. However, the retinopathy group still contained more individuals with proteinuria, neuropathy and cerebral and peripheral ischemia.

10.4.2. Plasma and serum viscosity

Plasma viscosity not only contributes to whole blood viscosity (and indeed correlates highly significantly with this variable in the context of bivariate analysis in groups of individual blood samples), but it is also an important determinant of blood flow through the microcirculation. The physiological relevance of serum viscosity measurements is less certain, but analysis of serum rheology does enable a careful evaluation of factors normally obscured by the presence of red cells and fibrinogen. Cogan et al [22], using a capillary viscometer, found serum viscosity to be increased in diabetics, but there was no difference between patients with and without retinopathy. By contrast, Mosora et al [60] using similar apparatus found serum viscosity to be decreased in diabetics despite an increase in total protein concentrations. The most comprehensive study of serum viscosity in diabetics was made by McMillan [61] using the Wells-Brookfield viscometer. He found that the acute phase globulins (haptoglobin, alpha-1-acid glycoprotein, alpha-1-antitrypsin, ceruloplasmin, C-reactive protein) and certain complement elements (C3c, C4, C3a) were increased considerably in diabetics when compared with control subjects. Alpha-2-macroglobulin, beta-2-glycoprotein 1 and hemopexin showed a moderate elevation, but the immunoglobulins (transferrin, Gc globulin and HS glycoprotein) showed little change. Albumin and prealbumin were marginally depressed in the diabetics. The levels of only three proteins; albumin, haptoglobin and beta-2-glycoprotein 1 were found to be related to clinically detectable microangiopathy. All three proteins were closely correlated with serum viscosity levels, whereas proteins unrelated to viscosity were also unrelated to microangiopathy. McMillan concluded that, except when associated with a serum viscosity increase, the widespread individual serum protein changes found in diabetics appeared to be unrelated to the development of microangiopathy. In a further study [62] the same author found progressively increasing concentrations of fibrinogen in controls, latent diabetics, diabetics with no complications and diabetics with microangiopathy respectively. He concluded that an elevation of fibrinogen might play a role in the pathogenesis of diabetic microangiopathy.

Plasma viscosity in diabetics was usually measured as an associated variable by researchers when evaluating whole blood viscosity in diabetes (Table 10.2), the main emphasis of the study being on the latter. Increases in plasma viscosity in diabetics were found frequently [36,44,49,51,63], whereas no differences between diabetics and non-diabetics were also reported [23,28,31,33,42]. In the largest study of plasma viscosity in diabetes significant elevations of this parameter were shown [49]. These were similar in males and females, in diabetics on insulin and on oral agents and in patients with and without various complications.

10.5. Microrheology of blood in diabetes

10.5.1. Red cell deformability

In capillary sized vessels, where many of the early complications of diabetes manifest, the physical properties of the red and white cells and the viscosity of plasma become more important than bulk viscosity in terms of flow determinants. The most spectacular studies in this area have probably been those of Brånemark and colleagues [64], who observed (through a light microscope) microcirculatory flow in vivo in titanium chambers mounted in the forearm of four diabetics. Erythrocytes were described as being biconcave with no morphological abnormalities and their disc shape was rapidly restored even after extreme deformation. The diabetic cells exhibited normal plasticity when passing narrow vascular segments and showed no signs of adherence to each other or to the endothelium. After three hours of artificially induced vascular stasis, the mass of red cells immediately broke up into separate cells with visually normal morphology and rheology. At low flow rates rouleaux formation occurred as in healthy volunteers. The red cells in the rouleaux did not adhere to each other with recognizably greater forces than in normals. The rouleaux broke up readily with increased flow without any tendency to block the microvessels or adhere to the endothelium. The influence of chylomicrons and the behavior of granulocytes, platelets and plasma were similar in diabetics and non-diabetics. Only a single abnormality was encountered and this occurred in one patient who during the period of examination had mild episodes of acidosis. When slow flow or circulatory standstill was induced during acidotic periods, platelets began to adhere to each other, a feature not shown during good metabolic control or in normals. The aggregates were loose, did not adhere to the endothelium and broke up again when the circulation was restored. It would appear, therefore, from these studies that functional rheological abnormalities are not a predominant event in the microcirculatory disturbance of diabetes. Valuable though this work is, there are two good reasons why it does not exclude hemorheological factors in the etiology of diabetic complications. Firstly, the evolution of diabetic microcirculatory disease is a gradual process, taking place over a period of years. Events are therefore infrequent and the development of lesions usually slow. In the present study only four individuals were examined (only one of whom had any significant complications) and these were examined over the comparatively short period of a few months. Secondly, observations were made on newly formed blood vessels that had vascularized freshly formed connective tissue laid down under a glass coverslip. Microvessels in other organs may present a different rheological challenge to circulating cells, particularly when the vessels have been long established and influenced or damaged by abnormalities in circulating metabolites and hormones for sustained periods. Indeed the histology of Brånemark's patients' newly formed capillaries seems likely to have shown considerable differences from that of, for example, retinal capillaries from a long standing diabetic with retinopathy. Clearly, further in vivo studies in animals and if possible, man are required to explore microcirculatory hemodynamics in the diabetic state.

A large number of in vitro studies of the flow properties of red cells have been made in diabetes; nearly all of them over the last decade. There are considerable difficulties in interpreting the available data, partially because of differences in methodology and partially due to differences in patient selection, which have included variations in therapy, age, duration of diabetes, degree of metabolic imbalance and the extent of complications. All variables might influence erythrocyte rheology in a particular group of diabetics. The majority of workers have examined the flow of erythrocytes (with or without other blood components) through polycarbonate Nuclepore sieves (usually pores with 5 μm diameter) as an index of erythrocyte deformability. Such methods are now generally accepted as measuring other variables as well as deformability and are best perhaps called filtration tests. Ditzel had reported impaired filtration of diabetic erythrocytes through Millipore filters in 1971 [65] and these initial results were later confirmed with similar filters [66] and by groups using Nuclepore filters [40,41]. Impaired filtration of either whole blood or erythrocyte suspensions in plasma or buffer were found in various populations of diabetics [40,53,63,67,68,69,76,77,78]. Others, using 5 μm Nuclepore filters [41], or using 3 μm filters [48], found no overall difference between diabetics and controls. Impaired filtration was found to be associated with microvascular and macrovascular complications by some groups [41,66,76,77], whereas others [40,48] detected no differences between diabetics with and without complications. Finally, impaired metabolic control was demonstrated to correlate with impaired filtration [40,70,69], while the absence of a correlation with fasting blood glucose (which is not a precise index of overall metabolic control in insulin dependent diabetes) was reported as well [41,48,63]. Details of different investigations of red cell rheology in diabetes are shown in Table 10.3.

Previous chapters have discussed the contaminating factors influencing blood filtration, which include pore clogging by white blood corpuscles, platelet aggregates, fibrin plugs and aggregates of erythrocytes (which may occur under the filter around the pore exit). It was pointed out that diabetics with impaired filration had raised white cell counts, but if these were standardized to match those of non-diabetics and plasma factors were minimized by examining cells suspended in buffer, the differences between diabetics and non-diabetics disappeared [53]. By contrast, others [52], using a slightly different filtration method, found that even after elimination of white cell, platelet and plasma effects, filtration remained slightly impaired in diabetics and the impairment correlated with metabolic control as assessed by HbA_1c.

In summary, most studies have found abnormalities of blood filtration in diabetics which many workers felt were more pronounced when patients either had widespread microcirculatory or macrocirculatory complications or when diabetes was badly controlled. Although differences between the mean values of filtration in diabetics and non-diabetics was often as much as 40% there was usually a big overlap between the groups, and the finding of an abnormal value of filtration in a given patient was probably not a reliable index of either the presence of complications or the degree of metabolic control in that individual. Filtration tended to remain abnormal in diabetics when red cells were suspended in buffer rather than native plasma, but the presence of raised white cell counts in the diabetics probably contributed towards this abnormality in many studies. Whether suspensions of pure red cells from diabetics in metabolically and hormonally normal suspending media would filter more slowly than those of non-diabetics remains undecided. As different laboratories filter red cells under widely varying conditions (pressure, temperature, pore size, suspending media, anticoagulant, etc.), the answer to this question is likely to remain contentious for some time.

A small number of workers have examined the rheological properties of individual red cells in diabetics using micropipettes. The advantages of these methods over filtration include the use of physiological pressure gradients, a longer cylindrical channel (often without the entry problems of filters) and the elimination of white cell and platelet effects. The main disadvantage of the methods is that they are time consuming and have difficulty in evaluating large numbers of cells. McMillan et al [71] oscillated red cells backwards and forwards in 4 μm diameter glass pipettes over a horizontal distance of 130 μm with a cycle time of 3 seconds. The pressure gradient required to maintain a constant oscillation was 50% higher in 9 diabetics than in 9 controls; similar differences were found between diabetic and normal rats. When diabetic red cells were ejected from the pipettes they took 50% longer to attain their discoid shape than did red cells from non-diabetics. Varying the glucose concentration in the suspending buffer had little influence on cell performance, and McMillan concluded that the reduced erythrocyte deformability in diabetics was due to an elevation of either intra-erythrocyte or membrane viscosity, possibly related to increased HbA_1c. Using similar apparatus Meiselman and LaCelle [1982, personal communication) were unable to find any difference between diabetic and normal red cells. Willars et al [92] again using McMillan's method, but at a constant temperature of 37°C, found only a 5% increase in flow resistance in 30 diabetics compared with 30 controls, the difference being present whether the cells were examined in buffer or native plasma. Using a pipette aspiration method, LaCelle [73] found no difference in red cell membrane properties between diabetics and non diabetics. Finally, employing flow chamber and micropipette techniques, Sewchand et al [82] found no difference between diabetics and controls in surface shear modulus of elasticity, membrane viscoelastic recovery time and membrane surface shear viscosity. Thus, with the exception of McMillan et al [71], laboratories using micropipettes methods have found either subtle or no abnormalities in the rheological properties of diabetic red cells.

Several hemorheologists have attempted to examine red cell deformability in diabetes using other methods. Dintenfass [42] derived values for the internal viscosity of the red cell from viscometry measurements of whole blood and plasma and found that five out of twelve diabetics had cells more rigid than the normal range. Oughton and Barnes [63], using a similar method, found no difference between diabetics and controls despite clearly impaired whole blood filtration in the diabetic group. Knight et al [70], assessing erythrocyte flexibility with a centrifugation method, reported that when plasma fibrinogen concentrations exceeded 3 g/l, diabetics showed impaired flexibility compared with controls. Oughton and Barnes [63], using a simplified version of the same method, found that diabetic red cells were more flexible than normal, but they made no correction for fibrinogen and did not specifically comment on patients with high levels of fibrinogen. Baba et al [72], using fluorescent polarization techniques to measure microviscosity of the lipid domain of the erythrocyte membrane, have reported increased viscosity in diabetic patients.

The varying methodology used over the past decade prevents a simple conclusion about whether diabetic red cells offer more resistance in their flow through the microcirculation than do normal cells. Data reporting that a given group of diabetic patients exhibited impaired red cell filterability, normal packed cell viscosity and better than normal deformability as assessed by centrifugation, underlines the critical importance of methodology in this area of research [63]. It would seem likely, however, that if red cells are intrinsically more resistant to flow in diabetes, this change is comparatively small in magnitude compared with the rigidity seen in sickled cells or in cells hardened with acetaldehyde or diamide.

Impaired erythrocyte deformability in diabetes could be due to changes in the intracellular hemoglobin, changes in the physical properties of the cell membrane or changes in the surface area to volume ratio of the cells. Hemoglobin A_1a, b and c concentrations are increased in diabetics, particularly during poor metabolic control. Although no differences in the viscosity of solutions containing varying amounts of glycosylated hemoglobins have been noted in one study [74], it remains possible that HbA_1c binds more avidly to the red cell membrane [93] with deleterious effects on its flexibility. Membrane flexibility is thought to be dependent upon several factors, including intracellular ATP and the chemical composition of the membrane. Reduced intracellular ATP in diabetes has been reported [77]. Improvement in metabolic control with an infusion of insulin led to a rise in red cell ATP and increased filtration of blood through Nuclepore sieves. It was demonstrated that the role of insulin in improving blood filtration was independent of changes in blood glucose (both in vivo and in vitro), and that the hormone also reversed enhanced platelet aggregation, an effect which seemed to be at least in part mediated by the presence of red cells [67-69]. Subsequently these authors have shown that administration of insulin via the artificial pancreas for a period of 24 hours to badly controlled diabetics partially reversed the increased cholesterol/phospholipid ratios and the abnormal phospholipid composition of their erythrocyte membranes, in parallel with improved filtration of both whole blood and red cell suspensions [94]. A number of abnormalities have been found in erythrocyte membranes in diabetes and have been reviewed elsewhere [95]. Several groups have now investigated the effect of insulin on red cell flow properties both in vitro and in vivo without agreement. Insulin was found to improve filtration by some workers [67,68,69,77] but the hormone was also shown to have no effect [96,97]. Demonstrating the importance of methodology in coming to conclusions in this area, one study showed that in vitro incubation of metabolically hardened red cells with insulin improved their flow characteristics in micropipettes, worsened erythrocyte flexibility as measured by centrifugation, and had no influence on filtration [97]. The third mechanism by which erythrocyte deformability might be abnormal in diabetes is a disturbance in the surface area to volume ratio. Although there is some evidence that MCV is reduced slightly in diabetics [31], others have found it to be increased [98,99] and errors may be due to the cell counter. It seems unlikely that the comparatively small changes found would fully account for the observed changes in erythrocyte deformability.

10.5.2. Red cell aggregation

Red cell aggregation has been studied in diabetes by several workers and found to be increased. The pathophysiological significance of these findings in terms of blood flow is not certain, but this abnormal aggregation seems likely to be a

Table 10.3. Summary of erythrocyte rheology studies in diabetes mellitus.

Author	Method	Diabetics	Controls	RBC Rheology in diabetics	Correlation with complications	Correlation with
Ditzel 1970 (65)	6 μm Millipore filters	6	None	Cells filtered during and after ketoacidosis	–	Metabolic control impaired in ketoacidosis
Ehrly & Köhler 1976 (66)	8μ Millipore filters	9	15	↓	In patients with occlusive arterial disease	–
Schmid-Schönbein & Volger 1976 (40)	5μ Nuclepore filters. 5 cm. H_2O pressure. 10% RBC in plasma	49 Varying comps. and metabolic control Rx not stated	22	(↓)	None	Yes, filtration improved when sugars improved
Barnes et al. 1977 (41)	5μ Nuclepore filters. 20 cm. H_2O pressure. Whole blood	64 Varying comps Rx-mainly insulin	61	No difference	Filtration impaired in patients with comps	None
Dintenfass 1977 (42)	Viscometric method (TK value)	12 Rx not stated Comps not stated	Not stated	5 out 12 diabetics had rigid red cells	–	–
Juhan et al. 1978, 1979, 1981 (67)(68)(69)	5μ Nuclepore filters. 20 cm H_2O pressure. Whole blood & washed	Not stated Rx insulin	Not stated	↓	–	Yes, insulin replacement not glucose lowering important
Knight et al. 1978 (70)	RBC in buffer Centrifugation	21 Rx various Comps not stated	Not stated	Impaired when fibrinogen > 300 mg/100 ml	–	–
McMillan et al. 1978 (71)	4μ micropipettes. Cell oscillation resistance, Shape restoration time. Cells in Tris buffer	9 Rx not stated Comps not stated	9	↓	–	No effect of varying exogenous glucose

1979 (72)	dipolarisation of RBC membranes	Rx insulin-7 Tabs/Diet-60		viscosity↑		impaired control
LaCelle 1980 (73)	Micropipette aspiration. Capillary flow	Not stated Rx not stated	Not stated	No difference	–	–
Boudart et al. 1981 (74)	5μ Nuclepore filters 20 cm H_2O pressure. Whole blood	20 Rx insulin 8 Tabs/Diet 12	none	–	–	Correlation between impaired control & impaired filtration
Drouin et al. 1981 (75)	5μ Nuclepore filters 20 cm H_2O pressure. Whole blood	11 Rx insulin No ketoacidosis dehydration or overt infection	44	Impaired rheology before Rx (artificial pancreas). Rx normalized rheology	–	Strict improvement of met. control normalized rheology
Isogai et al. 1981 (76)	5μ Nuclepore filters. RBC in Tris saline	44 Rx not stated	11	↓	Greater impairment in severe retinopathies	Impaired filtration correlated with HbA1c
Le Devehat et al. 1981 (77)	5μ Nuclepore filters. 20 cm H_2O pressure Whole blood	40 arteriopaths 20 non arteriopaths. Rx not stated	20	↓	Filtration worse in arteriopaths	Impaired filtration correlated with ↓ ATP and ↑ 2,3 DPG
McMillan et al. 1981, 1983 (79)(80)	RBC doublet formation	20	20	↓	–	–
Oughton & Barnes 1981 (63)	5μ Nuclepore filters. Whole blood. Viscometric method (Tk). Centrifugation	30 Rx insulin Mixed comps	28	Filtration impaired, viscometry no different, centrifugation improved	–	No method correlated with fasting glucose
Pozza et al. 1981 (81)	5μ Nuclepore filters. Whole blood	37 Rx insulin Mixed comps.	35	Impaired but improved with pentoxifylline	Yes	Yes
Rand et al. 1981 (48)	3μ Nuclepore filters 10 cm H_2O pressure. 0.6% solution RBC in buffer	42 Rx insulin 16 tabs/diet 26 Mixed comps	36	No difference	None	None

Table 10.3 (continued)

Author	Method	Diabetics	Controls	RBC Rheology in diabetics	Correlation with complications	Correlation with metabolic control
Williamson et al. 1981 (82)	Elongation index calculated from photos of cells under controlled stress	6 Rx not stated Comps not stated	5	Impaired rheology function of red cell age	–	–
Sewchand et al. 1982 (83)	Flow chamber Micropipettes Cells in buffered saline	14 Rx insulin Severe retinopathy	10	No abnorm. of surface shear modulus of elasticity, membrane viscoelastic recovery time or surface shear visc.		
Bryszewska & Leyko 1983 (84)	Flourescence depolarisation of RBC membrane	13 Rx insulin Mainly no comps	Not stated	–	–	Insulin increased fluorecent probe mobility in RBC membranes
Caimi 1983 (85)	5μ Nuclepore filters. 20 cm H_2O pressure. Whole blood 5% sol. RBC RBC in plasma (def index)	45 Rx insulin 10 diet-tabs 26 Mixed comps	37	Whole blood filtration imp. Deformability index not different	Whole blood filtration most abnormal in presence of comps. Deformability index no different	–
Hanss 1983 (86)	5μ Nuclepore filters	200 Rx insulin 100 diet/tabs. 100	Not stated	Impaired in diabs but only if heparin used as anticoag. c.f. EDTA	–	–

Kamada & Otsuji 1983 (87)	Electron spin resonance	16 + 45 Rx insulin 6 + 19 7 + 16 tabs 3 + 10 diet mixed comps.	14	↓	No	No
Stuart et al. 1983 (53)	5μ Nuclepore filters. Constant flow, RBC in buffered saline	55 Rx insulin 38 tabs 17 Mixed comps	37	Impaired deform. eliminated when corrected for WBC	–	–
Leiper et al. 1984 (52)	5μ Nuclepore filters. Constant flow Pi/Pb. Low shear stresses	22 Rx insulin Mainly comp free	22	Impaired Different types insulin did not alter rheology	–	Impaired filtration correlated with HbA1c
Caimi et al. 1985 (88)	5μ Nuclepore 20 cm H_2O pressure 1. whole blood 2. 5% RBC in plasma under gravidity	36 Rx insulin		Not related to HLA status	–	–
Ritchie 1985 (89)	5μ Nuclepore Constant flow RBC in buffered saline	20 Rx insulin Mainly no comps		No change when differences in WBC count eliminated	–	None

– = not tested.

Other papers published on red cell deformability and diabetes mellitus include those by Rouselle et al. 1980 (54), Vague et al. 1980 (90), Sacks et al. 1981 (91) and Volger et al. 1981 (92).

major cause of the raised low-shear blood viscosity and yield stress found in studies of whole blood viscosity. It is probable that flow would be most affected in areas of low shear stress such as the post-capillary venules.

Early clinical observations initiated the interest in this area [100], red cell aggregates being observed in the conjunctival vessels of diabetics. Results suggested that the tendency to aggregation was due to a coating of the erythrocyte which was related to elevated plasma fibrinogen and globulin levels. Using syllectometry as a measure of red cell aggregation, abnormal results in diabetics were found, which correlated with plasma concentration of fibrinogen, alpha-2-globulin, and to a lesser extent beta-globulin. There were no significant differences in red cell aggregation between patients with and without retinopathy. Later these data were confirmed, showing that aggregates formed faster in diabetics, were larger than in non-diabetics, and had a higher resistance to dispersion by shear forces [40]. Again, no differences were found between patients with or without retinopathy, although the presence of complicating infections, such as pyelonephritis, in the diabetics led to further elevations of red cell aggregation. Differences in metabolic control did not seem to influence aggregation. Subsequent data were in line with previous work, but a correlation between the extent of aggregation and the severity of diabetic retinopathy was found [101,102]. More recently, others found the velocity of red cell aggregation to be significantly correlated with not only the extent of retinopathy, but also with the degree of metabolic control as assessed by HbA_1c [103]. It is of interest to examine these studies against the background of Brånemark's work [64] discussed above. His group found that red cell aggregates artificially induced by vascular stasis in vivo in diabetics always broke up when the pressure cuff was released. However, it remains possible that over more sustained periods of time and in damaged microvessels, red cell aggregation might participate in the etiology of vascular occlusion.

10.5.3. Red cell adhesion

In capillaries, red cell flow is dependent not only on the intrinsic properties of the red cells and the plasma layer, but also on many other factors including the surface properties of the endothelial cells, which are known to be abnormal in diabetes. The findings of increased adhesion of erythrocytes to endothelial cells in diabetes [104] is, therefore, of particular interest. Increased adhesion was related to the extent of vascular complications but did not correlate with HbA_1c. Both fibrinogen and fibrinectin enhanced adhesion in diabetics and controls. The adhesion of diabetic red cells to cultured human fibroblasts and to plastic surface was also increased. As most observations of red cell flow properties have involved the exposure of cells to non-physiological surfaces, these investigations represent a new dimension in rheological studies and will doubtless stimulate more research in the future.

10.6. Implications

10.6.1. Whole blood viscosity and large vessel disease

The literature seems to be in reasonable agreement that whole blood viscosity (corrected and uncorrected for hematocrit) is raised in diabetes, particularly at low shear rates. Although the average increase in viscosity was about 5-10% at high shear rates and 15-25% at low shear rates, viscosity values tended to have a skewed distribution, and a number of diabetics showed increases of over 30% at high shear rates and 60% at low shear rates, making these individuals an important sub-group for further study. During episodes of poor metabolic control, blood viscosity levels could be expected to become even more abnormal. What would be the hemodynamic consequences of these findings and what might be their pathophysiological effect on the patient? The hemodyamic changes resulting from these modest increases in viscosity are likely to be complex and will depend upon factors other than viscosity itself. These include variations in prevailing blood pressure, circulating and local metabolites, the presence or absence of morphological changes in conducting vessels as well as others; furthermore, the effect of such changes will vary from organ to organ. It is also likely that the implications of hyperviscosity mediated by increases in acute phase proteins will differ from that due to relative or absolute polycythemia. A number of biochemical and physiological studies (mainly in non-diabetics) are pertinent to this area but their results do not present a uniform picture. These are discussed in relation to the three organs most strikingly affected by large vessel disease in diabetes, namely the lower limb, the brain and the heart.

A significant rise in blood flow in the lower limb of patients prior to surgery was found by lowering the viscosity through reducing hematocrit with various intravenous fluids [105]. A 12% fall in high-shear viscosity (230 s^{-1}) was accompanied by a 30% increase in flow. Despite initially disappointing results following venesection in patients with intermittant claudication the same group [106] found that venesection to a much lower hematocrit of 0.35 not only led to a 170% rise in peak calf flow, but also a 111% rise in hemoglobin delivery [107], which was accompanied by an increased walking distance. In contrast, others found that reducing the hematocrit of polycythaemic patients from 0.57 to 0.47 (50% fall in low shear viscosity at 0.1 s^{-1}) led to insignificant changes in resting leg blood flow and only an 18% increase in peak flow after post occlusion hyperemia [108]. Due to the concomitant fall in hematocrit overall hemoglobin delivery actually fell by 23% at rest and 10% at peak flow. The conflicting message emerging from these two studies is perplexing, but in the latter hematocrit was not lowered as extensively as in the former and probably more importantly, there was no documented evidence of peripheral vascular disease the polycythemic group [108], whereas in the former study [107] the presence of large vessel narrowing may well have increased the power of blood viscosity as a flow determinant. Reduction of blood viscosity in a different way, by reducing fibrinogen with ancrod, was found to benefit intermittant claudication by some workers [109] but not by others; here hematocrit remained constant following therapy. What do these studies mean for the diabetic leg? In the absence of significant arterial narrowing it is likely that even those diabetic patients with the highest levels of blood viscosity can compensate for the latter by adjustments in vessel diameter at the level of the microcirculation. However, in patients with significant occlusion of their lower limb vessels by atheroma, blood viscosity could be a flow-limiting factor, particularly if local oxygen requirements were elevated by concurrent poor metabolic control. In this situation normalizing hyperviscosity by venesection, plasma exchange or drugs might confer a moderate but clinically significant benefit to patients with claudication or ischemia of the toes or feet. One study is of particular interest in the context of the diabetic lower limb [110]. It was found that preoperative hemoglobin (and presumably viscosity) was significantly lower in diabetics whose amputations subsequently healed than in patients whose limbs showed failure of healing. Prospective studies of reducing hematocrit prior to surgery in diabetics are now indicated to see if this manoeuvre will improve the outcome of surgery for gangrene of the lower extremities. The practical implications of such a study could be very important in patient management.

It is possible that sustained elevations of blood viscosity and plama fibrinogen concentrations over long periods may be factors promoting hemostasis and enhancing the deposition of fibrin and lipid in atheromatous plaques in the arteries of the lower limb and indeed elsewhere. However, this hypothesis remains speculative and careful prospective epidemiological surveys (some of which are now in progress) are required to dissect out candidate risk factors for the etiology and evolution of diabetic large vessel disease. Raised viscosity might also be one factor promoting intravascular thrombosis in diabetics. Although there is no good evidence of a greater risk of venous thrombosis in ambulant diabetic outpatients, in ketoacidosis and hyperosmolar nonketotic coma where blood viscosity levels are extremely high, cerebral and visceral thromboses are well recognized [112-114].

The relationship between blood viscosity and cerebral blood flow has received considerable attention in the past decade and may have a bearing on the higher prevalence of cerebrovascular disease in diabetes mellitus [15,17]. Clinical observations [115-118] have convincingly shown a raised hematocrit to be a risk factor in a variety of cerebrovascular disorders and it would seem appropriate to investigate the hemodynamic effects of alterations in hematocrit on the cerebral circulation. Cerebral blood flow in several studies was found to be reduced in relative and absolute polycythemia compared with the normal values [119,120] and reverted back to normal after venesection [120]. In the latter study, a fall in whole blood viscosity of 31% at low shear rates (0.75 s^{-1}) and 20% at higher shear rates (91 s^{-1}) was accompanied by a rise in cerebral blood flow of 84%

[120]. In contrast to these results, reduction of plasma viscosity by plasma exchange (hematocrit kept constant) in normal individuals was not accompanied by any significant changes in cerebral blood flow [121]. It is well known that the cerebral circulation has considerable powers of autoregulation, with which it protects the metabolic environment of the brain from changes in systemic blood pressure, blood viscosity and oxygen availability. These studies suggest that whilst changes in blood viscosity may play a compensatory role in maintaining cerebral oxygenation following a fall in hematocrit, under normal circumstances viscosity changes can be over-riden, if necessary, by local adjustment of vascular geometry. Does this mean that the high levels of whole blood viscosity exhibited by some diabetics are of little consequence? The short answer is probably "no", because raised blood viscosity was found to be a risk factor in the clinical studies described above. Autoregulation has been found to be disturbed in a proportion of diabetics [21], since they were unable to respond to hypercapnia by increasing their cerebral blood flow. After a stroke autoregulatory mechanisms may also be disrupted. In these circumstances blood viscosity may exert a greater influence as a rheological factor and high levels of this variable may be undesirable. Changes in viscosity may also affect flow in the collateral supply to an area of infarction after a stroke if there is maximum vasodilation or vasoparalysis due to ischemia [116].

In view of the near-maximum oxygen extraction in the coronary circulation under normal conditions, the relationship between blood viscosity (especially hematocrit) on the one hand and coronary hemodynamics and myocardial metabolism on the other is of special interest. Following hemodilution with Dextran, several investigators have shown that coronary blood flow is affected by whole blood viscosity [122,123]. More detailed studies have recently been carried out [124,125]. Following isovolumetric exchange with plasma or red cells in normotensive dogs, coronary blood flow and cardiac output varied inversely with hematocrit. The range of optimum hematocrit for maximum oxygen transport was wider in the coronary circulation (0.20-0.60) than in the systemic circulation (0.40-0.60), coronary vasodilation occurring outside the range of hematocrit 0.20-0.60. Oxygen consumption was essentially constant over this range; in the coronary circulation the arteriovenous oxygen extraction ratio was unchanged over the range of hematocrit studied, suggesting that oxygen consumption was primarily determined by coronary oxygen transport. In contrast, maintenance of total body oxygen consumption was attributable also to variations in arteriovenous oxygen extraction. Subsequent experiments in hypotensive dogs (arterial pressure 50 mmHg) revealed a rather different situation. Here maximum oxygen consumption occurred at a hematocrit of 0.25 in the myocardium and over a range of 0.25-0.45 in the total body, which fell when hematocrit was moved outside these ranges. In summary, when blood pressure is normal and the morphology of the coronary arteries intact, changes in blood viscosity within the range found in diabetics probably have little influence on myocardial metabolism. However, when the pressure falls, e.g. after hemorrhage or myocardial infarction, or indeed when narrowing of the coronary arteries occurs, alterations in blood viscosity may assume a much greater degree of significance. The importance of elevated blood viscosity in the etiology of coronary artery disease, angina of effort, myocardial infarction and in myocardial function during shock or during exertion remains to be evaluated by clinical studies on diabetics. Both epidemiological investigations and evaluation of viscosity-lowering agents or procedures are clearly indicated.

10.6.2. Red cell deformability, plasma viscosity and microangiopathy

Whilst whole blood viscosity is a prime determinant of blood flow in large and medium sized vessels, in the microcirculation, plasma viscosity and erythrocyte deformability assume greater importance. As previously stated, it was the retinal microcirculation that first drew attention to the possible involvement of hemorheological factors in diabetic complications. Several studies showed a mean increase in plasma viscosity in diabetics of about 10% (Table 10.2). Although it is possible that this in itself might retard capillary flow, the effects of this modest rise in viscosity would appear to be insufficient to cause diabetic retinal changes by itself, particularly as other patients (e.g. those with rheumatoid arthritis) who show a similar rheological abnormality do not get retinopathy. Indeed patients with hyperviscosity syndrome and retinopathy have markedly higher levels of plasma viscosity than diabetics.

The importance of erythrocyte deformability as a flow determinant in capillaries has been demonstrated by cinephotographic studies of the microcirculation. In sickle cell disease, occlusion of retinal capillaries by rigid cells may lead to proliferative retinopathy. Could the same be true for diabetes? Unfortunately, despite the large number of studies carried out purporting to measure erythrocyte deformability in diabetics, it is not yet possible to make a definitive comment on whether this variable is abnormal in diabetes or not. The majority of studies (Table 10.3) were carried out using Nuclepore polycarbonate filters which are susceptible to many artifacts which are discussed in detail in chapter 2 of this book. If there are abnormalities in erythrocyte flow properties in diabetes, they are likely to be much less marked than in sickle cell disease - whether such subtle changes are able to participate in the genesis of retinal hypoxia or in capillary occlusion must remain speculative at present. The coexistence of other abnormalities in the microcirculation in diabetes might, however, magnify the importance of relatively small changes in red cell rheology. Abnormalities of the endothelial cells themselves and the increased adhesion potential of erythrocytes to the endothelial cell surface are two examples. Furthermore, abnormalities in the flow behavior of circulating white cells as a factor in capillary occlusion requires evaluation, and in vitro investigations of white cell deformability are topics of present research in several centers. An interesting hypothesis [71] was that a 50% elevation of erythrocyte deformability in diabetics might lead to sustained increases in pressure on capillary walls which might in turn result in basement membrane thickening. This pressure would, of course, be enhanced by the rise in blood flow often reported in diabetes.

Studies of red cell survival in diabetes provide some indirect evidence that erythrocyte deformability may be impaired in diabetes. Increased cell rigidity with ageing has been put forward as the predominant mechanism determining red cell survival due to the trapping of the less flexible, aged cells by the splenic sinuses. Red cell survival was found to be reduced in diabetics with poor metabolic control, this abnormality reverted towards normal when good control was resumed [127].

It is pertinent to examine any hemorheological changes in diabetes mellitus in relation to other hemodynamic parameters which might be relevant to microcirculatory events. Proximal arterial stenosis may protect the ipsilateral retina or kidney from microvascular damage [128,129]; similarly unilateral glaucoma may reduce the severity of retinopathy in the affected eye, suggesting that reduction of capillary flow or pressure in diabetics may be favourable under certain circumstances. Increases in retinal [2], muscle, fat and skin blood flow [130] and renal plasma flow [131] occur early on in diabetes. There is evidence that the reflex fall in skin blood flow to the lower extremities following standing, which is present in normal individuals, is impaired in diabetics [132]. Furthermore, capillilary hypertension has been found in the dependent diabetic foot [133] and is worse in the presence of poor metabolic control. Microvascular overperfusion is, therefore, an early feature of diabetes and appears to precede clinically detectable microangiopathy. The potential relationships between overperfusion and the early microvascular changes of diabetes have recently been discussed [134].

With the progression of diabetes, there is evidence that vascular underperfusion occurs. This is most readily demonstrable as a limitation of maximum perfusion under stress conditions. Impaired cerebral blood flow in response to hypercapnia [21], diminished peripheral blood flow after ganglion blockade [135], impaired skin flow following heat or trauma [136] and blunting of peak nailfold capillary flow velocity following arterial occlusion [137] are some of the observations indicating limitation of vascular and microvascular perfusion in diabetics under stress conditions. The relative importance of the vascular and neural components of this limited dilatation is still under debate. Further evidence of underperfusion comes from the falloff of local blood flow as retinopathy progresses [2] and the decline in renal plasma flow with the advance of nephropathy [138].

Loss of autoregulation in the microcirculation is another of the hemodynamic disturbances of diabetes. The extent to which this contributes to over or under perfusion is currently a matter for speculation. Impairment of retinal vascular responses to breathing oxygen [139], the loss of constancy of glomerular filtration in the face of variations in perfusion pressure [140] and the failure of constancy of skin flow to alterations in limb posture [141] are all pieces of evidence pointing to defective autoregulation in diabetes.

Elevation of plasma viscosity and impaired deformability of red cells might have several effects on the microcirculation. In the overperfused state they may contribute to rises in perfusion pressure and increase the shear stress on small vessel walls, a factor thought to be a stimulant to basement membrane thickening of capillaries [142,143]. A further consequence of raised capillary hydrostatic pressure might be increased transudation of fluid into the extravascular space [144], a phenomenon well known in diabetes and clearly visible in the diabetic eye as enhanced escape of dye into the vitreous following fluorescein angiography. In the underperfused state, particularly if loss of autoregulation occurs, more rigid red cells and more viscous plasma could lead to reduced red cell velocity [144], local reductions in capillary hematocrit [145] and possibly a predilection to capillary occlusion, three situations predisposing to tissue hypoxia.

Research in the area of erythrocyte flow properties and diabetic microcirculatory disease is currently impaired by deficiencies in methodology and by the large number of different methods being used by various groups of workers; this making results difficult to compare. The large amount of research presently being carried out by basic scientists into new and improved methods of measuring the flow characteristics of red and white cells will hopefully form a basis for future clinical work. More information is also required on the hemodynamics of blood flow in the microcirculation in diabetics, although tissue accessability remains a major problem. Indeed, the studies by Brånemark et al [64] and investigations of capillary flow in nailbeds [134] have already provided valuable information in this area.

10.6.3. Blood rheology relation to other etiological candidates of diabetic complications

Many variables other than rheology have been found to be abnormal in cross sectional studies of diabetic patients, and a number of them have shown correlations with the presence of different complications. These include growth hormone excess, insulin deficiency, abnormalities of platelet aggregation and fibrinolysis, elevated circulating lipids and lactic acid, and irregularities of sorbitol accumulation to name a few. The etiology of the macro- and microcirculatory disease in diabetes is therefore now wideley regarded as being multifactorial. It is clearly beyond the scope of this chapter to discuss this in more detail, and the reader is referred to recent reviews [146,147].

The relative importance of such variables can be assessed more critically by prospective longitudinal studies in which candidate risk factors are evaluated in relation to their temporal association with the evolution of circulatory and microcirculatory disease. Such studies are now beginning to be mounted, but they are time consuming and costly, especially if a large number of factors are being evaluated simultaneously; furthermore, objective monitoring of microcirculatory events (especially in the retina) although possible is difficult and intricate. An alternative approach to evaluate the power of rheological and other candidate factors is administration of carefully chosen therapies to selectively normalize one or more factors. In this context it is notable that improvement in metabolic control has been reported to favourably influence many of the risk factors found in diabetics, including rheological variables. The results of present ongoing studies seeking to evaluate the effectiveness of improved metabolic balance by continuous subcutaneous infusion of insulin on microangiopathy may provide valuable indirect information concerning the etiological importance of blood rheology in diabetes.

10.7. References

1. Keen H., Jarrett J. (eds) 1982: 2nd edition: Complications of diabetes. Edward Arnold, London.
2. Kohner E.M., McLeod D., Marshall J. 1982: Diabetic eye disease. In: Complications of diabetes. Eds. Keen H., Jarret J. Edward Arnold, London pp. 19-108.
3. Ashton N. 1974: Vascular basement membrane changes in diabetic retinopathy. Montgomery lecture 1973. Br. J. Ophthal. 58, 344-366.
4. Vracko R., Benditt E.P. 1975: Restricted replicative life-span of diabetic fibroblasts in vitro: its relation to microangiopathy. Fed. Proc. 34, 68-70.
5. Ashton N. 1953: Arteriolar involvement in diabetic retinopathy. Br. J. Ophthal. 37, 282-292.
6. Wise G.N. 1956: Retinal neovascularisation. Trans. Amer. Ophthal. Soc. 54, 729-826.
7. Butterfield W.J.H., Whichelow M.S. 1965: Peripheral glucose metabolism in control subjects and diabetic patients during glucose, glucose-insulin and insulin sensitivity test. Diabetologia 1, 43-53.
8. Alexander K., Teusen R., Mikzkat H.J. 1968: Vergleichende Messungen der Extremitätendurchblutung bei Diabetikern und Stoffwechselgesunden. Klin. Wschr. 46, 234-238.
9. Christensen N.J. 1970: A reversible vascular abnormality associated with diabetic ketosis. Clin. Sci. 39, 539-548.
10. Thuesen L., Christiansen J.S., Jensen N.F. 1984: Reduced cardiac output following improved metabolic control in type 1 (insulin-dependent) diabetic patients. Diabetologia 27 (2), Abs 527, 338A.
11. Nair K.S., Webster J., Garrow J.S. 1984: Effects of glucose intolerance and diabetes on energy expenditure. Diabetologia 27 (2), Abs 379, 314A.
12. Ireland J.T., Viberti G.C., Watkins P.J. 1982 2nd edition: The kidney and renal tract. In: Complications of Diabetes. Eds Keen H., Jarrett J. Edward Arnold, London, pp. 137-178.
13. Bell E.T. 1952: Post mortem studies of vascular disease of diabetics. Arch. Pathol. 53, 444-445.
14. Thomas P.K., Ward J.D., Watkins P.J. 1982 2nd edition: Diabetic neuropathy. In: Complications of diabetes. Eds. Keen H., Jarrett J. Edward Arnold, London, pp. 109-136.
15. Garci M.J., McNamara P.M., Gordon T., Kannell W.B. 1974: Morbidity and mortality in diabetics in the Framingham population. Diabetes 23, 105-111.

16. Liebow I.M., Hallerstein H.K., Miller M. 1955: Arteriosclerotic heart disease in diabetes mellitus. Am. J. Med. 18, 438-447.
17. Haywood R.E., Lucena B.C. 1965: An investigation into mortality of diabetics. J. Institute of Actuaries. 91, 286-336.
18. Bell E.T. 1950: Incidence of gangrene of the extremities in non diabetic and in diabetic persons. Archs. Path. 49, 469-473.
19. Watkins P.J., Edmonds M.E. 1983: Sympathetic nerve failure in diabetes. Diabetologia 25, 73-77.
20. Jarrett R.J., Keen H., Chakrabarti R. 1982: Diabetes, hyperglycemia and arterial disease. In: Complications of diabetes. Eds. Keen H., Jarrett J. Edward Arnold, London, pp. 179-203.
21. Dandona P., James I.M., Newbury P.A., Woollard M.L., Beckett A.G. 1978: Cerebral blood flow in diabetes mellitus: evidence of abnormal cerebrovascular reacitivity. Br. Med. J. 2, 325-326.
22. Cogan D.G., Merola L., Laibson P.R. 1961: Blood viscosity, serum hexosamine and diabetic retinopathy. Diabetes 10, 393-395.
23. Skovborg F., Nielsen A.V., Schlichtkrull J., Ditzel J. 1966: Blood viscosity in diabetic patients. Lancet 1, 129-131.
24. Mausolf F.A., Mensher J.H. 1973: Experimental hyperviscosity retinopathy: preliminary report. Ann. Ophth. 5, 205-209.
25. Ring C.P., Pearson T.C., Sanders M.D., Wetherley-Mein G. 1976: Viscosity and retinal vein thrombosis. Br. J. Ophthal. 60, 397-410.
26. Kornerup T. 1955: Studies in diabetic retinopathy. An investigation of 1000 cases of diabetes. Acta Med. Scand. CLIII 81-111.
27. The Kroc Collaborative Study Group 1984: Blood glucose control and the evolution of diabetic retinopathy and albuminuria. A preliminary multicentre trial. New Engl. J. Med. 331, 365-372.
28. Langer L., Bergentz S.E., Bjure J., Fagerberg S.E. 1971: The effect of exercise on haematocrit, plasma volume and viscosity in diabetes mellitus. Diabetologia 7, 29-33.
29. Gordon W. 1969: The effect of ingested glucose and intravenous injections of glucose on the viscosity of whole blood in man. Clin. Sci. 36, 25-39.
30. Swank R.L. 1959: Blood viscosity in cerebrovascular disease. Effects of low fat diet and heparin. Neurology 9, 553-560.
31. Skovborg F. 1974: Blood viscosity in normal and diabetic subjects. A clinical and haemorheological study. FADL's Forlag, København, Århus, Odense.
32. Rees S.B., Simon L., Peltier G.A., Gleason R., Balodimos M., Marble A., Merrill E.L.O. 1967: Hemorheologic studies during the progression and remission of diabetic retinopathy. Biorheology 4, 102-103.
33. Ditzel J. 1968: Whole blood viscosity and related components in diabetes mellitus. Dan. Med. Bull. 15, 49-53.
34. Zingg W., Sulev J.C., Morgan C.D., Ehrlich R.M. 1971: Blood viscosity in diabetic children. Diabetologia 7, 461-462.
35. Bollinger A., Berchtold P., Berger W. 1969: Untersuchungen der Blutviskosität bei Diabetikern. Praxis 35, 1104-1107.
36. Isogai Y., Ichiba K., Iida A., Chikatsu I., Abe M. 1971: Viscosity of blood and plasma in various diseases. In: Theoretical and clinical hemorheology. Proc. 2nd Int. Conf. Haemorheology, Heidelberg 1969. Eds. Hartert H., Copley A.L. Springer Verlag, Berlin, Heidelberg, New York 326-332.
37. Isogai Y., Iida A., Michizuki K., Abe M. 1976: Hemorheological studies on the pathogenesis of diabetic microangiopathy. Thromb. Res. 8, Suppl. 2, 17-24.
38. Labib M.A.M., Higazi A.M., El-Ebrashy N., El-Ashmawy S., Madkoor M.K., Barhooma G.A. 1971: Studies on diabetic retinal vascular changes with special reference to blood coagulation and viscosity. Bull. Ophthalmol. Soc. Egypt. 64, 457-482.

39. Hoare E.M., Barnes A.J., Dormandy J.A. 1976: Abnormal blood viscosity in diabetes and retinopathy. Biorheology 13, 21-25.
40. Schmid-Schönbein H., Volger E. 1976: Red cell aggregation and red cell deformability in diabetes. Diabetes 25, Suppl. 2, 897-902.
41. Barnes A.J., Locke P., Scudder P.R., Dormandy T.L., Dormandy J.A., Slack J. 1977: Is hyperviscosity a treatable component of diabetic microcirculatory disease? Lancet 2, 789-791.
42. Dintenfass L. 1977: Blood viscosity factors in severe non diabetic and diabetic retinopathy. Biorheology 14, 151-157.
43. Dintenfass L., Davis E. 1977: Genetic and ethnic influences on blood viscosity and capillaries in diabetes mellitus. Microvas. Res. 14, 161-172.
44. Lowe G.D.O., Lowe J.M., Drummond M.M., Reith S., Belch J.J.F., Kesson M., Wylie A., Foulds W.S., Forbes C.D., MacCuish A.C., Manderson W.G. 1980: Blood viscosity in young male diabetics with and without retinopathy. Diabetologia 18, 359-363.
45. McMillan D.E., Utterback N.G., Stocki J. 1980: Low shear rate viscosity in diabetes. Biorheology 17, 355-362.
46. Paisey R.B., Harkness J., Hartog M., Chadwick T. 1980: The effect of improvement in diabetic control on plasma and whole blood viscosity. Diabetologia 19, 345-349.
47. Barnes A.J. 1981: Blood viscosity in diabetes mellitus. In: Clinical aspects of blood viscosity and cell deformability. Eds. Lowe G.D.O., Barbenel J.C., Forbes C.D. Springer Verlag, Berlin, Heidelberg, New York 151-162.
48. Rand P.W., Norton J.M., Barker N.D., Richards A.L., Lacombe E.H., Pirone L.A. 1981: Effects of diabetes mellitus on red cell properties. Clin. Hemorheology 1, 373-385.
49. Stoltz J.F., Gaillard S., Drouin P. 1981: Hemorheology and diabetes mellitus. Verh. Dtsch. Ges. Inn. Med. 87, 1302-1312.
50. Hill M.A., Court J.M., Mitchell G.M. 1982: Blood rheology and microalbuminuria in type 1 diabetes mellitus. Lancet 2, 985.
51. Poon P.Y.W., Dornan T.L., Orde-Peckar C., Mullins R., Bron A.J., Turner R.C. 1982: Blood viscosity, glycaemic control and retinopathy in insulin dependent diabetes. Clin. Sci. 63, 211-216.
52. Leiper J.M., Lowe G.D.O., Anderson J., Burns P., Cohen H.N., Manderson W.G., Forbes C.D., Barbenel J.C., MacGuish A.C. 1982: Effects of diabetic control and biosynthetic human insulin on blood rheology in established diabetics 1984. Diabetes Res. 1, 27-30.
53. Stuart J., Kenny M.W., Aukland A., George A.J., Neumann V., Shaprio L.M., Cove D.H. 1983: Filtration of washed erythrocytes in atherosclerosis and diabetes mellitus. Clin. Hemorheology 3 (1), 23-30.
54. Rousselle D., Gaillard S., Voisin P., Pointel J.P., Debry G., Drouin P., Stoltz J.F. 1980: Blood viscosity and erythrocyte filterability in diabetic patients controlled via an artificial pancreas. In: Hemorheology and diseases. Proceedings of the 1st Europ. Conf. on Clin. Hemorheology. Eds. Stoltz J.F., Drouin P. (Doin Editeurs Paris) 411-418.
55. Reubi F.C. 1953: Glomerular filtration rate, renal blood flow and blood viscosity during and after diabetic coma. Circulat. Res. 1, 410-413.
56. Skovborg F., Nielsen A.V. 1969: Variation in whole blood and plasma viscosity in acidotic diabetics. Bibl. Anat. 10, 145-152.
57. Barnes A.J. 1978: Blood rheology in diabetes mellitus. MD thesis University of London 134-148.
58. Barnes A.J., Locke P., Dormandy T.L., Dormandy J.A. 1977: Blood viscosity and metabolic control in diabetes mellitus. Clin. Sci. Molec. Med. 52, 24.
59. DeSilva S.R., Shawe J.E.H., Patel H., Cudworth A.G. 1979: Plasma fibrinogen in diabetes mellitus. Diabetes Metab. 5, 201-205.
60. Mosora N., Baciu T., Vincze J. 1972: The viscosity of the serum, haematocrit and fibrinogen in diabetes mellitus and their relationship with diabetes mellitus. Diabetologia 8:59.
61. McMillan D.E. 1974: Disturbance of serum viscosity in diabetes mellitus. J. Clin. Invest. 53, 1071-1079.

62. McMillan D.E. 1975: Two roles for plasma fibrinogen in the production of diabetic microangiopathy. Diabetes 24, Suppl. 2, 438.
63. Oughton J., Barnes A.J. 1981: Red cell filterability in diabetes mellitus: it's relation to other methods of measuring deformability and to blood viscosity. Scand. J. Clin. Lab. Invest. 41, Suppl. 156, 147-150.
64. Brånemark P.I., Langer L., Fagerberg S.E., Breine U. 1971: Studies in rheology of human diabetes mellitus. Diabetologia 7, 107-112.
65. Ditzel J. 1970: Changes in rheology and oxygen transport function of the erythrocytes in diabetes. Microcirculatory approaches to current therapeutic problems. Symposia 6th European Conf. Microcirculation, Aalborg. 123-131. Karger, Basel.
66. Ehrly A.M., Kohler H.J. 1976: Altered deformability of erythrocytes from patients with chronic occlusive arterial disease. Vasa 5, 319-322.
67. Juhan I., Bayle J., Vague Ph., Juhan C. 1978: Déformabilitié des hématies chez les diabétiques. Nouv. Presse Med. 7, 759-760.
68. Juhan I., Buonocore M., Vovan L., Durand F., Calas M.F., Moulin J.P., Vague P. 1979: Filterabilié des hématies chez les diabétiques. Influence de la glycémie et variations aprés connection 'a un pancréas artificiel. Nouv. Presse Med. 8, 4083-4085.
69. Juhan I., Vague Ph., Buonocore M., Moulin J.P., Calas M.F., Vialettes B., Verdot J.J. 1981: Effects of insulin on erythrocyte deformability in diabetics: relationship between erythrocyte deformability and platelet aggregation. Scand. J. Clin. Lab. Invest. 41, Suppl. 156, 159-164.
70. Knight K., Rampling M.W., Sirs J.A. 1978: Erythrocyte flexibility in blood from patients with diabetes mellitus. Biorheology 15, 51-52.
71. McMillan D.E., Utterback N.G., LaPuma J. 1978: Reduced erythrocyte deformability in diabetes. Diabetes 27, 895-901.
72. Baba Y., Kai M., Kamada T., Setoyama S., Otsuji S. 1979: Higher levels of erythrocyte membrane microviscosity in diabetes. Diabetes 28, 1138-1140.
73. LaCelle P.L. 1980: Behavior of abnormal erythrocytes in capillaries. In: Erythrocyte mechanics and blood flow. Eds. Coklet G.R., Meiselman H.J., Brooks D.E. Alan R. Liss, New York, 195-209.
74. Boudart D., Ozanne P., Leloup R., Chupin M. 1981: Déformabilité érythrocytaire et hémoglobins glycosylées chez le diabétique. La Nouvelle Presse Médicale 10 (11), 910.
75. Drouin P., Rousselle D., Stoltz J.F., Guimont C., Gaillard S., Vernhes G., Debry G. 1981: Study of blood viscosity and erythrocyte parameters in diabetic patients using the artificial pancreas. Scand. J. Clin. Lab. Invest. 41, Suppl. 156, 165-169.
76. Isogai Y., Mochzuki K., Maeda T. 1981: Red cell filterability in diabetes. Scand. J. Clin. Lab. Invest. 41, Suppl. 156, 171-173.
77. Le Devehat C., Lemoine A., Cirette B., Ramet M. 1981: Red cell filterability and metabolic state in diabetic subjects with macroangiopathy. Scand. J. Clin. Lab. Invest. 41, Suppl. 156, 155-158.
78. McMillan D.E., Utterback N.G., Sparks L.L., Bramwell P.C. 1981: Impaired erythrocyte doublet formation in diabetes. Diabetologia 21, 575-578.
79. McMillan D.E., Utterback N.G., Mitchell T.P. 1983: Doublet formation of diabetic erythrocytes as a model of impaired membrane viscous deformation. Microvas. Res. 26, 205-220.
80. Pozza G., Cordaro C., Carandente O., Margonato A. 1981: Study on the relationship between erythrocyte filtration and other risk factors in diabetic angiopathy. La Ricerca Clin. Lab. 11, Suppl. 1, 317-326.
81. Williamson J.R., Kilo C., Sutera S.P., Gardner R.A., Boylan C.W., Chang K.C. 1981: Shear induced deformation of red cells: decreased elongation and membrane rotation in diabetes mellitus. Horm. metab. Res. Suppl. 11, 103-104.
82. Sewchand L.S., Hampel W.L., Diddie K.R., Meiselman H.J. 1982: Membrane mechanical properties of erythrocytes from patients with diabetic retinopathy. Microcirculation 1, 361-380.
83. Bryszewska M., Leyko W. 1983: Effect of insulin on human erythrocyte membrane fluidity in diabetes mellitus. Diabetologia 24 (5), 311-313.

84. Caimi G. 1983: Blood viscosity and erythrocyte filterability: Their evaluation in diabetes mellitus. Horm. Metab. Res. 15, 467-470.
85. Hanss M. 1983: In: Red cell deformability and filterability. Ed. Dormandy J. Martinus Nijhoff, Boston, The Hague, Dordrecht, Lancaster p. 189.
86. Kamada T., Otsuji S. 1983: Lower levels of erythrocyte membrane fluidity in diabetic patients. A spin label study. Diabetes 32, 585-591.
87. Caimi G., Galluzzo A., Giordano C., Caruso C., Capobianco D., Sarno A. 1985: Genetic pattern and haemorheological determinants in type 1 diabetics. Clin. Hemorheology 5, 155-158.
88. Ritchie D.M. 1985: Filtration of dilute erythrocyte suspensions as a measure of erythrocyte deformability and it's relationship to blood glucose control in diabetes mellitus. Clin. Hemorheol. 5, 257-268.
89. Vague P., Juhan I., Buonocore M., Moulin J.P., Vovan L. 1980: Normalisation of erythrocyte filterability after correction of hyperglycaemia by an artificial endocrine pancreas in insulin-dependent diabetics. In: Hemorheology and Diseases. Proc. 1st Europ. Conf. Clin. Hemorheol. Eds. Stoltz J.F., Drouin P. (Doin Editeurs, Paris), 425-429.
90. Sacks A.H., Bradley M., North P. 1981: Filtration measurements to determine the effects of red cell rigidity and aggregation on resistance to flow. Microvasc. Res. 22, 331-344.
91. Volger E. 1981: Effect of metabolic control and concomitant diseases upon the rheology of blood in different states of diabetic retinopathy. Horm. Metab. Res. Suppl. 11, 104-107.
92. Willars E.J., Hunt W.B., Clark P.A., Barnes A.J. 1985: Micropipette studies in diabeties mellitus. Proc. 4th Europ. Conf. Clin Hemorheol., Siena 1985.
93. Paulsen E.P., Koury M. 1976: Hemoglobin AIc levels in insulin-dependent and -independent diabetes mellitus. Diabetes 25, 890-896.
94. Juhan-Vague I., Rahmani-Jourdheuil D., Mourayre Y., Aillaud M.F., Vague P., Mishal Z. 1985: Study of red blood cell membrane fluidity in insulin-dependent diabetics using fluorescence polarization. Effect of insulin. Proc. 4th Europ. Conf. Clin. Hemorheol. Siena 1985.
95. Outsuji S., Baba Y., Kamada T. 1981: Erythrocyte membrane microviscosity in diabetes. Horm. Metab. Res. 2, (Suppl.) 97-102.
96. Voisin Ph., Kolopp M., Rôusselle D., Gaillard S., Pointel J.P., Stoltz J.F., Debry G., Drouin P. 1982: Influence du controle métabolique sur la viscosité sanguine et l'activité plaquettaire chez les diabétiques insulino-dépendants. Nouv. Rev. Fr. Hematol. 24, 187-190.
97. Willars E.J., Barnes A.J., Oughton J., Clark P.A. 1983: Effect of incubation hardening and insulin on normal red cells: a comparitive study using four different methods for measuring deformability. Clin. Hemorheol. 3 (3), 268.
98. Davidson R.J.L., Evan-Wong L.A., Stowers J.M. 1981: The mean red cell volume in diabetes mellitus. Diabetologia 20, 583-584.
99. Morse E.E., Kalache G., Germino W., Stockwell R. 1981: Increased electronic mean corpuscular volume induced by marked hyperglycaemia. Ann. Clin. Lab. Sci. 11, 184-187.
100. Ditzel J., Moinat P. 1959: Changes in serum proteins, lipoproteins and protein bound carbohydrates in relation to pathological alterations in the microcirculation of diabetic subjects. J. Lab. Clin. Med. 54, 843-859.
101. Van Haeringen N.J., Oosterhuis J.A., Terpstra J., Glasius E. 1973: Erythrocyte aggregation in relation to diabetic retinopathy. Diabetologia 9, 20-24.
102. Little H.L., Sacks A.H. 1977: Role of abnormal blood rheology in the pathogenesis of diabetic retinopathy. Tr. Am. Acad. Ophth. and Otol. 83, 522-534.
103. Satoh M., Imaizumi K., Bessho T., Shiga T. 1984: Increased erythrocyte aggregation in diabetes mellitus and it's relationship to glycosylated haemoglobin and retinopathy. Diabetologia 27, 517-521.
104. Wautier J.L., Paton R.C., Wautier M.P., Pintigny D., Abadie E., Passa P., Caen J.P. 1981: Increased adhesion of erythrocytes to endothelial cells in diabetes mellitus and its relation to vascular complications. New Eng. J. Med. 305, 237-242.

105. Dormandy J.A. 1970: Clinical significance of blood viscosity. Ann. Roy. Coll. Surg. Engl. 47, 211-228.
106. Ford T.F., Berent A., Speed K., Rose M.S., Dormandy J.A. 1978: Symptomatic and objective effects of venesection on patients with intermittant claudication. Br. Med. J. 1, 1189.
107. Yates C.J.P., Berent A., Andrews V., Dormandy J.A. 1979: Increase in leg blood flow by normovolaemic haemodilution in intermittant claudication. Lancet 2, 166-168.
108. Milligan D.W., Tooke J.E., Davies J.A. 1982: Effect of venesection on calf blood flow in polycythemia. Br. Med. J. 284, 619-620.
109. Dormandy J.A., Goyle K.B., Reid H.L. 1977: Treatment of severe intermittant claudication by controlled defibrination. Lancet 1, 625-626.
110. Bailey M.J., Johnston C.L.W., Yates C.J.P., Somerville P.G., Dormandy J.A. 1979: Preoperative haemoglobin as predictor of outcome of diabetic amputations. Lancet 2, 168-170.
111. Hobin F.P., Maraist F.B. 1973: Diabetic hyperosmolar non-ketoacidotic coma complicated by mesenteric thrombosis. J. Fla. Med. Assoc. 60, 25-26.
112. Timperley W.R., Preston F.E., Ward J.D. 1974: Cerebral intravascular coagulation in diabetic ketoacidosis. Lancet 1, 952-956.
113. Tchertkoff V., Nayak S.V., Kamath C., Salomon M.I. 1974: Hyperosmolar non ketotic diabetic coma: vascular complications. J. Amer. Ger. Soc. 22, 462-466.
114. Ramon J.S., Daroca J.C., Perez J.F.C., Frances J.M.C., Gorina A.B. 1975: Complicaciones cardiovasculares del coma diabético hipersmolar. Estudio de cuatro observaciones. Rev. Clin. Española. 137, 521-526.
115. Pearson T.C., Weatherley-Mein G. 1978: Vascular occlusive episodes and venous haematocrit in primary proliferative polycythemia. Lancet 2, 1219-1222.
116. Harrison M.J.G., Pollock S., Kendall B.E., Marshall J. 1981: Effect of haematocrit on carotid stenosis and cerebral infarction. Lancet 2, 114-115.
117. Pearce J.M.S., Chandrasekera C.P., Ladusans E.J. 1983: Lacunar infarcts in polycythemia with raised packed cell volumes. Br. Med. J. 287, 935-936.
118. Lowe G.D.O., Jaap A.J., Forbes C.D. 1983: Relation of atrial fibrillation and high haematocrit to mortality in acute stroke. Lancet 1, 784-786.
119. Humphrey P.R.D., DuBoulay G.H., Marshall J., Pearson T.C., Ross Russell R.W., Symon L., Weatherley-Mein G., Zilkha E. 1979: Cerebral blood flow and viscosity in relative polycythemia. Lancet 2, 873-876.
120. Thomas D.J., DuBoulay G.H., Marshall J., Pearson T.C., Ross Russell R.W., Symon L., Weatherley-Mein G., Zilkha E. 1977: Cerebral blood flow in polycythemia. Lancet 2, 161-163.
121. Brown M.M., Marshall J. 1982: Effect of plasma exchange on blood viscosity and cerebral blood flow. Br. Med. J. 284, 1733-1736.
122. Murray J.F., Escobar E., Rapaport W. 1969: Effects of blood viscosity on haemodynamic responses in acute normovolemic anemia. Am. J. Physiol. 216, 638-642.
123. Restorff W.V., Höfling B., Holtz J., Bassenge E. 1975: Effect of increased blood fluidity through haemodilution on coronary circulation at rest and during exercise in dogs. Pflüg. Arch. 357, 15-24.
124. Jan K.M., Chien S. 1977: Effect of haematocrit variations on coronary hemodynamics and oxygen utilization. Am. J. Physiol. 233, H106-H113.
125. Jan K.M., Heldmann J., Chien S. 1980: Coronary hemodynamics and oxygen utilization after hematocrit variations in hemorrhage. Am. J. Physiol. 239, H326-H332.
126. Grigoleit H.G., Lehrach F., Multer R. 1973: Diabetic angiopathy and blood viscosity. Acta Diab. Lat. 10, 311-324.
127. Jones R.L., Peterson C.M. 1981: Hematologic alterations in diabetes mellitus. Am. J. Med. 70, 339-352.
128. Behrendt T., Duane T.D. 1970: Unilateral complications in Diabetes retinopathy. Trans. Am. Acad. Ophth. Ot. 74, 28-32.

129. Berkman T., Rifkin H. 1973: Unilateral nodular diabetic glomerulosclerosis (Kimmelstiel-Wilson). Report of a case. Metab. Clin. Exp. 22, 715-722.
130. Gundersen H.J.G. 1974: Peripheral blood flow and metabolic control in juvenile diabetes. Diabetologia 10, 225-231.
131. Christiansen J.S., Gammelgaard T., Tronier B., Svendsen P.A., Parving H.-H. 1982: Kidney function and size in diabetics, before and during initial insulin treatment. Kidney International 21, 683-688.
132. Rayman G., Hassan A., Spencer P.D., Wise P.H., Tooke J.E. 1984: Vascular responses to postural change in the diabetic neuropathic foot. Diabetologia 27, 324 (Abstract number 440).
133. Rayman G., Williams S., Hassan A., Gamble T., Tooke T.E. 1985: Capilllary hypertension and overperfusion in the feet of young diabetics. Diabet. Medicine abst. (in press).
134. Tooke J.E. 1986: Microvascular haemodynamics in diabetes mellitus. Clin. Sci. 70, 119–125.
135. Megibow R.S., Megibow S.J., Pollack H., Boorkman J.J., Osserman T. 1953: The mechanism of accelerated peripheral vascular sclerosis in diabetes mellitus. Am. J. Med. 15, 322-329.
136. Rayman G., Spencer P.D., Smaje L.H., Wise P.H. 1984: Relationship of cutaneous blood flow to duration and control of diabetes. Int. J. Microcirc. Clin. Exp. 3, 285 (Abstract).
137. Fagrell B., Hermansson I.-L., Karlander S.-G., Ostergren J. 1984: Vital capillary microscopy for assessment of skin viability and microangiopathy in patients with diabetes mellitus. Acta Med. Scand. 687, 25-28.
138. Mongensen C.E., Christensen C.K., Vittinghus E. 1983: The stages in diabetic renal disease. Diabetes 32, Suppl. 2, 64-78.
139. Grunwald J.E., Riva C.E., Sinclair S.H., Brucker A.V. 1983: Altered retinal vascular response to 100% O2 breathing in diabetes mellitus. Microvasc. Res. 25, 236 (Abstract No 35).
140. Parving H.-H., Kastrup H., Smidt U.M., Andersen A.R., Feldt-Rasmussen B.F., Sandahl Christiansen J. 1984: Impaired autoregulation of glomerular filtration rate in type I (insulin-dependent) diabetic patients with nephropathy. Diabetologia 27, 247-252.
141. Faris I., Vagn Nielsen H., Henriksen C., Parving H.-H., Lassen N.A. 1983: Impaired autoregulation of blood flow in skeletal muscle and subcutaneous tissue in long-term Type I (insulin-dependent) diabetic patients with microangiopathy. Diabetologia 25, 486-488.
142. Williamson J.R., Kilo C. 1977: Current status of capillary basement membrane disease in diabetes mellitus. Diabetes 26, 65-72.
143. Longhurst J. Capone J.R., Zelis R. 1975: Evaluation of skeletal muscle capillary basement-membrane thickness in congestive heart failure. Chest 67, 195-198.
144. Simpson L.O. 1985: Intrinsic stiffening of red blood cells as the fundamental cause of diabetic nephropathy and microangiopathy: a new hypothesis. Nephron 39, 344-351.
145. Gaehtgens P., Pries A., Albrecht K.H. 1979: Model experiments on the effect of bifurcations on capillary blood flow and oxygen transport. Pflügers Arch. 380, 115-120.
146. McMillan D.E. 1975: Deterioration of the microcirculation in diabetes. Diabetes 24, 944-957.
147. Alberti K.G.M.M., Press C.M. 1982: The biochemistry of the complications of diabetes. In: Complications of diabetes. Eds. Keen H., Jarret J. Edward Arnold, London, pp. 231-270.

11
Other syndromes associated with impaired blood flow and rheology

S. Forconi *, D. Pieragalli *, E. Ernst **
** Institute of Special Medical Pathology, University of Siena, Italy*
*** Clinic for Physical Medicine, University of Munich, Federal Republic of Germany*

11.1. Introduction

While the preceding chapters have dealt extensively with ischemic diseases, diabetes, thrombosis, hematological and gynecological aspects of hemorheology, a variety of other disease entities associated with hemorheological deficits have been left untouched. It is therefore the aim of this chapter to briefly summarize the hemorheological findings in this range of largely unrelated diseases and to discuss their possible pathophysiological significance.

11.2. Shock

In 1872 Samuel Gross described shock as a "manifestation of a crude unhinging of the machinery of life" [2]. Since then we have learned more about the fundamental mechanisms involved, enabling us to design regimes of treatments. However, a total understanding of the complex sequence of deleterious events that results from a prolonged deficiency of tissue perfusion has not been achieved at present. This deficiency in microcirculatory flow can be brought about by a number of etiologies, each of which leads to characteristic sequaele. Moreover, each form of shock results in secondary changes of almost all body systems.

Microcirculatory flow is regulated by a number of morphological, biochemical or physiological factors which interact (see chapter 4). Their exact functional interrelationship is not fully understood and may vary in different vascular beds. A large variety of physical, chemical, hemodynamic, and immunological mechanisms can jeopardize the microcirculation and lead to hypoxia. The slightest degree of injury to the endothelium can result in platelet adhesion [2] and an inflammatory reaction with leukocyte sticking [3]. At the beginning of this chain of events, there might be vasodilatation mediated by local vasoactive chemicals (histamine, kinins, serotonin, prostaglandins, etc.) and hence a rise in local blood flow. Some of these vasoactive substances also increase vascular permeability and can therefore lead to fluid loss and blood viscidation. Later, vascular resistance will increase, locally due to more cells adhering to the vessel wall or to each other, and systemically due to loss in blood volume, resulting in decreased flow. This process may easily be perpetuated with further adhesion and aggregation of blood cells [4], leading to reduced flow forces which results in even further cell sticking. This would bring about tissue hypoxia with pH changes, red cell rigidification, and alterations in blood clotting. Finally a disruption of the integrity of the vessel wall and other complex alterations in cell function [5] may take place with increased permeability, fluid leakage, local intravascular hemoconcentration, and hyperviscosity [6]. The possible role of white cells and their rheology in capillary obstruction and endothelial damage is only just emerging. In the course of these events which may differ from one form of shock to another, the normal responsiveness of the microvasculature to neurohumoral regulatory stimuli may be diminished or lost completely [7], leading to the irreversibility of the microcirculatory failure. Thus, during the final stage of shock, the distal vasculature can behave like a passive structure without active adjustments to circulatory demands. Even though this progressive failure of the microcirculation is rarely primary in the development of shock, it is crucial in the perpetuation of low flow states.

A variety of compensatory mechanisms, the most prominent of which are increased sympathoadrenal discharge and vasoconstriction, are designed to maintain adequate perfusion to the vital organs. Thus, blood flow to the heart and to the brain are preserved as long as possible. This compensation is a purposeful mechanism in the short term; however, it operates at the expense of the blood flow to virtually all other organs, the most important of these non-vital circulation being of course the kidney. Moreover it may well induce hemorheological impairement: norepinephrine was shown to decrease deformation of red cells for a given shear stress [8]. Such alterations could perpetuate the disturbance of microcirculatory flow. Another homeostatic response is the conservation or expansion of plasma volume: under the influence of aldosterone and anti-diuretic hormones, sodium and water excretion in the kidney can be reduced.

It seems likely that the rheological behavior of blood plays a key role in the development of the shock syndromes. By virtue of the shear dependence of blood, it is possible that a "vicious viscous cycle" establishes itself. Diminished shear forces, which may exist in shock locally or systemically for a variety of reasons, will result in red cell aggregation, pre-stasis, and hypoxia. Hypoxia in turn can lead to a further deterioration of the flow properties of blood. Therefore, in shock from trauma, burns, sepsis, toxins or hemorrhage, hemorheology can have an important contributory part in inducing and perpetuating the stagnation of flow, leading to the progression of microcirculatory failure and finally to decompensation [9]. This mechanism can be amplified when rheological deficits develop under certain conditions. The following will deal more specifically with the characteristic rheological changes in different forms of shock.

11.2.1. Traumatic shock

The pioneering work of Gelin and his colleagues helped to elucidate the hemorheological alterations which occur in response to trauma [20,11]. As a reaction to local injury, there is an invasion of leukocytes which can temporarily obstruct the terminal vasculature [21,12], an increase in acute phase proteins, and a consequent increase in red cell aggregation [23]. All this will lead to a rise in blood [23,14] and plasma [23,15] viscosities, contributing to an increase in peripheral resistance [26]. The rheological changes take place independent of alterations in hematocrit [26].

11.2.2. Hemorrhagic shock

A common feature of all shock syndromes is a marked drop in microcirculatory tissue perfusion. In hemorrhagic shock this is due to a decrease in cardiac output as a result of the decline in circulating blood volume. The obvious cause of blood loss is bleeding, but the circulating volume may be further decreased by the effects of kinins and histamine, which increase vascular permeability. Compensatory mechanisms aim at restoring blood flow to vital organs: for instance the replacement of intravascular fluid from the extravascular space to a rate up to 2 ml/min [27] and an increase of catecholamines to values of 20 times the normal [28] with subsequent vasoconstriction. If more than 25% of the total intravascular volume is lost, persistent and refractory hypotension and malperfusion may develop. At the microcirculatory level this will result in maldistribution of nutritive flow [29], brought about at least in part by microrheological changes [26,20,21,22]. In addition, the vasomotor activity will cease to function, if the pressure head falls below a critical value. The microcirculatory dysfunction induced in hemorrhagic shock can be observed by intravital microscopy [23]. Because of the influx of the extravascular fluid, the hematocrit falls in hemorrhage; this would result in a decrease in blood viscosity if the flow conditions were normal. Within the microcirculation, where local hematocrit differs from the venous hematocrit, the viscosity of the red cell suspension might still increase even with a lowering of systemic hematocrit [26,24]. In experimental hemorrhagic shock, changes in shape and deformability of red cells [25,26] and leukocytes [22,6] have been observed, and these may contribute to the plugging of exchange vessels. Correction of blood loss and volume replacement are the logical first measures in the prevention and treatment of hemorrhagic shock. In this respect, albumin and dextran 40 seem to be more effective than other colloids [27]. Dextran 40 has the advantage of a strong volume effect because of its high oncotic pressure, while albumin solutions exhibit a lower intrinsic viscosity. In order to maintain cellular function, precursors of ATP synthesis or ATP itself could prove to be beneficial.

11.2.3. Burns

While in other forms of shock there might be an initial hemodilution, in burns, anaphylactic shock, and septic shock, hemoconcentration can be a prominent early feature, causing hemorheological deterioration. In these syndromes a rapid loss of plasma proteins, predominantly albumin, due to venular leakage has been described in the early phase of shock [28]. Protein loss leads to decreases of oncotic pressure and intravascular water. The resulting hemoconcentration is associated with increases of red cell aggregation and blood viscosity [20]. Another detrimental mechanism might be a decrease in red cell deformability [29]. Microcirculatory changes in major burns have been shown to respond to prednisolone [30]. Possibly this is helped by the drug's action on decreased blood cell deformability [31]. The combination of adverse rheological changes may well perpetuate microcirculatory dysfunction by the mechanisms outlined above.

11.2.4. Septic shock

A variety of synonymous names are used for this form of shock which usually results from gram-negative organisms [32]: endotoxic, gram-negative, bacterial shock. Endotoxins have been shown to have profound effects on coagulation, complement, platelets, leucocytes, and endothelial cells [33]. Again, protein loss will be a prominent feature. These alterations may have direct or indirect effects on blood rheology resulting in a loss of blood fluidity [34]. Disseminated intravascular coagulation is a prominent and devastating event in septic shock syndromes [35], resulting in microthrombi and a rise of fibrin-fibrinogen degradation products in the plasma [36]. This may have adverse effects on the rheological properties of blood cells as described recently. It has been suggested that the development of disseminated intravascular coagulation might be favoured by rheologically mediated stasis or pre-stasis [38].

11.2.5. Anaphylactic shock

Here again the loss of plasma proteins [28] is the most important cause for hemorheological changes. This, in combination with local acidosis, will lead to red cell rigidification and viscidation of blood contributing to the sequence of events detailed above. Recently it was reported that red cells become rigidified in shock (etiology not further defined) [39]. The mortality of shocked patients correlated with filterability results ($r = 0.81$, $p < 0.001$). It was postulated that the rheological damage might be a consequence of shock, leading to its aggravation, which possibly could be used as an index for its severity. Red cell rigidification could well be brought about by local acidosis which must not neccessarily be overt in the systemic circulation and which was termed "hidden acidosis" early on in shock research [40].

This brief discussion suggests that a loss of the fluidity of blood (local or systemic) is a common feature (early or late) in the development of shock

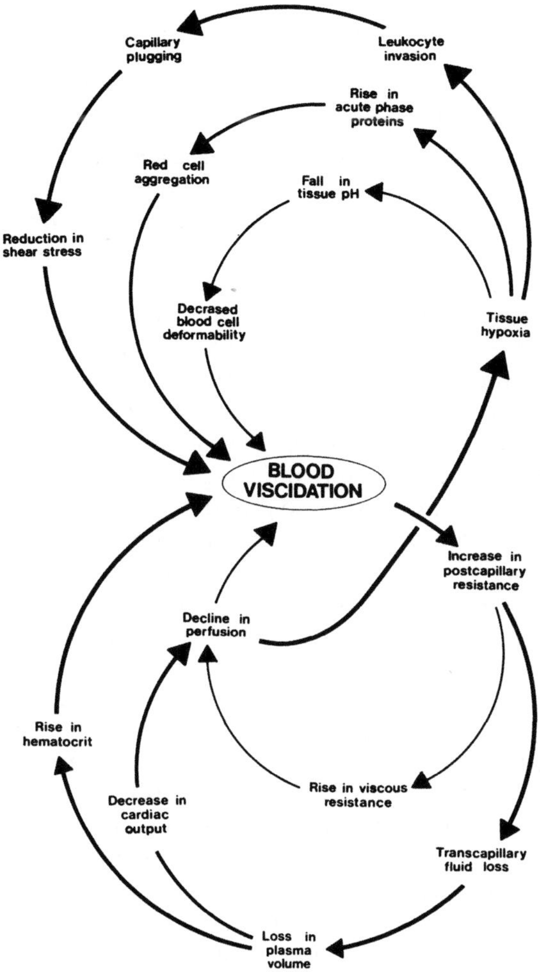

Figure 11.1. Schematic outline of possible feedback loops capable of amplifying rheological deficits that may lead to decompensation of shock. Depending on the specific etiology, the feedback may be started from different links within a chain of events (modified from [15]).

syndromes. Based on these considerations, various feedback loops can be implicated [25], as shown in Fig. 11.1. From this point of view it would seem that optimizing hemorheological factors might be an important contribution in preventing and treating shock. This aspect is dealt with in more detail in Chapter 12.

11.3. Surgery and anesthesia

Surgery may represent a major cause of hemorheological deficits. The question as to what part anesthesia plays in this, is unsolved at present. Existing data do not suggest that medications used in anesthesia exert significant influences on the flow properties of blood [41]. The same applies to the overnight fast before an operation [42]. In surgery and anesthesia, situations may develop in which blood viscosity can either be reduced or increased. Both the increase and the reduction depend upon the type of operation, the amount of intra- and postoperative blood loss and medication or infusion regime. The hematocrit may fall sharply due to the operation or postoperative infusions. Plasma viscosity may rise through reactive changes in fibrinogen [43,44]. Infusions of albumin or low molecular weight dextran may also be responsible for variations in blood viscosity and its determinants. Albumin tends to reduce plasma viscosity; 10% low molecular weight dextran produces a transient elevation in plasma viscosity immediately after administration, before it can extract sufficient water from the tissue due to its hyperoncotic nature. Blood cells may be affected in various ways. Erythrocyte deformability is diminished following changes in osmolarity of the suspending medium or when the acid-base balance is disturbed [45]. Hypoxia may also be a stimulus for erythrocyte rigidification, while hyperoxygenation may enhance deformability. Clinical studies have shown red cell filterability to decrease after minor and major surgical interventions [46,47,48].

Summarizing the available data, there is a varying degree of hyperviscosity and hypercoagulability, following surgery. The extent of the abnormality will depend on the extent, localization, and duration of the trauma and is mediated by modifications of the plasma protein pattern. The frequency with which postoperative thrombosis particularly in the veins occur, might be associated with disturbances in the rheological behavior of blood (see chapter 7). An elevation in blood viscosity might unfavourably affect the circulation by rising vascular resistance [49]. Several groups have pointed out that the prognosis of an operation is linked to hemorheological variables [50,51] and can indeed be ameliorated by enhancing blood fluidity before the operation [52]. Presently, it has become more and more accepted that a low hematocrit of around 30% is sufficient or even beneficial for oxygen delivery. Pre-operative hemodilution is associated with a number of other advantages such as availability of own blood postoperatively, reduction of cost and risk of transfusions [53].

11.4. Rheumatic disease

Hemorheological alterations in rheumatic diseases have been recognized for a long time [54,55,56,57]. At least in part the loss of blood fluidity is due to the effects that the proteins of inflammation exert on the flow properties of blood [58]. Increased plasma and serum viscosity have been reported in experimental arthritic disease [59,60,61] as well as in patients with rheumatic fever, rheumatoid arthritis, subacute infective polyarthritis, Sjoegren Syndrome, Felty Syndrome, cryoglobulinemia, polymyalgia rheumatica, and polymyositis [62,63]. In most of these studies rheology is not evaluated from a circulatory point of view, but as an index of disease activity comparable to the erythrocyte sedimentation rate [64]. Paired measurements of plasma and serum viscosity have been shown to improve the diagnostic value of this [65]. Lane [66] has described the sludging of blood in the conjunctival blood vessels of patients with rheumatoid arthritis and attempted to correlate this finding with the activity of the disease and with the increase in erythrocyte sedimentation rate. In 1970 Jasin [67] studied two patients with rheumatoid arthritis who showed symptoms which he interpreted as signs of a "Hyperviscosity Syndrome". Both patients had bleeding gums and epistaxis with clinical signs of congestive heart failure. Jasin suspected hyperviscosity to be due to the interaction of IgG complexes which resulted in the formation of large molecular conglomerates. The patients showed no signs of vasculitis but evidence of minor disturbances in peripheral circulation, such as palmar erythema attributable to hyperviscosity. Blaylock [68] described a case of a 47-year-old black woman with Sjoegren syndrome and high titres of rheumatoid factors. Ultracentrifugal studies showed complexes of rheumatoid factors with IgG in the blood. The patient was followed up for 2 years. She was hospitalized several times for various symptoms (epistaxis, headache, dizziness, blurred vision) possibly related to a hyperviscosity. Plasmapheresis relieved the symptoms, and the final recovery of this patient was associated with the normalization of serum viscosity. Similar cases were described by Pope [69] as well as by Kosaka and Solomon [70]. A case of rheumatoid arthritis with Felty's syndrome and hyperviscosity [71] is of considerable interest because it demonstrated that plasma hyperviscosity does not result from the action of one single protein but presumably from the interaction of protein factors such as IgG-IgG self-associating polymers and IgG-IgM complexes.

Clinical manifestations due to hyperviscosity are probably quite rare in rheumatic diseases. In practice rheumatoid arthritis, even when very acute, is not generally accompanied by overt evidence of a "Hyperviscosity Syndrome". In a study of 21 patients with rheumatoid arthritis in the active stage, carried out by the Siena group, an increase in the viscosity of plasma and serum, a slight elevation of fibrinogen and a slight decrease in whole blood filterability was demonstrated. Due to a reduction in hematocrit, native blood viscosity was normal (Tab. 11.1]. None of these patients had symptoms which might suggest a "Hyperviscosity Syndrome". A recent study [72] in the same disease carried out in Munich, confirms these findings. It also shows that hematocrit-standardized blood viscosity and red cell aggregation were significantly above normal. When measuring repeatedly some patients, there was an association between extent of hemorheological abnormality and acuteness of subjective symptoms which was most evident with red cell aggregation (Fig. 11.2). Interestingly, in this study the differences were more pronounced in women than in men. Others also find impaired red cell filterability (washed cells) and aggregation; the aggregation seems to correlate closest with the clinical state [73]. This relationship was even

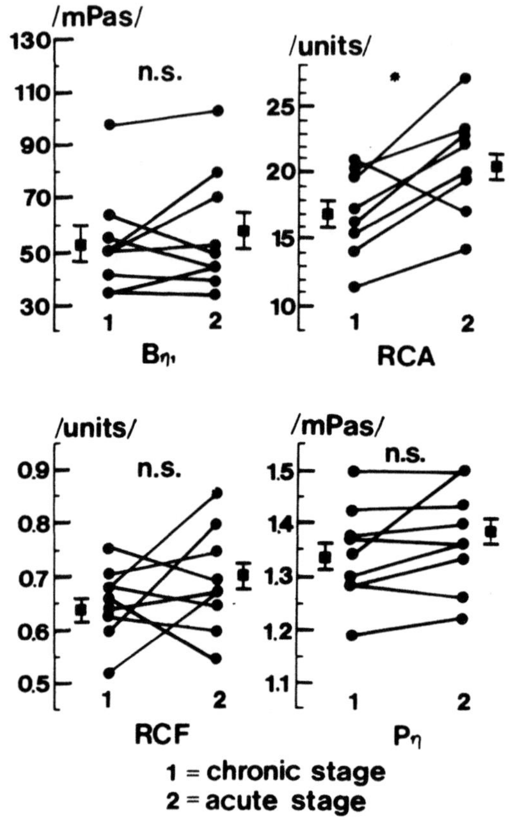

Figure 11.2. Longitudinal study on 8 patients suffering from rheumatoid arthritis. Only red cell aggregation (RCA) changes in parallel with acuity of disease, whole blood viscosity ($B\eta_1$), red cell filterability (RCF) and plasma viscosity reveal only minor changes which do not reach significance ($p > 0.05$).

more significant when low measuring temperatures were employed. Yet another study stresses the pathologically altered red cell filterability in rheumatoid arthritis [74]. Patients suffering from ankylosing spondylitis were recently shown to exhibit a deficit of all determinants of blood fluidity: elevations in blood plasma and serum viscosities, red cell aggregation and filterability, and hematocrit [75].

Clinical symptoms of hypoperfusion due to rheological abnormalities depend critically on the co-existance of abnormalities in the flow conditions of blood. Hence it is not surprising that most rheumatic patients do not present clinical symptoms of hyperviscosity. Nevertheless the rheological deficit could have some pathological relevance. It might contribute to local hypoperfusion in the micro-vascular bed of the diseased tissues where flow conditions might be altered unfavourably [76]. If this were true, the transport of pharmacological substances to their place of action and the washout of metabolite waste products and pain mediators might be hindered. Clearly this hypothesis needs further experimental testing.

11.5. Renal disease

11.5.1. Nephrotic syndrome

On the one hand there is evidence that red cell deformability is reduced in renal diseases [77]; on the other, it has been suggested that the impaired deformability of red cells, for instance in malaria [78] or sickle cell disease [79] may lead to renal insufficiency or occlusion of the vasa recta. Renal failure is associated with abnormalities in a number of blood viscosity factors; a varying degree of dehydration may lead to increased red cell aggregation and blood hyperviscosity. Thus it seems possible that rheological deficits may be both a cause and a consequence of renal diseases.

Red cell filterability (washed erythrocytes) has been reported to be reduced in renal insufficiency and the extent of this abnormality correlates with the levels of urea, nitrogen, and creatinin levels [80]. Animal experiments show that blood and plasma viscosity rise when renal failure is acutely induced by glycerol [81]. These findings could be related to the known hematological abnormalities like mild hemolytic anemia with decreased red cell life span [82].

This data seems to suggest that the rheological properties of the red cell are altered as a result of a breakdown in the fluid, electrolyte, and acid-base balance. Red cell filterability worsens both in acidosis and alkalosis, as well as in hypo- and hyperosmolarity [83]. These changes, along with retention of nitrogen and uremic toxins (the so-called middle molecular weight toxins), not only affect circulating red cells altering the properties of leukocytes and platelets, but also change the colloid oncotic pressure of plasma. This may contribute to a rise in blood viscosity even though hematocrit values are usually low. It has been suggested recently that nephrotic syndromes due to a number of different pathologies are associated with abnormal whole blood filtration and blood viscosity [84], and elevated red cell aggregation [85]. Blood filtration and viscosity results correlated with the incidence and severity of the evolution of nephrotic syndromes. It is postulated that the hemorheological abnormalities lead to the progression of the disease and contribute to concomitant thrombotic events, which could be prevented by hemorheological therapy. Others [86] have speculated that minimal change nephrosis is partly the result of impaired glomerular blood flow due to mildly elevated blood viscosity; intraglomerular pressure would rise leading to albumin extrusion into Bowman's space. Hence hemorheological therapy was proposed as an alternative to steroid treatment in minimal change nephrosis [86].

There is a high incidence of hyperlipidemia in nephrotic syndrome [87]. It has been suggested on the basis of in vitro experiments that high plasma viscosity is the stimulus to enhanced lipogenesis in this disease [88]. However, no correlations between plasma viscosity and plasma cholesterol, total triglyceride, and VLDL triglyceride were found in patients [89], making this hypothesis unlikely. Another study confirms the elevation of the plasma viscosity in nephrotic syndrome, due to an increase of plasmatic macroproteins [90].

11.5.2. Dialysis

There is considerable controversy regarding the effects of dialysis on the rheological behavior of the blood. A significant reduction in erythrocyte sedimentation rate after dialysis has been reported and there is evidence that whole blood filterability decreases after both hemodialysis and peritoneal dialysis [91,92]. In uremic patients under intermittent hemodialysis, a relationship between decreased red cell filterability and premature elimination from the circulation could be demonstrated [93]. Others, however, attribute red cell rigidification under such conditions not to dialysis but to the presence of uremia [94]. These findings require confirmation. As dialysis causes marked changes in blood volume and compromises the colloid oncotic, electrolyte, and acid-base balance of plasma and blood cells, the hemorheological consequences may be complex and variable. When studying 36 individuals with compensated chronic renal failure not treated whith dialysis, an increase in plasma viscosity as well as fibrinogen, and a decrease in whole blood filterability can be found (Table 11.1). Native venous blood viscosity is not significantly altered as hematocrit levels are subnormal.

The data suggests that renal failure may cause rheological deficits. On the other hand, there is evidence that hyperviscosity may affect renal function. Blood flow in the kidney varies in different regions. Hydrostatic pressure is high in glomerular and low in peritubular capillaries. The blood in the efferent arteriole, having lost 20% of its plasma volume, will flow out of the Bowman's capsule with a greatly elevated hematocrit and is submitted to shear stresses which are probably the lowest of the whole arterial system. Therefore rheological changes may affect blood flow in the kidney in a very significant way. Animal experiments show red cell accumulation in ischemic acute renal failure, which might have an important role in medullary ischemia seen under such conditions [95]. Any further impairment of blood fluidity will decrease kidney function. Hence renal dysfunction is a frequent consequence of the classical "Hyperviscosity Syndromes", polycythemia and paraproteinemia. Specific glomerular lesions are present in polycythemia vera and secondary polycythemias in congenital cardiomyopathies. The renal lesions in serum hyperviscosity syndromes are complex and chiefly attributable to deposits of immunocomplexes and paraproteins or their fragments at the level of the basal membrane. Reduction in

Table 11.1.

	Controls (n = 140)	Rheumatoid arthritis (n = 21)			Renal failure (n = 36)			Neoplastic disease (n = 47)		
	Mean ± S.D.	Mean ± S.D.	"t"	p	Mean ± S.D.	"t"	p	Mean ± S.D.	"t"	p
Blood viscosity 150 s-1	4.68 ± 0.66	4.40 ± 0.55	1.22	n.s.	4.42 ± 1.15	1.70	n.s.	4.22 ± 1.31	1.24	n.s.
Plasma viscosity 150 s-1	1.69 ± 0.13	1.75 ± 0.18	2.40	*	1.84 ± 0.31	4.27	***	1.85 ± 0.19	5.78	***
Serum viscosity 150 s-1	1.50 ± 0.12	1.56 ± 0.16	2.20	*	1.55 ± 0.22	1.72	n.s.	1.56 ± 0.14	2.74	**
Haematocrit %	42.4 ± 4.81	38.5 ± 4.50	2.20	*	36.5 ± 7.28	5.92	***	31.2 ± 7.53	5.04	***
Fibrinogen mg%	284 ± 103	339 ± 96	2.60	*	389 ± 131	4.93	***	342 ± 90	2.60	*
Whole blood filterability	0.449 ± 0.443	0.345 ± 0.06	9.40	**	0.343 ± 0.056	18.04	***	0.341 ± 0.06	16.4	***

Rheological parameters in rheumatoid arthritis, renal failure, neoplastic disease, in comparison with a control group.
Statistical analysis was performed using Student's "t"-test.
Mean ± S.D.; * $p < 0.05$; ** $p < 0.01$; *** $p < 0.001$; n.s.: not significant.
Methods: Viscosity: Wells-Brookfield cone plate viscometer, shear rate (blood, plasma and serum) 150 s^{-1}.
Hematocrit: Wintrobe method.
Fibrinogen: M Partigen Radial Immunodiffusion Behringwerke.
Whole blood filterability (V_{BC}) by Reid and Dormandy's method (Reid et al. 1976) modified for temperature of 37 °C (Forconi et al. 1983).

the glomerular filtration rate is also a result of hypoperfusion due to elevated blood viscosity. In sickle cell disease and sickle cell trait, renal tissue injury is primarily caused by recurring disturbance of the renal circulation, principally in the medulla due to pathological red cell rigidity [96].

As outlined in Chapter 6, hypertension is associated with abnormalities in viscosity factors. The renal involvement in this is largely speculative at present. However, it has been shown in animal experiments that increasing blood viscosity due to a rising hematocrit results in afferent arteriolar vasodilatation, which in turn stimulates renin release [97]. Hence an indirect role of blood fluidity in hypertension is conceivable, via the renin-angiotensin axis.

11.6. Neoplastic disease

Hemorheological deficits have repeatedly been reported in neoplastic diseases. It is well known that the incidence of thrombophlebitis, especially recurrent thrombophlebitis or thrombophlebitis migrans, is high in malignant diseases. This fact directed investigations towards studies of coagulation and hemorheology.

Based on animal experiments it has been suggested that red cells are poorly deformable in cancer and that this deficit may prevent adequate drug delivery to tumor cells [98]. These studies also indicate that treatment could be optimized if red cell deformability was restored prior to chemotherapy. This resulted in a 70% prolongation of survival rates in leukemic experimental animals.

Dintenfass [63] speculated that the formation, localization, and multiplication of cancer metastases may be influenced by rheological factors. This theory is based on the notion that blood flow is impaired in patients with cancer as a result of elevated plasma viscosity and red cell aggregability predominantly due to elevations in fibrinogen levels. This might cause a displacement of blood borne cancer cells from the axial flow towards the vessel wall, as is more thoroughly described in the case of white cells (see chapter 4). Consequently the probability of cancer cell trapping might increase. This theory is apparently supported by experiments showing that high molecular weight dextran enhances metastasis formation primarily due to increasing aggregation of circulating blood cells [99]. Platelet hyperaggregability, hyperfibrinogenemia, and a general tendency towards hypercoagulability could aggravate this process.

Dintenfass [100] has devoted particular attention to hemorheological abnormalities in malignant melanoma and has demonstrated a higher viscosity in patients with metastasis than in those without. Furthermore he could demonstrate that the extent of the abnormality correlates with the prognosis [101]. Of course, this could simply mean that the sicker the patient, the more pronounced his hemorheological abnormality. This, in fact, is supported by a clinical study on patients with lung cancer, showing that individuals with one or two organ system involvement had normal, those with 3 or more organ system involvement had pathological, red cell filterability [102]. Others have shown hemorheological changes in different neoplastic diseases [103]. It has been suggested that anemia in cancer is partly due to decreased red cell deformability and that normal or even better than normal filterability can be achieved by medication of prostaglandin synthesis inhibitor [104]. Similar data emerged from a study made on 47 subjects with various malignancies. This population exhibited a rise in plasma and serum viscosity, an impairment of whole blood filterability, and a decrease in hematocrit and native blood viscosity (Table 11.1). Recently 25 patients with various forms of lung cancer were compared to controls. Fibrinogen and red cell aggregation were evaluated. Both parameters were significantly increased in patients [105].

Notwithstanding these findings, the hypothesis that hemorheological factors may facilitate metastasis needs confirmation. At present it seems more likely that hemorheological abnormalities are a consequence rather than a cause of the metastatic process. Fascinating information emerges from the studies of the rheology of the malignant tissue cell itself [106]. This, however, is bio-, rather than hemorheology and exceeds the scope of this review.

11.7. Miscellaneous

Hemorheological abnormalities have been observed in a number of further diseases: Scleroderma [107], Multiple sclerosis [108], systemic lupus erythematosus [109], systemic sclerosis [110], Behcet's disease [111], parodontopathic disorders [112], and alcoholic liver disease [113]. In hyperthyroidism, blood and plasma viscosities are lower [114], in hypothyroidism higher [115] than normal, which can be normalized by adequate treatment. Micro- or macrovascular involvement, local or sytemic, is common in all these diseases, and it can be speculated that hemorheology has a part - most certainly secondary - in this. However, the pathophysiological relevance of altered hemorheology in these diseases can only be evaluated when further basic research has been carried out.

11.8. Summary and conclusion

Primary blood hyperviscosity syndromes are well defined alterations of blood fluidity, causing a decrease in blood flow, particularly at the microcirculatory level. Even in the absence of vascular abnormalities they can result in hypoperfusion of tissues leading to specific symptoms. In secondary blood hyperviscosity Syndromes, that is in ischemic vascular diseases, hyperviscosity is, at least in part, a consequence or a marker of ischemia. Here hyperviscosity can initiate or maintain vicious circles resulting in an inevitable increase of ischemia. The diseases listed in this chapter are also characterized by hemorheological deficits.

These are, however, not usually involved in the development of characteristic symptoms. Hence they are probably of less pathophysiological relevance. Nevertheless these secondary changes could interfere in the disease processes in ways which are only little understood at present. Important exceptions may be the various shock syndromes where hemorheological factors could well play a key role in the evolution, perpetuation, and irreversibility of microcirculatory failure.

11.9. References

1. Gross S.G. 1872: System of Surgery: Pathological Diagnostic, Therapeutic and Operative. Lea and Febinger, Philadelphia.
2. Berman H.J., Fulton G.P. 1961: Platelets in the peripheral circulation. In: Henry Ford Hospital International Symposium, Blood Platelets. S.A. Johnson, Little, Brown, Boston.
3. Block E.H. 1956: Microscopic observations of the circulating blood in the bulbar conjuctive in man in health and disease. Ergeb. Anat. Entwicklungsgesch. 35, 1.
4. Kinsely M.H., Eliot T.S., Block E.H. 1945: Sludged blood in traumatic shock. I. Microscopic observations of the precipitation and agglutination of blood flowing through vessels in crushed tissues. Arch. Surg. 51, 220.
5. Mela L., Bacalzo L.V., Miller L.D. 1971: Defective oxidative metabolism of rat liver mitochondria in hemorrhagic and endotoxin shock. Am. J. Physiol. 220, 571-577.
6. Wilson J.W. 1972: Leucocyte segmentation and morphologic augmentation in the pulmonary network following hemorrhagic shock and related to forms of stress. Adv. Microcirc. 4, 197.
7. Zweifach B.W. 1973: Microvascular aspects of tissue injury. In: The Inflammatory process. Zweifach B.W., Graut L., McCluskey R.T. (eds). Vol. II, pp. 3-46, Academic Press, New York.
8. Pfafferott C., Volger E., Meiselman H.J. 1985: High local norepinephrine concentrations: a possible cause for impaired red blood cell microrheologic behaviour in myocardial infarction. Proc. 4th Europ. Conf. Clin. Hemorheol. Siena.
9. Gelin L.E. 1970: Reaction of the body as a whole to injury. J. Trauma 10, 932-939.
10. Gelin L.E. 1956: Studies in anemia of injury. Acta Chir. Scand. Suppl. 210.
11. Bergentz S., Gelin L., Rudenstam G., Zederfeld B. 1965: The viscosity of whole blood in trauma. Acta Chir. Scand. 126, 289-293.
12. Bagge U., Amundson B., Lauritzen C. 1980: White blood cell deformability and plugging of skeletal muscle capillaries in hemorrhagic shock. Acta Physiol. Scand. 108, 159-163.
13. Yao S.T., Shoemaker W.C. 1966: Plasma and whole blood viscosity changes in shock and after dextran infusions. Ann. Surg. 164, 973-984.
14. Dawidson I., Gelin L.E., Haglind E. 1980: Blood viscosity and red cell aggregation changes after hemodilution in vivo and in vitro: A comparison between different plasma substitutes. Biorheology 17, 9-16.
15. Long D.M., Rosen A.L., Malone L.V.W., Meier M.A. 1972: Blood rheology in trauma patients. Surg. Clin. N. Am. 52, 19-30.
16. Chien S. 1969: Blood rheology and its relation to flow resistance and transcapillary exchange with special reference to shock. Adv. Microcirc. 2, 89-103.
17. Moore F.D. 1965: The effects of hemorrhage on body composition. N. Engl. J. Med. 273, 567.
18. Jakschik B.A., Kourik J.L., Needleman 1974: Prostaglandin metabolism and release by the lung during hemorrhage. Pharmacologist 16, 197.
19. Nickerson M. 1970: Vascular adjustments during the development of shock. Can. Med. Ass. J. 103, 853-859.
20. Lofstrom B. 1966: Changes in the flow properties of blood related to nutritive blood flow. Acta Anaesth. Scand. (suppl) 25, 305.

21. Dintenfass L. 1968: Blood viscosity, internal fluidity of the red cell, dynamic coagulation and the critical capillary radius as factors in the physiology and pathology of circulation and microcirculation. Med. J. Anst. 1, 688.
22. Goldstone J., Schmid-Schoenbein H., Wells R.E. 1970: The rheology of red blood cell aggregates. Microvasc. Res. 2, 273-286.
23. Zweifach B.W. 1958: Microcirculatory derangements as a basis for the lethal manifestation of experimental shock. Brit. J. Anaesth. 30, 446.
24. Ehrly A.M. 1971: Rheologische Probleme beim Schock. Med. Welt 22, 1167-1168.
25. Baeckström P., Folkow B., Kovach A.G.B., Loefving Olberg B. 1971: In: Proc. 6th Conf. Microcirculation. J. Ditzel, D.H. Lewis: pp. 16-22, Karger, Basel.
26. Braasch D. 1971: Red cell deformability and capillary blood flow. Physiol. Rev. 51, 679-701.
27. Gelin L.E., Dawidson I. 1982: Plasma expanders and hemodilution in the treatment of hypovolemic shock. In: Pathophysiology of Shock, Anoxia and Ischemia. R.A. Cowley, B.F. Trum (eds). Williams and Wilkins, Baltimore.
28. Dawidson I. 1980: Hemodilution, oxygen consumption and recovery from shock: An experimental study on the relative effectiveness of various fluid infusions. Ph.D. Dissertation. University of Gothenborg, Sweden.
29. Braasch D., Gossling G. 1966: Erythrozytendeformierung und Quellung durch Plasmafaktoren nach schweren Verbrennungen. Pflüg. Arch. 289, 1.
30. Eriksson E., Plym-Forshell, Robson M.C. 1981: Distant microcirculatory changes after a major burn: effects of methyl prednisolone, Dextran 40, heparin and normal saline. Burns 7, 158.
31. Ernst E. 1982: Microcirculatory changes after burns (letter). Burns 8, 150.
32. Berry L.J. 1977: Bacterial toxins. C.R.C. Crit. Rev. Toxicol. 5, 239-318.
33. Morrison D.C., Ulevitch R.J. 1978: The effects of bacterial endotoxins on host mediation systems. Am. J. Pathol. 93, 526-617.
34. Chien S. 1965: Hematocrit changes in endotoxic shock. Proc. Soc. Exp. Biol. Med. 127, 982.
35. Hardaway R.M. 1951: Disseminated intravascular syndromes. Arch. Surg. 83, 842.
36. Graeff H., Ernst E., Bocaz J., von Hugo R., Hafter R. 1976: Evaluation of hypercoagulability in septic abortion. Hemostasis 5, 285-294.
37. Sueiski K., Nanno S., Tanaka K. 1981: Permeability enhancing and chemotactic activities of lower molecular weight degradation products of human fibrinogen. Thromb Hemost. 45, 90.
38. Dintenfass L. 1985: Blood viscosity. MTP Press, Lancester, pp. 246-256.
39. Poraicu D., Stefanesen G.K. 1985: Rigid blood cells related to shock. Proc 4th Europ. Conf. Clin. Hemorheol. Siena.
40. Bergentz S.E., Carlstein A., Gelin L.E., Kreps J. 1969: Hidden acidosis in experimental shock. Ann. Surg. 169, 227-230.
41. Aronson H.B., Magora F., London M. 1970: The influence of Droperidol on blood viscosity in man. Brit. J. Anaesth. 42, 1089-1092.
42. Aronson H.B., Sharon R. 1981: Blood viscosity in the fasting surgical patient. Clin. Hemorheol. 3, 251-255.
43. Harvey-Kemble J.V., Hickman J.A. 1972: Postoperative changes in blood viscosity and the influence of hematocrit and fibrinogen. Brit. J. Surg. 59, 629.
44. Scholz P.M., Kinney J.M., Chien S. 1975: The effects of major abdominal operations on human blood rheology. Surgery 77, 351-359.
45. Charm S.E., Kurland G.S. 1974: Blood flow and microcirculation. Wiley and Sons, New York 243.
46. Mathews N. 1981: Surgery and post-operative thrombosis. In: Clinical Aspects of Blood Viscosity and Cell Deformability. G.D.O. Lowe, J.C. Barbenel, Forbes C.D. Springer.
47. Ernst E., Rose M. 1985: Transoperative Veränderungen der Blutfluidität. Intensivmedizin 22, 45.
48. Burke A.M., Chien S., McMurry J.G., Quest I.O. 1979: Effects of low molecular weight dextran on blood viscosity after craniotomy for intracranial aneurysma. Surgery, Gyn. Obst. 148, 9-15.

49. Scholz P.M., Karis J.H., Gunp F.E., Kinney J.M., Chien S. 1975: Correlation of blood rheology with vascular resistance in critically ill patients. J. Appl. Physiol. 39, 1008-1011.
50. Bailey M.J., Johnston C.L.W., Yates C.J.P., Somerville P.G., Dormandy J.A. 1979: Preoperative hemoglobin as predictor of outcome of diabetic amputations. Lancet 2, 168-170.
51. Bouhoutsos J., Morris T., Chavatzas D., Martin P. 1974: The influence of hemoglobin and platelet levels on the results of arterial surgery. Brit. J. Surg. 61, 984-986.
52. Parker M.C. 1984: Haemodilution in peripheral vascular surgery. Arch. Emergency Med. 1, Suppl., 31.
53. Messmer K. 1981: Stabilisation of the circulation by hemodilution in elective cardiac surgery. In: Effros R.M., Schmid-Schönbein H., Ditzel J. (eds). Microcirculation. Academic Press, p. 299-313.
54. Huston J., Whittington R.B., Cowan J.C., Harkness J. 1949: The plasma viscosity in pulmonary tubercolosis and rheumatic diseases. J. Clin. Invest. 2, 752.
55. Cowan J.C., Harkness J. 1947: Plasma viscosity in rheumatic diseases. Brit. Med. J. 2, 686.
56. Fahey J.L., Barth W.F., Solomon A. 1965: Serum hyperviscosity syndrome. JAMA 192, 464-468.
57. Jasin H.E., Lo Spalluto J., Ziff M. 1970: Rheumatoid hyperviscosity syndrome. Am. J. Med. 49, 484-493.
58. Roudaut M.F., Freyburger G., Louit F., Boisseau M.R. 1985: Proteins of inflammation and rheology. Proc. 4th Europ. Conf. Clin. Hemorheol. Siena.
59. Görög P., Kovacs J.B. 1976: Thrombosis, formation, hemostasis, adhesiveness of leucocytes and morphological abnormalities in the microcirculation of adjuvant arthritic rats. Agents and Actions 6, 607-612.
60. Görög P., Kovács J.B. 1980: Impaired red cell deformability in established adjuvant arthritic disease in rats. Agents and Actions 10, 427-430.
61. Seiffge D., Kremer E. 1983: Hemorheological long term study of adjuvant arthritic disease in rats. Clin. Hemorheol. 3, 469-480.
62. Shearn M.A., Epstein W.V., Engleman E.P. 1963: Serum viscosity in rheumatic disease and macroglobinemia. Arch. Int. med. 112, 98.
63. Dintenfass L. 1976: Rheology of blood in diagnostic and preventive medicine. Butterworths, London.
64. Pickup M.E., Dixon J.S., Hallett C., Bird H.A., Wright V. 1981: Plasma viscosity - a new appraisal ot its use as an index of disease activity in rheumatoid arthritis. Ann. Rheum. Dis. 40, 272-275.
65. Alexander G.J.M., Blake D.R., Holman R.L., Bacon P.A. 1981: Predictive value of paired plasma and serum viscosity in early rheumatic conditions. Brit. Med. J. 282, 1198.
66. Dintenfass L. 1971: Blood microrheology - viscosity factors in blood flow, ischemia and thrombosis. Butterworths, London, chapter 5.
67. Jasin H.E., Lo Spalluto J., Ziff M. 1970: Rheumatoid hyperviscosity syndrome. Am. J. Med. 49, 484-493.
68. Baylock W.M., Waller M., Normasell D.E. 1974: Sjögren's Syndrome: Hyperviscosity and intermediate complexes. Ann. Int. Med. 80, 27.
69. Pope R.M., Fletcher M.A., Mamby A., Shapiro M. 1975: Rheumatoid arthritis associated with hyperviscosity syndrome and intermediate complex formation. Arch. Int. Med. 135, 281-285.
70. Kosaka M., Solomon A. 1980: Hyperviscosity syndrome associated with an idiopathic monoclonal IgA rheumatoid factor. Am. J. Med. 69, 145-154.
71. Clinopathologic Conference 1981: Rheumatoid Arthritis with Felty's Syndrome, hyperviscosity and immunologic hyperactivity 70, 89.
72. Thies W., Schöps P., Seichert N., Ernst E. 1985: Hemorheology in rheumatoid arthritis. Proc. 4th Europ. Conf. Clin. Hemorheol., Siena.
73. Becker H.G., Simon R., Genth E., Hartl W., Teitel P. 1983: Hemorheological abnormalities in patients with rheumatoid arthritis. Clin. Hemorheol. 3, (3), 326.

74. Nashel D.J., Petrone D.L., Ulmer C.C. 1984: Diminished red blood cell deformability in rheumatoid arthritis. Clin. Hemorheol. 4, 567.
75. Ernst E., Roloff Ch., Magyarosy I., Matrai A. 1985: Hemorheological abnormalities in ankylosing spondylitis. Clin. Hemorheol. 5, 109.
76. Spector W.C., Willoughby D.A. 1968: The pharmacology of inflammation. Grune and Stratton, New York.
77. Wells R.E., Schmid-Schönbein H. 1968: Effects of red cell deformability upon capillary flow. Circ. Res. 38, 205.
78. Kibyhamuskoke J.W. 1968: Nephrotic Syndrome and chronic renal disease in the tropics. Brit. Med. J. 2, 33.
79. Akinkugbe O.O. 1967: Renal papillary necrosis in sickle cell hemoglobinopathy. Brit. Med. J. 3, 283.
80. Kikuchi Y., Koyama T., Koyama Y., Tozawa S., Arai T., Horimoro M., Kakiuchi Y. 1982: Red blood cell deformability in renal failure. Nephron 30, 8-14
81. Kurtz T.W., Slaviceck J.M., Hsu C.H. 1982: Blood viscosity in experimental acute renal failure. Nephron 30, 348-351.
82. Kokko J. 1982: Chronic renal failure. In: Cecil, Textbook of Medicine, Wyngaarden J.B., Smith L.H. (eds). Saunders, Philadelphia p. 501.
83. Mohandas N., Clark M.R., Jacobs M.S., Groner W., Shohet S.B. 1980: Ektacytometric analysis of factors regulating red cell deformability. Blood Cells 6, 329-334.
84. Canavese C., Stratta P., Colla L., Salomone M., Pernigotti L., Neirotti M. 1985: Hyperviscosity in nephrotic syndromes: progression factor in renal impairment and primary agent of glomerular lesion. Proc. 4th Europ. Conf. Clin. Hemorheol. Siena.
85. Ozanne P., Francis R.B., Meiselman H.J. 1983: Red blood cell aggregation in nephrotic syndrome. Kidney Int. 23, (3), 519-525.
86. Simpson L.O. 1981: Increased blood viscosity as the pathogenic agent in minimal change nephrosis: a new hypothesis. Med. Hypotheses 7, 1421-1429
87. Baxter J.H., Goodman H.C., Havel R.J. 1960: Serum lipid and lipoprotein alterations in nephrosis. J. Clin. Invest. 39, 455.
88. Yedgar S., Weinstein D.B., Patsch W., Schonfeld G., Casanada F.E., Steinberg D. 1982: Viscosity of culture medium as a regulator of synthesis and secretion of very low density lipoproteins by cultured hepatocytes. J. Biol. Chem. 252, 2188-2192.
89. Appel G.B., Blum C.B., Chien S., Kunis C.L., Appel A.S. 1985: The hyperlipidemia of the nephrotic syndrome. Relation to plasm albumin concentration oncotic pressure and viscosity. N. Engl. J. Med. 312, 1544.
90. Mc Ginley E., Lowe G.D.O., Boulton-Jones M., Forbes C.D., Prentice C.R.M. 1983: Blood viscosity and haemostasis in the nephrotic syndrome. Thromb. Haemost. 49, 155-157.
91. Udden M.M., O'Rear E.A., Kegel H., Mc Intire L.V., Lynch E.C. 1984: Decreased deformability of erythrocytes and increased intracellular calcium in patients with chronic renal failure. Clin. Hemorheol. 4, 473.
92. Pretolani E., Zoli I., Battistini G., Salvi P., Turci F., Docci D., Salvi G. 1983: Blood filterability in patients on regular hemodialysis. Clin. Hemorheol. 3, (3), 324.
93. Fröber R., Halbhuber K.J., Unger J., Linss W., Stein G., Speerschneider H., Stoll W., Geyer G. 1981: Untersuchungen zur Genese von Mikrocyten bei Hämodialysepatienten mit chronischer Urämie. Gegenbaurs Morphol. Jahrb. 127, 654-658.
94. Inauen W., Stäubli M., Descoeudres C., Galeazzi R.L., Straub P.W. 1982: Erythrocyte deformability in dialysed and non-dialysed uraemic patients. Eur. J. Clin. Invest. 12, 173-176
95. Karlberg L., Källskog O., Nygren K., Wolgast M. 1982: Erythrocyte and albumin distribution in the kidney following warm ichemia. A study in rats. Scand. J. Urol. Nephrol. 16, 173-177.
96. Gassock R.J. 1982: Mechanisms of renal injury. In: Cecil, Textbook of Medicine. Wyngaarden J.B., Smith L.H. (eds). Saunders, Philadelphia p. 454.

97. McDonald K.M. 1974: Effect of hematocrit and colloid induced changes in blood viscosity on renal hemodynamics and renin release in the dog. Circ. Res. 34, 112-122.
98. Cohen M.H. 1981: Cure of advanced L 1210 leukemia after correction of abnormal red blood cell deformability. Cancer Chemother. Pharmacol. 5, 175-179.
99. Invarson L. 1976: Pulmonary metastasis formation after trauma: an experimental study on the relevance of rheological disturbances of blood. Acta Chir. Scand. 142, sup: 463, 46.
100. Dintenfass L. 1978: Elevation of plasma viscosity and of aggregation of red cells in melanoma metastasis. Biorheol. 15, 99-110.
101. Dintenfass L., Milton G.W. 1973: Blood viscosity factors and prognosis in malignant melanoma. Med. J. Aust. 1, 1092-1094.
102. Cohen M.H. 1981: Influence of tumor burden on red blood cell deformability in small cell lung cancer patients. Ann. Clin. Res. 13, 387.
103. Isogai Y., Iida A., Chikatsu I., Fuhada E., Abe M. 1973: Dynamic viscoelasticity of blood during clotting in health and disease. Biorheol. 10, 411-424.
104. Merckie C.E. 1981: Anaemia in patients with solid tumors and the role of erythrocyte deformability. Brit. J. Cancer 44, 425-432.
105. Poggio M., Agosti R., Scapellato L. 1985: Plasma fibrinogen level and erythrocyte aggregation in patients with lung cancer. Proc. 4th Europ. Conf. Clin. Hemorheol. Siena.
106. Brooks D.E. 1984: The biorheology of tumor cells. Biorheology 21, 85-91.
107. Freitas J.P., Nunes J. Santos M.D. et al 1985: Hemorheology, capillary microscopy and oxygen transport in cleroderma patients. Proc. 4th Europ. Conf. Clin. Hemorheol. Siena.
108. Seaman G.V., Swank R., Tamblyn C. 1980: Plasma origin of red cell membrane changes in multiple sclerosis. Lancet 1, 938.
109. Gadenne C., Hatron P.V., Vinckier L. et al 1985: Erythrocyte filterability and connective tissue disease. Proc. 4th Europ. Conf. Clin. Hemorheol., Siena.
110. Kovacs J.B., Rustin M.H.A., Meyrick-Thomas R.H. et al 1985: The plasma or serum from patients with systemic sclerosis alters behavior of normal erythrocytes. Proc. 4th Europ. Conf. Clin. Hemorheol. Siena.
111. Souza-Ramalho P., Santos M.D., Cardoso L. et al 1985: hemorheological changes in Behčet disease. Proc. 4th Europ. Conf. Clin. Hemorheol. Siena.
112. Gaillard S., Lotter R., Stoltz J.F., Ritchie D.M. 1985: Blood viscosity and parodontopathic disorders. Clin. Hemorheol. 5, 251.
113. Driss F., Gueguen M., Delamaire D., Durand F., Darcet Ph. 1985: Abnormalities of erythrocyte deformability and membrane lipid composition in alcoholic liver diseases. Proc. Clin. Hemorheol. 5, 245.
114. Selerte S.B., Adamo S., Bozzetti A., Viola C., Ferrari E. 1985: Reduced blood and plasma viscosity in patient with severe clinical hyperthyroidism. Proc. 4th Europ. Conf. Clin. Hemorheol. Siena.
115. Larsson H., Vademarsson S., Hedner P., Odeberg H. 1985: Acta Med. Scand. 217, 67.

12
Hemorheological treatment

Edzard Ernst
Hemorheology Research Laboratory, Clinic for Physical Medicine, University of Munich, 8000 München 2, Ziemssenstr. 1, Federal Republic of Germany

12.1. Introduction

"Doctors, like other men, are creatures beguilded by fashion - so that every treatment has its day. The pattern is predictable: each treatment provokes an initial wave of enthusiasm when it is applied to every possible disease, only for this to be followed by utter rejection and despondency when it is said to be good for nothing. Eventually, we hope, it finds its level: specific for this, useful for that, to be used in such and such when all else fails" [1]. This aphorism applies perfectly well to hemorheological treatment which presently enjoys increasing popularity in several fields of medicine.

Hemorheological therapy can be defined as a medical intervention to increase the fluidity of blood, or its components, to prevent or improve ischemia. Hemorheological therapy should not be seen in isolation. Numerous physiological and pathological events can affect blood rheology; thus many therapeutic principles to be discussed in this chapter affect not solely the rheological properties of blood, but also other determinants of blood flow. A single causal relationship between rheological effect and clinical efficacy is often difficult or impossible to establish. In order to verify whether a certain modification of blood rheology ameliorates a specific clinical situation directly, several conditions should be fulfilled:

- temporal relationship between the rheological change and the clinical effect,
- dose-effect-relationship,
- predictability of the clinical result from the rheological change in a qualitative and quantitative manner,
- independence of clinical efficacy from non-rheological effects,
- explicability of the mode of action in theoretical terms.

This, of course, represents the ideal rather than reality. None of today's "rheological treatments" fulfill all of these conditions.

Blood fluidity is determined by cytocrit, plasma viscosity, and the microrheological properties of the blood cells. Modifications of any of those factors will therefore have marked effects. Such alterations can be achieved by hemodilution, apheresis, defibrinogenation, oral medications lowering plasma fibrinogen levels, or drugs to increase blood cell deformability. These forms of treatment will now be considered in detail.

12.2. Hemodilution

"In the times when antiphlogistic treatment was still in fashion and the whole field of practical medicine could be packed into a nut-shell, a fast pulse was taken as a sufficient sign of fever. Where there was fever, there was inflammation and where there was inflammation blood letting was the cure. In each disease venesection had to be done. If the patient died, the question was: Did you do blood letting and how often? If the answer was *ten times*, the criticism would be: *one should have done it an eleventh time*." (Schoenleins Klinische Vorträge 1842, cited by [2]).

Hemodilution is certainly one of mankind's oldest remedies. "Blood letting" was, and still is, used in almost all cultures of the world [2]. When humoral medicine became obsolete, blood letting disappeared from the orthodox therapeutic repertoire except for a few, rare indications. With the birth of hemorheology as a medical science, venesection was re-introduced, first as a method to treat and prevent certain forms of circulatory shock [3] and later as a way to increase perfusion in a number of organs, reported as early as 1913 [4]. Hemodilution became more widely used, during the 1960s when Dextrans became available [5].

12.2.1. Forms of hemodilution

Depending on the volume balance three principal forms can be distinguished.

Hypovolemic hemodilution is similar to venesection and only indicated when hypervolemia is a prominent feature. This may be the case in congestive heart failure, secondary hyperparathyroidism, obstructive lung disease, and polycythemia. One important beneficial effect of hemodilution is the increase of the stroke volume (see below), but this cannot be achieved in the presence of hypovolemia. Therefore therapeutic success of hypovolemic hemodilution may be jeopardized. Withdrawing relatively small amounts of blood more frequently might be a practical, effective way of achieving hypovolemic hemodilution and at the same time avoiding the potentially hazardous effects of severe hypovolemia. Using this technique, good results in terms of neurological symptoms have been obtained, for instance, in polycythemic patients [6].

Isovolemic hemodilution, a combination of venesection and infusion therapy, results in a nearly constant blood volume. Strictly speaking, however, normovolemia is an aim seldomly achieved if the infused fluid is not iso-oncotic, because the infused liquid equilibrates with the extravascular space. The hyperoncotic nature of most plasma expanders leads to volume expansion when blood is exchanged on an equal volume basis. If this is taken into account and proportionally less plasma expander is infused, the continuous excretion and metabolism of the artificial colloids will lead to hypovolemia at a later stage.

In *hypervolemic hemodilution* the effects outlined above are supplemented by blood volume expansion. Taking into account the distensibility of the vascular tree, Guyton has derived a formula quantitatively describing the control of venous return [13].

$$Q = \frac{MCFP - RAP}{VR + (AR/26)} \tag{1}$$

where VR is venous resistance and AR is arterial resistance. According to this equation the cardiac output (Q), which in a steady state equals the venous return, is proportional to the difference between the mean circulatory filling pressure ($MCFP$) and mean right arterial pressure (RAP). Thus the extra filling in hypervolemic hemodilution, by raising $MCFP$, leads to a more pronounced increase in cardiac output than in normovolemic dilution. Because the venous resistance (VR) has an effect 26 times greater than the arterial resistance (AR), the formula suggests that rheological flow improvements should aim at decreasing blood fluidity at shear stresses acting in the venous rather than in the arterial side. Because of the possible side effects of hypervolemia, this form of hemodilution is potentially more hazardous than the isovolemic hemodilution. The danger is greatest when the oncotic pressure of the plasma substitute employed is high or when the patient's excretion or metabolism of the colloids is impaired (as in renal insufficiency). On the other hand, some patients may be dehydrated, in which case a slight hypervolemic effect might be advantageous (hyperoncotic fluids, however, would further decrease extracellular volume).

12.2.2. Mode of action

The consequences of isovolemic hemodilution are complex [7]. Enhanced blood fluidity leads to a rise in venous return [8], which causes an increase in stroke volume through a rise in filling pressure [9]. Heart rate and mean arterial pressure remain essentially constant, oxygen consumption of the heart increases marginally, due to the extra-myocardial work load [10]. The heart is possibly the only organ to which (isovolemic) hemodilution may not be beneficial in terms of oxygen transport rate. Oxygen consumption increases due to higher work de-

Table 12.1.

Isovolemic hemodilution

a. Schematic outline of chain of effects leading to increased perfusion.

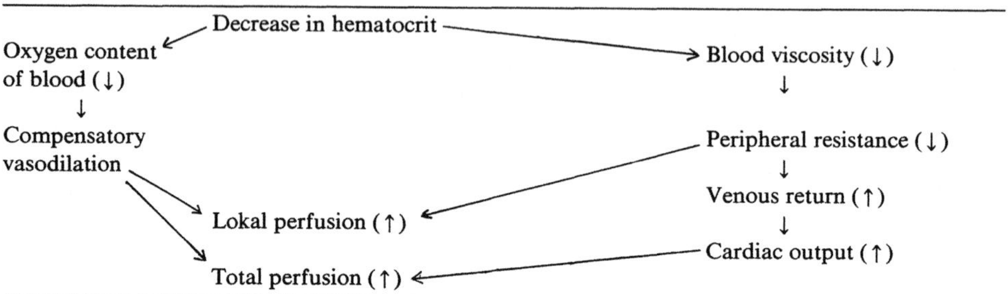

b. Schematic outline of opposing effects on oxygen availability.

Hematocrit (↓)	O_2 content of blood (↓)	→ decrease	of O_2 availability
	Oxygen extraction of tissue (↑)	→ increase	
	Right shift of O_2 dissociation curve	→ increase	
	Perfusion (↑)	→ increase	
		net increase (within certain limits of hematocrit)	

mands and coronary reserve may be limited. This could unfavourably influence the balance between oxygen demand and supply. Blood flow to most other organs, however, is definitely improved following hemodilution with dextran [11] (Table 12.1a). In terms of oxygen availability there are opposing effects resulting in an overall increase in most cases (Table 12.1b).

Theoretically, oxygen transport should reach a peak at a certain red cell concentration. This "optimal hematocrit" has been (and still is) the subject of extensive discussion. It depends on a variety of factors as described in Chapter 5. There have been conflicting results in the literature concerning the optimal hematocrit. Most discrepancies may be explained on grounds of experimental differences. The optimal value will depend on whether it has been calculated, obtained on the basis of in vitro experiments or measured in a particular vascular bed. Most workers agree that the optimal hematocrit in low flow states is below the physiological [12].

An additional effect of hemodilution, independent of oxygen availability, is the increased wash-out of metabolites from the peripheral tissues. This is, of course, a result of enhanced perfusion (especially when hypervolemic hemodilution is used) and may be an important contribution to the therapeutic success. In hypoperfused tissues this phenomenon might lead to a reduction of ischemic pain.

12.2.3. Clinical evidence

Cerebral ischemia

As outlined in Chapter 8, all forms of polycythemia are associated with a high incidence of vascular complications which are related to blood hyperviscosity. Cerebral blood flow (CBF) is low when hematocrit is high and vice versa. It is presently accepted by the majority of workers that the oxygen content of blood and the blood viscosity are independent variables in the control of CBF (details see Chapter 6]. Possibly viscosity exerts a stronger influence. Hemodilution therefore seems a promising approach to increase CBF.

Looking back on 13 years of experience in hemodilution as a routine measure after stroke, Gottstein [14] summarized his results as follows. For the patients over 70 years of age there was a 19% fall in mortality after the introduction of hypervolemic hemodilution and a drop of 27% when continuous isovolemic hemodilution was used during the first ten days or longer. In the younger patients, total mortality declined by 10% and in the older patients by 33%. The number of patients who were asymptomatic on discharge rose by 16.5%. Such strong evidence is impressive, but since "nothing ameliorates the quality of an innovation more than the lack of controls" [15], controlled, preferably double blind, randomized, placebo controlled trials are of special interest (and will be attributed particular attention throughout this Chapter).

In an early report of a randomized controlled single blind study on 100 patients with thromboembolic stroke low molecular weight dextran (LMWD) was tested against an equal volume of saline infusions for 3 days after the acute event [16]. After 10 days mortality decreased by 10.5% in the treatment group. These results are in keeping with an animal study showing that hemodilution can minimize the size of the necrosis after experimental occlusion of the middle cerebral artery [17]. In one single blind prospective study, clinically homogeneous groups of patients were randomized to be treated during 3 days either with glucose or LMWD infusions [18]. In patients suffering from complete hemiplegia treated with LMWD, the mortalities at 3 weeks and 6 months were lower by 35% and 18% respectively. With incomplete hemiplegia these values were 7% and 6% respectively (not significant). Considering that most authors would favour longer treatment periods, these results are strikingly good, indicating beneficial short term effects especially in severely affected patients. Another prospective randomized trial using a combination of LMWD and venesection ($n = 52$) versus non treatment ($n = 50$) yielded similar results [19]. Hematocrit was lowered from 0.43 to 0.37 resulting in a 40% decline of blood viscosity at a shear rate of 23 s^{-1}. Short term clinical improvement (neurological scoring) was seen 20% more frequently, and lack of improvement was 15% less in the LMWD group ($p < 0.05$). 3 months' mortality was 3% lower in these patients (not significant). Long term clinical follow-up was significantly more favourable in the treated group. Subsequently a multicenter trial with a similar design was initiated. Surprisingly the results were negative (Asplund, personal communications). Finally in a prospective randomized trial with 40 patients suffering from acute hemiplegia due to internal carotid or middle cerebral obstructions [20] cerebral blood flow (xenon technique) and the clinical course were assessed. Again LMWD was tested against glucose infusions, this time daily for 2 weeks. CBF and the neurological score rose in parallel in the LMWD patients, while it changed only insignificantly in the glucose group. These results provide evidence for hemodilution being of great value in the treatment of acute stroke. This is now accepted in many centers and hemodilution is gradually becoming a routine treatment following stroke [21,22,23].

It has been shown that venesection enhances alertness in patients with high hematocrits [24]. It has also been demonstrated that blood fluidity is abnormal in the rehabilitation period after stroke [25]. So far there is no conclusive evidence whether hemodilution also ameliorates symptoms of such patients or whether it is helpful in other clinical situations associated with cerebral hypoperfusion like transient ischemic attacks. Furthermore, possible long term effects of regular hemodilution (e.g. depletion of iron and a number of other blood constituents, microcytosis and its rheological consequence, etc.) have not been studied extensively.

Peripheral ischemia

Based on a concept similar to the one outlined above, hemodilution has been advocated as a conservative treatment in all symptomatic stages of peripheral vascular disease. The majority of workers reports an increase in peak and resting blood flow of the calf muscle and the forefoot after hemodilution, leading to symptomatic improvements (see Chapter 6). Results of open studies seem promising, taking into account that there is frequently a negative selection of patients who did not respond to other remedies. Our own group recently demonstrated clinical benefits of isovolemic hemodilution in patients suffering from claudication in a randomized, placebo controlled, double blind, cross-over trial [26]. Patients were treated with hemodilution following a period of "sham" dilutions or vice versa. During the treatment period a significant improvement of walking distance, as compared to the "sham" period, was noted. The final results of this trial suggest that patients presenting a hemodynamic situation in which the shear stress can be calculated to be low will benefit from hemodilution while those with high shear stress will not increase their walking distance (unpublished data). With hemodilution, double blind controlled trials are especially difficult to carry out, but judgement of hemodilution in peripheral vascular disease will be only possible on the basis of such studies.

Myocardial ischemia

Based on observations describing a worsening of blood viscosity parameters after myocardial infarcts (see Chapter 6), it was suggested by uncontrolled open studies that hemodilution might be of benefit in this disease [27,28]. This concept is apparently supported by animal studies showing an increase in coronary perfusion [29] and a reduction in the size of necrosis following coronary ligation [30] after the hematocrit was artificially lowered.

Single [31-33] as well as double blind studies, however, indicate no clinical efficacy of hemodilution in acute myocardial infarcts. The only randomized trial showing clinical improvement is the one by Langsjoen from 1968 [34], where the mortality of the hemodiluted patients is 13% as opposed to 32% in the controls ($p < 0.05$). In contrast, three published double blind studies [35-37] reveal higher mortality in the treated groups (by 15%, 26% and 25%, respectively). This suggests that hypervolemic hemodilution with LMWD in daily doses ranging from 500 to 1500 ml during the acute stage of infarction cannot be recommended. Whether hemodilution therapy is ineffective, contraindicated, or whether dilution with adequate volume adjustment (hypervolemic in hypohydrated, hypovolemic in hypervolemic patients) would lead to better results, cannot be answered at present.

Some of the above findings might be explainable in terms of the mechanisms operational in hemodilution. The oxygen demand of the myocardium increases as the stroke volume rises. This may well outweigh the beneficial effect of increased perfusion and oxygen delivery through narrowed coronaries. Blood volume expansion might put an additional strain on to the heart. In the presence of restricted coronary reserve (as in myocardial ischemia) this could have detrimental effects on myocardial function. Hence most workers express their caution when discussing hemodilution in ischemic heart disease [38]. Likewise there is uncertainty as whether to employ hemodilution for other indications when there are signs of concomitant heart disease. There again, the principal danger would be to unfavourably disturb the balance of myocardial oxygen supply and demand. In order to answer these questions further studies, monitoring central venous pressure, would be of interest.

Polycythemia

High hematocrit, hyperviscosity, low cardiac output, as well as decreased tissue perfusion and oxygen supply, together with high risk of thromboembolic events are the common features of polycythemia. As outlined in Chapter 8, reduction of hematocrit is followed by marked clinical improvement. The form of hemodilution used should aim at normalizing blood volume.

Surgery

Pre- and transoperative hemodilution is widely and successfully used in general and cardiac surgery. There are many advantages; banked blood can be saved and the risks of transfusion reduced [39,40]. When hypothermia must be used in cardiac surgery, dilution minimizes the otherwise inevitable viscidation of blood [41]. In addition, the thromboprophylactic effects of transoperative hemodilution in general surgery have been pointed out [42]. With correct indications, hematocrit can be lowered safely down to values of 0.23-0.27. This will lead to an increase in tissue oxygen supply and faster postoperative recovery [43]. This has recently been established in a controlled trial. Parameters like healing tendency and frequency of postoperative complications improved significantly when using preoperative hemodilution in general surgical patients [44].

Pre-eclampsia
Promising results employing hemodilution have been obtained in pre-eclampsia. The therapeutic aims are the normalisation of hypovolemia and the improvement of placental blood perfusion, with the purposes of improvement of fetal nutrition and prolongation of the threatened pregnancy. Pathophysiologic and therapeutic aspects in this disease are discussed in Chapter 9.

Shock
A common feature of shock, independent of its etiology, is hypoxia mediated by microvascular failure. In this hemorheology may play an important role [45]. The characteristic rheological feature of shock is the decline of perfusion pressure with a subsequent rise in blood viscosity and the unmasking of abnormal blood cell rheology. Thus blood rheology may indicate "vicious viscous circles" perpetuating microcirculatory failure.

In septic and anaphylactic shock and shock due to burns, there may be a substantial loss of intravascular fluid [46] and hemoconcentration. In all other forms of shock there will be a varying degree of hemodilution [47]. Hemodilution seems to be a feature of the early stages of shock due to decreased filtration forces [47]. As microcirculatory failure proceeds, local acidosis will lead to vasodilatation, with a reversal of the above phenomena and hemoconcentration [48]. Thus hemoconcentration, early in some and late in others, occurs in most forms of shock. Possibly the only exception to this rule is hemorrhagic shock, where hemodilution persists and blood rheology interfers only to a minor degree in the pathogenesis [49]. Additional rheological abnormalities differ depending on the etiology of the shock. In traumatic shock fibrinogen levels and red cell aggregation are increased [50], leading to a rise in blood viscosity [51,52]. In severe burns, increased red cell aggregation [3] and rigidity [53] have been reported. In septic shock there is a significant deterioration of plasma viscosity and red cell rheology [54] (see Chapter 11).

In view of these results, hemodilution seems to be a logical approach for the treatment of some forms of shock. Normalizing blood volume in hypovolemic shock may stabilize the threatened microcirculation [3]. There is surprisingly little data on the rheological treatment of shock, but it seems that good clinical results can be obtained by hemodilution when hemoconcentration and/or hypovolemia are present [50]. It is, however, mandatory to always consider the specific etiology of shock when initiating hemodilution for its treatment.

12.3. Apheresis

Since its introduction in 1914 [55], apheresis therapy has been used for an increasing number of diseases. Blood withdrawn from the patient is anticoagulated and separated into its constituents (plasma, red cells, leukocytes, platelets). One or more of these can be discarded while the rest will be reinfused with or without a volume substitute. This technique reached its present popularity (about 150 different diseases have been subjected to this form of treatment) through the development of highly sophisticated machines separating cells and plasma by means of centrifugation or filtration.

With increasing interest in hemorheology, plamapheresis or plasma exchange, erythrapheresis, and leukapheresis have gained some importance. The domaine of apheresis therapy lies, however, in the treatment of diseases where rheological aspects are of secondary importance (immunology, poisonings, rheumatic diseases, leukemias). Generally speaking, apheresis requires a demonstrable and removable factor in the blood which is directly related to a group of defined clinical manifestations. Whenever possible, concomitant causal therapy is mandatory.

12.3.1. Plasma exchange

Plasmatic hyperviscosity can be treated by exchanging plasma containing abnormally high amounts of proteins of a molecular weight above 150,000 daltons, such as paraproteins, fibrinogen, IgM, IgG, lipoproteins, and others, with a fluid of more favourable rheological properties. As a result, not only plasma viscosity, but all other hemorheological parameters measured ex vivo like blood viscosity, red cell aggregation and deformability, will improve. This can lead to enhanced blood flow and symptomatic improvement. However, pathological plasma proteins will rapidly be replaced by the body, making therapeutic effects temporary. The speed of replacement will depend on the nature and activity of the disease as well as the nature of the protein.

Paraproteinemias have long been treated successfully with plasma exchange [56] and there is little doubt about its clinical efficacy [57]. Paraproteinemias are frequently associated with ocular and neurological symptoms responding well to plasma exchange therapy when truly related to hyperviscosity [58,59] (Details see Chapter 8).

In familial hypercholesterolemia, a condition associated with abnormal blood rheology, cerebral blood flow could be significantly improved, even after only one exchange of 40% of total plasma volume [60]. The effect persisted 7 days after one treatment. In a mixed group of hyperlipoproteinemias with circulatory disorders, plasma exchange resulted in marked but short lasting rheological effects and subjective clinical benefits. The latter, however, could not be verified by objective methods [61].

In patients suffering from Raynaud's disease, plasma exchange was shown to improve blood rheology and to be clinically effective. This is dealt with in detail in Chapter 6. Plasma exchange may also be of clinical value in peripheral vascular disease [62,63]. However, at present the available data is scarce and more work is needed to allow even a preliminary conclusion. Some promising results have been obtained in coronary ischemia [64]. In symptomatic patients (angina) with normal arteriogram and without evidence of increased myocardial oxygen demand or reduction of oxygen availability, coronary function could be improved in parallel with blood rheology by repeated plasma exchange [64]. Again this is still at the experimental stage.

Plasma exchange is associated with a number of side effects and potential hazards such as syncope, chills, vomiting, hypovolemia, hypothermia, hypotension, hypocalcemia, anaphylaxia, hypervolemia. The incidence of such events is reported to lie between 5% and 22%. Hence it may be wise to employ it with strict indications and when other treatments have failed. There are many variables in plasma exchange, for instance the volume and frequency of exchange, plasma substitue (see below), underlying disease, the possibility of rebound phenomena, the time needed to replace a certain protein, the efficacy of removal of plasma components by the various techniques available, the unintentioned removal of plasma factors resulting in coagulation, immunological and other changes, the anticoagulant used, concomitant therapy, and placebo effects. The data available today are insufficient to adequately consider all these variables from a hemorheological point of view.

12.3.2. Erythrapheresis

Erythrapheresis is a therapeutic measure to rapidly reduce the hematocrit, minimizing the risk of hypo- or hypervolemia. The effects are similar to those of isovolemic hemodilution. Good clinical results have been obtained in sickle cell disease, when rapid exchange of rheologically abnormal sickle cells with normal erythrocytes is required [65]. Erythrapheresis is effective in terms of subjective improvement, exercise tolerance, maximal walking distance, and mental function in primary and secondary polycythemia [66,67]. Compared to hemodilution, erythrapheresis seem to have some advantages. It leads to relatively fast and pronounced hematocrit reduction, avoiding frequent venesections. The loss of plasma proteins can be reduced. It is, however, less thoroughly investigated and, of course, more expensive as well as less available.

12.3.3. Leukopheresis

Removing leukocytes can be of hemorheological relevance in leukemias. Owing to their relatively slower and limited ability to deform passively (see Chapter 3) leukocytes may represent a temporary obstacle in the microcirculation when present in excessively large numbers. There has been one report where such patients have benefited in terms of neurological signs paralleled by the reduction of the white cell count [68]. However, this approach is clearly experimental at present.

Many of the serious side effects of apheresis therapy might be avoided by more elaborate techniques. For instance, achieving the selective elimination of just one plasma protein fraction might prevent deprivation of other essential plasma factors. Cascade filtration using the removal criterium of protein size [69] and immunoadsorption with the removal criterium of protein immunogenity [70] could prove to take us a long way to make this treatment more efficient and safe. Using apheresis techniques available today for the sole purpose of improving blood rheology might be described by Francis Bacon's remark, "The remedy seems worse than the disease".

12.4. Plasma substitutes

Both apheresis and hemodilution require the use of plasma substitutes. Therefore it seems appropriate to briefly discuss the principal substances from a hemorheological point of view. Generally, the ideal solution should be pharmacologically inactive, remain intravascular for a reasonably long time, and have rheological properties which induce positive effects on blood fluidity. While crystalloid solutions do not fulfill these criteria, either homologous or heterologous colloids approximate this ideal (Table 12.2).

12.4.1. Albumin

For plasma exchange 3.5% human albumin, plasma or serum solutions are frequently recommended [71]. Their use minimizes hypoproteinemia due to large volumes of plasma exchange. It may be wise to add 2.5-5 g/l IgG in order to counterbalance the immundeficiency that can exist in patients considered for plasmapheresis [71]. The two major disadvantages are the danger of anaphylactic reactions and the possiblity of transmitting infectious diseases.

12.4.2. Dextrans

Dextrans are known to induce red cell aggregation and elevate plasma viscosity. This effect is a function of the molecular size, being more pronounced with high molecular weight dextrans. When first introduced, dextrans were thought of as "flow improvers", with specific beneficial effects on blood rheology [72]. Subse-

Table 12.2 A. Rheological and other characteristics of plasma substitutes

	Molecular configuration	Subunits	Molecular weight *	Relative * viscosity	Effect on RCA	Oncotic pressure (mmH_2O)	Volume effect	In vivo distribution	Halflife	Safety	Cost
Albumin	globular	amino-acids	65 000	1.9–2.3	–	350–400	–	intra + extravasal	19 days	–	+ +
Dextran 40	linear	mono-saccarides	40 000	5.4	+	2400	+ + +	intravasal	3–4 h	+	+
Dextran 70	linear	mono-saccarides	70 000	3.4	+ +	800	+ +	intravasal	6–8 h	+	+
HES 450	globular	mono-saccarides	450 000	4.6	+	330	+(+)	intravasal	3–4 h	+ +	+
HES 200	globular	mono-saccarides	200 000	5.1	+	800	+ +	intravasal	3–4 h	+ +	+
Gelatines	globular	amino-acids	35 000	1.8–2.1	?	390	–	intravasal	1–2 h	+ +	(+)

RCA = red cell aggregation * there may be product specific differences

Table 12.2 B. Some advantages and disadvantages of colloidal plasma substitutes

Advantages	Possible disadvantages
no infections hazard	no O_2 transport capacity
availability	protein depletion
stability	dextrans: bleeding
cost	kidney function
little effect on clotting	RCA (↑)
thromboprophylaxis (dextrans)	accumulation
independent of blood groups	side effects possible

quently it became clear, however, that improvement of blood rheology was achieved mostly by blood volume expansion and hemodilution [73]. In terms of volume expansion, dextrans seem to be superior to alternatives [74]. This is due to their strong hyperoncotic nature, depending on molecular size [75]. Dextran 40 was shown to delay plasmatic coagulation [76]. Since the introduction of its low molecular weight hapten, dextran has become much safer. Anaphylactic reactions are now extremely rare. To avoid accumulation and hyperhydration it is advisable to monitor the kidney function of patients under treatment.

12.4.3. Hydroxyethyl starch (HES)

The rheological properties of HES are somewhat controversial at present. At low concentrations it seems to enhance red cell aggregation, while higher amounts may inhibit it [74]. HES has also been shown to inhibit platelet aggregation [76]. The incidence of anaphylactic reactions after HES infusions is lower than with dextran [78]. Like with dextrans, the elimination of HES from the body can be delayed, leading to accumulation with the danger of hypervolemia [79]. Hence the need for frequent checks on the creatinine level.

12.4.4. Gelatins

Gelatin solutions show a relatively small volume effect and, furthermore, remain only for a short time in the intravascular compartment [77]. Therefore their use in hemorheology is limited.

At present there is no plasma substitute available which is without any risk. Whenever the therapeutic aim is to enhance tissue oxygenation, the new and presently still experimental concept of employing cell-free liquids capable of carrying oxygen [80,81] might let us advance towards this goal.

12.5. Defibrinogenation

In 1963 it was observed that victims bitten by the Malayan Pit Viper (Agkistrodon rhodostoma) presented symptons not dissimilar to hereditary hypofibrinogenemia [82], including a generalized bleeding tendency 30 min. after the bite. The subsequent clinical course proved to be benign, with complete recovery after about two weeks. The venoms of this and another snake (Bothrops atrox) were investigated, the enzyme responsible for splitting fibrinogen was isolated, biologically standardized, and hence called ancrod and defibrase respectively [83].

12.5.1. Mode of action

Defibrinogenating enzymes (*D.E.*) show thrombin-like activity, catalyzing the hydrolysis of an arginine-glycine link within the fibrinogen molecule and splitting off the A-chain [83]. In contrast, thrombin also liberates the B-chain allowing a stable fibrin clot to be formed (Fig. 12.1). *D.E.* lead to the formation of des-A-fibrin-monomers, which polymerize into non-crosslinked (no factor XIII activation), mechanically and biochemically unstable structures capable of forming an atypical fibrin clot. These clots are plainly visible in the test tube when performing in vitro experiments and may also develop in the microcirculation [84]. Physiologically, however, these clots are readily lysed while developing by endogenous plasminogen and eliminated by the reticuloendothelial system.

By and large fibrinogen is the only coagulation factor affected by *D.E.* [85]. There is, however, also an effect on platelet count and aggregation. Probably due to both the low fibrinogen and the raised fibrinogen degradation products, platelet aggregation is inhibited [86]. Platelet numbers decline temporarily, possibly as a result of being trapped in microclots [87]. Furthermore, there is some evidence that *D.E.* provide a stimulus for the fibrinolytic system [88]. Recently there have been reports that *D.E.* increase the tissue plasminogen activator. *D.E.* have a biological half life of 3-10 hours in man; they are metabolized in the reticuloendothelial system as well as excreted via the kidneys. Summarizing its pharmacological activity, defibrinogenation leads to blood coagulation [89] with a fall in fibrinogen and a rise in fibrinogen degradation products. Since the resulting clots are normally immediately lysed by fibrinolysis, *D.E.* act as an anticoagulant by depriving the reaction fibrinogen-fibrin of its substrate.

Lowering fibrinogen levels will limit red cell aggregation and reduce plasma

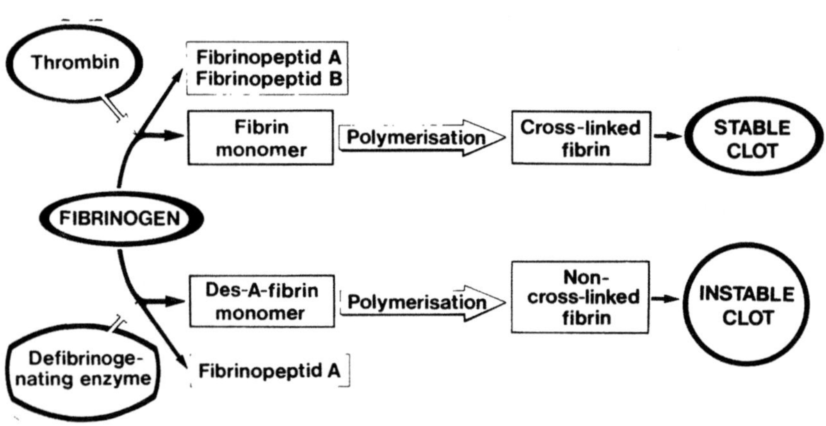

Figure 12.1. Comparison of mechanisms of action of defibrinogenating enzymes (*D.E.*) and thrombin. In contrast to thrombin, *D.E.* induce an unstable fibrin clot, which is readily lysed and destroyed mechanically in the normal circulation.

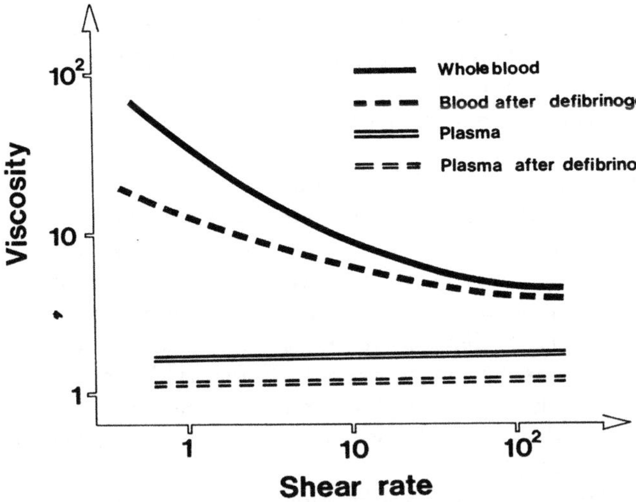

Figure 12.2. Effect of defibrinogenation on blood and plasma viscosity, plotted as a function of shear rate. Through the inhibition of red cell aggregation blood is rendered more Newtonian. Through the lowering of its fibrinogen content plasma is rendered more fluid.

and blood viscosity [90]. Therefore it renders blood a less non-Newtonian fluid. Fig. 12.2 also shows that the viscosity-lowering effect is more pronounced at low shear. Theoretically this could mean that perfusion can be enhanced mostly where the driving forces are low, as in poststenotic areas or on the venous side of the circulation. The effect of *D.E.* on red cell filterability is controversial. Looking only at results obtained in filtration systems, no effect has been reported using 8 μm pores [91] but *D.E.*-induced red cell rigidification was suggested employing 5 μm filters [92].

12.5.2. Guidelines for medication

Indications will be dealt with under section 5.3. of this chapter. In principle intravenous, intramuscular, and subcutaneous administrations of *D.E.* are possible. To prevent a sudden drop of fibrinogen with the possible risk of microthrombi, most experts advocate subcutaneous injections. A fixed treatment schedule has been suggested (1 unit/kg for the initial 4 days and 4 units/kg thereafter), but it seems more reasonable to monitor fibrinogen levels and to adjust the dosage aiming at fibrinogen levels between 0.5 and 1.0 g/l. Animal experiments suggest caution with excessively high doses, which might result in microcirculatory blockade [93].

After a variable time of 4-6 weeks, antibodies will develop against the enzyme, making the medication increasingly ineffective. Fibrinogen levels can still be kept low for some days by increasing the dosage, but eventually *D.E.* cease to have any effect. If required, the other available enzyme can be given subsequently, as there is no cross-antigeneity. The literature is contradictory as to whether antibodies persist for life or whether treatment can be re-introduced at a later stage.

The most frequent side effect is bleeding. There is some evidence that it occurs mostly when *D.E.* are given intravenously. Bleeding may be spontaneous but is more commonly precipitated by trauma. Recently significant intraoperative bleeding was reported when ancrod was given preoperatively via the subcutaneous route at dosages well short of defibrinogenation [96]. Allergic complications, pyrexia, hypotension, respiratory depression, headache, and drowsiness are all rarely recorded adverse reactions. Several workers have reported venous and arterial thromboses (including myocardial infarction) during medication of *D.E.* [94]. It is presently not clear whether this is truly related to hypofibrinogenemia or to a dissemination of microthrombi.

Contraindications are similar to those for anticoagulant therapy: coagulation abnormalities, ulcers of the digestive system, acute brain or heart infarcts, systolic blood pressure above 200 mmHg, shock, retinal bleeding (diabetic retinopathy). Relative contraindications are inadequate liver or kidney function, pregnancy, and malignant diseases. Therapy with ancrod can be interrupted acutely by an antitoxin. In cases of severe bleeding it may be advisable to additionally give human fibrinogen. The simple discontinuation of the treatment will result in spontaneous normalization of fibrinogen after a few days.

12.5.3. Clinical evidence

There are several hundred published reports dealing with this subject. The following aims at giving a brief overview summarizing the most important information. As outlined above, the principal actions of *D.E.* are enhancement of blood perfusion through blood fluidification and anticoagulation, with the possible benefit of preventing venous and perhaps arterial thrombosis. Defibrinogenation has the greatest rheological effect at low shear, and therefore it may be clinically most effective in low flow areas. This hypothesis is supported by evidence from various vascular provinces.

Peripheral ischemia

Animal studies suggest improvement of arterial flow with and without the introduction of experimental proximal stenoses [97,98]. In patients with severe peripheral vascular disease, *D.E.* were first tried with promising clinical results in the early 1970's [99,100]. Subsequently this was confirmed in open studies by many authors. Both subjective (pain free walking distance, relief of pain, healing tendency) and objective parameters (plethysmographic measurements, Doppler pressure ratio, muscle pO_2, xenon clearance from skin or muscle, subsequent amputation frequency, and reduction in analgesic medication) have been often, but not unanimously, shown to be influenced favourably during and after treatment with *D.E.* In most of these studies 50-80% of the patients with severe peripheral vascular disease benefit from the treatment. A minimum systolic ankle pressure of around 40 mmHg seems to be a precondition for therapeutic success.

Peripheral vascular diseases may be associated with an extremely variable spontaneous clinical course and are prone to pronounced placebo effects. Controlled studies are therefore of special interest, if not mandatory. In stage III peripheral vascular disease, intravenous ancrod has been compared first to subcutaneous heparin and then to the combination of oral anticoagulation plus a vasodilator. Both parts of the study were controlled but not double blind. The results were significantly in favour of *D.E.* [101]. Similarly, when stage III or IV patients were given first subcutaneous ancrod and then vasodilator, the former treatment yielded better results [102]. This controlled data may be misleading, however, as vasodilators are generally accepted to induce a negative steal effect.

Placebo-controlled, double blind trials should provide a conclusive answer. At present three such studies have been published [103,104,105], none of which could demonstrate that *D.E.* had clinical effects more beneficial than placebo. This issue becomes even more confused when one considers the criticism that can be put forward against each of these three trials (Table 12.3).

In summary, there is no conclusive evidence that defibrinogenation is of clinical value in severe leg ischemia. Considering more than 20 years of investigation, apparently well defined effects of *D.E.*, and the comprehensible theoretical background (lower viscosity and better perfusion), this fact seems surprising. On the basis of experimental findings, it has been suggested [106] that *D.E.* can lead to microthrombi and occlusion of exchange vessels when mechanical forces and fibrinolytic activity are low as in the affected tissues of peripheral vascular disease. Possibly this may be a clue to the explanation of the discrepancies.

Myocardial infarction

If *D.E.* promote blood flow, it could in principle be used to increase the oxygen supply to the heart. Only a few studies have dealt with this problem. It has repeatedly been postulated [95] that some of the therapeutic success of streptokinase in myocardial infarction might be due to its rheological effects which are similar to those of *D.E.* An investigation of *D.E.* in heart infarcts might therefore be considered relevant. So far this has not been done in humans, but animal studies show no effect in terms of infarction size or coronary perfusion [107,108,109].

Angina pectoris

Beneficial symptomatic effects have been reported in patients with typical angina, employing a double blind design with subcutaneous ancrod against

Table 12.3. Placebo-controlled trials with defibrinogenating enzymes (DE) in peripheral vascular disease (PVD).

Author	PVD stage	DE	N	Duration of treatment	Parameter	Result	Comment
Martin 1976	II	Batroxobin	10	21 days	Walking distance ankle pressure	D.E. no better than placebo	Not double-blind
Tonnesen 1978	III + IVa	Ancrod	21	21 days	Ankle pressure rest pain healing tendency	D.E. induced sign. increased in ankle pressure, but no clinical benefit	Strong placebo effect
Lowe 1981	III + IVa	Ancrod	14	8 days	Ankle pressure analgetics consumption rest pain	No clinical benefit, placebo slightly better	Treatment too short strong placebo effect

placebo [110]. Nitroglycerine consumption was reduced by 63% in the treated group and only by 39% in the placebo group. Finally 10 patients with severe unstable angina and high fibrinogen levels were treated with ancrod to reduce fibrinogen down to 1.4 g/l for 4 weeks [111]. In 7 of these patients angina disappeared instantly even before fibrinogen had fully dropped to therapeutic levels. In the remaining 3 patients nitroglycerine consumption was reduced and angina became stable. Both were long term effects which might also be due to a concomitant exercise program aimed at enhancing collateral vessel growth. These few studies, on small numbers of patients, seem promising and imply a good clinical effect of *D.E.* in angina pectoris. It seems surprising that this field has not been investigated more actively.

Prevention of venous thrombosis

Deep vein thrombosis is still one of the most frequent and dangerous complications of surgery. Various ways of minimizing the risk have been described. Heparin is used most widely, generally with good results; however, in certain situations, such as surgery on the hip joints, it is unsatisfactory [112]. There is some evidence that *D.E.* yield better results than heparin in this condition [112,113,114]. In a placebo-controlled double blind trial, subcutaneous ancrod was shown to reduce the frequency of venographically verified deep vein thrombosis following reconstructive surgery for hip fractures [113]. In a similar study following hip replacement surgery, it was demonstrated that ancrod minimized the extent of major thrombi in the femoral vein, while the incidence of deep vein thrombosis was not reduced significantly [114]. *D.E.* was safe in terms of bleeding and other postoperative complications. The underlying danger in postoperative deep vein thrombosis is, of course, a potentially lethal pulmonary embolism. The few studies available indicate that pulmonary embolism might be less frequent with *D.E.* than with placebo [112,113]. This is also supported by an animal study showing decreased severity and mortality when *D.E.* were used prior to pulmonary embolism induced experimentally [115]. Similary, there are some indications that *D.E.* are of value in the treatment of central retinal vein thrombosis [116,117]. A controlled trial would be needed for more conclusive evidence. The treatment of manifest deep vein thrombosis with *D.E.*, however, seems to be unsuccessful [118]. *D.E.* may prevent thrombosis by affecting at least two of the components of the classical triad of Virchow - blood coagulability and blood flow. There is a remarkable association between blood rheology and venous thrombosis [119], suggesting indirectly that "blood fluidication" might play a role independent of *D.E.*-induced hypocoagulability (see also Chapter 7).

Miscellaneous

If *D.E.* promote macro- and microcirculatory perfusion, they may be expected to have beneficial effects on wound healing. Indeed this could be demonstrated in two uncontrolled studies. Healing of skin flaps after leg amputations for peripheral vascular disease [120] and the other after plastic surgery [98] was suggested to be promoted. This is an intriguing new aspect where the natural time limitation of defibrinogenation would not be disadvantageous.

There are several uncontrolled reports suggesting that artificial venous [121] and arterial [120] grafts remain patent more frequently and for longer periods when patients are defibrinogenated. Again, both the enhanced blood flow and *D.E.*'s anticoagulant properties might be the mechanisms responsible. In experimental glomerulonephritis *D.E.* reduced glomerular fibrin deposits and its long term sequela [122]. Similar results were obtained in a small pilot study in man [123]. Finally, the list of human diseases experimentally treated by *D.E.* with some success comprises renal allograft failure [124], priapism [125], sickle cell crisis [126], tumor metastases [127], progressive scleroderma [128], Bürger's disease [129], systemic lupus erythematosus [130].

Scanning the available data on *D.E.* in man, one cannot help being fascinated by the possibilities of these drugs. And yet too little clinical work has so far been performed. Much is still at the experimental stage. No doubt this is partly due to the expense of the drugs and the limited duration of the therapeutic effect. Adverse effects of fibrinogen degradation products [131] have hardly been investigated. Some of the drawbacks could be overcome, if other defibrinogenating enzymes [132] were made available or a synthetic product could be developed. Fibrinolytic therapy with urokinase or streptokinase has pronounced hemorheological effects [133,134], similar to defibrinogenation, and part of its clinical success may be rheologically mediated [135].

12.6. Oral drugs

In our time "therapy" has become almost synonymous with pharmacotherapy, the vast majority of which is constituted by oral medications. This is also essentially true for hemorheological treatment. Publications on this subject are innumerable. A list of substances with possible beneficial effect on "red cell deformability" includes 47 medications [136]. The attempt for a fully comprehensive review is therefore impossible. The aim of this section is thus to depict the important drugs, to outline some of the existing problems, and to suggest possible future developments.

It is difficult to categorize oral drugs with hemorheological effects as they belong to many different pharmacological classes and may affect blood fluidity by different mechanisms. However, most drugs either affect the plasmatic macroproteins and lead to a reduction of plasma viscosity (with additional effects on red cell aggregation and blood viscosity) or they are thought to restore abnormal blood cell deformability. Frequently there is an overlap between these two categories.

12.6.1. Oral drugs decreasing plasma viscosity

Clofibrate

Several workers have shown that clofibrate not only affects serum lipids, but also reduces abnormally high fibrinogen levels [137]. Indeed it has been suggested that this effect might be of paramount clinical relevance [138]. Clofibrate reduces blood viscosity by lowering fibrinogen, possibly leading to a prolongation of pain-free walking distance in claudicants [139,140] and an increase in cerebral blood flow in hyperfibrinogenemic patients [141]. Unfortunately it has a number of potentially dangerous side effects. An extensive double-blind randomized study under the guidance of the WHO showed an excessive non-cardiovascular mortality in the clofibrate-group which was clearly related to the treatment period [142]. Hence rheological treatment with this compound requires caution. Etofibrat, a combination of clofibrate and nicotinic acid, incorporates similar pharmacological actions and is said to cause less side effects. The fibrinogen lowering [143] property and the rheological activity of this compound could be shown in hyperlipoproteinemic patients [144]. Further studies are needed before this drug can be recommended for hemorheological therapy.

Stanozolol

This anabolic steroid may induce fibrinolytic activity. Several groups have reported a drop in fibrinogen and consequently plasma viscosity [145]. The drug might therefore have some potential for hemorheological therapy. Its effect on blood viscosity is, however, neutralized by its hematocrit-raising property (anabolic action). In Raynaud's disease some clinical benefit of stanozolol may be due to its rheological effect [146]. The normal transoperative fibrinogen increase, however, could not be minimized in a double-blind trial using intramuscular stanozolol [147]. Similar effects may be attributed to ethylestrenol [148] and furazabol [149], two anabolic compounds also capable of reducing fibrinogen levels in man by its fibrinolytic activity. Possibly owing to their serious side effects, these drugs have not been examined in detail for their hemorheological potential.

Ticlopidine

Ticlopidine was developed for its strong anti-platelet action [150], but has additional effects on fibrinogen [151] and/or blood cell deformability [152]. In diabetics it normalizes plasma viscosity as well as red cell filterability [153], and in cerebral vascular disease it reduces fibrinogen levels when given orally for one year [154]. Although some of these rheological effects have been demonstrated in double-blind, placebo-controlled trials [152], their association to clinical efficacy is still unclear - even more so since white cells may play an important role [152,153] (see also section 6.2. of this Chapter).

Suloctidil
This anti-platelet, anti-thrombotic vasodilator was shown to be effective in peripheral vascular disease both experimentally [155] and clinically [156]. Blood viscosity fell at high shear when suloctidil was given orally for 5 months in a double-blind, placebo-controlled trial. Although the precise mechanism of this effect remains somewhat obscure, the results imply that it was mediated by a drop in plasma viscosity caused by a fall in fibrinogen [157].

Calcium-dobesilate
Calcium dobesilate given to diabetic patients induces changes in plasma protein pattern, leading to a reduction in plasma and blood viscosity [158]. It was also shown to normalize pathologically low red cell filterability in claudicants [159]. In a small but placebo-controlled, double-blind, cross-over trial, no significant effect on blood viscosity was seen, although normalization of red cell filterability was confirmed [160]. It was also reported that this drug lowers blood- and plasma viscosity when given to diabetic patients in a double blind, controlled trial [161].

Hydroxychloroquine
This anti-malaria, anti-rheumatic medication was shown to reduce the incidence of postoperative deep vein thrombosis [162]. A subsequent placebo-controlled, blind trial on its hemorheological properties showed no change in volunteers, but demonstrated a transoperative fall in plasma viscosity and other rheological parameters. In the placebo group there was the usual worsening of blood rheology subsequent to surgical trauma. Fibrinogen levels rose equally in both groups, but plasma viscosity showed a significant increase only in the placebo group, suggesting not a quantitative but a qualitative change in fibrinogen induced by hydroxychloroquine [163]. No doubt this preliminary study requires confirmation and evaluation of its possible clinical relevance.

12.6.2. Oral drugs to normalize red cell deformability

"When a lot of remedies are suggested for a disease, that means it can't be cured"

Anton Chekhov

Since the time of Leuvenhoek it has been known that human red cells deform when passing through the exchange vessels. A partial loss of this quality might therefore be harmful in terms of oxygen supply. Three further assumptions were subsequently based on this fundamental axiom. Firstly, it is supposed that red cell deformability can be quantified by blood filtration methods. Recent data casts doubt on this, suggesting that leukocyte rheology might have played an important interfering role in early filtration systems. Secondly, it is assumed that a reduction in red cell deformability is a causative factor in disease. Thirdly, it is postulated that red cell rigidification can be treated successfully by pharmacotherapy. The following will mainly evaluate this last hypothesis. The validity of the aforementioned assumptions will not be questioned in detail, but the reader is referred to the preceeding Chapters in this book.

In recent years there has been an increasing interest in the pharmacotherapy of red cell deformability [164]. However, the number of open questions is growing in line with new experimental data. Several possible mechanisms of improving red cell deformability have been suggested mostly on theoretical grounds - intracellular adenosin triphosphate, membrane-plasma interactions, red cell surface and charge, red cell proteins, and modification of transmembraneous electrolyte transport [165]. There is little experimental evidence for any of these possibilities. Therefore, none of the medications discussed below are associated with a precise and well described mechanism of rheological action.

It has become increasingly evident that interpretations of the early blood filtration results are far from being straight forward. While investigators assumed that results obtained by filtering either whole blood, washed or unwashed red cell suspensions in fact reflected the rheological properties of red cells, it was later shown that filter blockade by white cells had a strong influence on the result. (It is only until recently that one can distinguish between red cell transit and filter clogging in filtration systems). Even more recently it was demonstrated that drugs famed for increasing "red cell deformability" actually changed white cell rheology and had little influence on red cells, when leukocytes were carefully and completely discarded. Many studies show the clinical relevance of filtration tests. Thus its value might be considerable. The question to what extent it really quantifies red cell deformability, however, seems unanswered at present. Taking these recent developments into account, many of the reported results on "red cell deformability" probably should be referred to as "blood cell deformability" or "blood cell filterability".

Pentoxifylline

Pentoxifylline, a xanthine derivative with a wide spectrum of pharmacological actions, is the most extensively studied and publicized drug in the list of substances modifying deformability. Although it was originally designed as a vasodilator, pentoxifylline inhibits phosphodiesterase and platelet aggregation, and it enhances fibrinolytic activity, prostacyclin-synthesis and glycolysis. It decreases plasma and blood viscosity as well as red cell aggregation by lowering fibrinogen levels. Its most prominent feature is said to be the normalization of the filterability of rigidified red cells (review see [166]). This is believed to be mediated by an increase in cytoplasmatic adenosine triphosphate [167] and possibly 2,3 diphosphoglycerate levels [168] and/or by red cell membrane stabilization [168]. Its effect on red cell filterability has been shown by several groups in vitro with or without various "stress models" [169] and in vivo in different groups of patients suffering from vascular diseases [170].

Table 12.4 Pentoxifylline: double blind studies in peripheral vascular disease (PVD).

1st author	Year of publication	Reference medication	Number of patients	Stage of disease	Daily oral dose and duration	Main endpoints	Comment: in all studies Pent, was superior to Ref.
Kellner	1976	placebo	40 20 Pent. 20 Ref.	II–IV	1200 mg 7–8 weeks	walking distance rest pain	stages of disease not uniform
Schubotz	1976	placebo	50	(diabetics) I–III	800 mg 6–8 weeks	walking distance rest pain	treatment of diabetes may induce uncontrolled
Bollinger	1977	placebo	19 10 Pent. 9 Ref.	II	600 mg 8 weeks	walking distance ankle pressure	groups differed in terms of medical history
Feine-Haake	1977	3 × 2.4 mg adenosine	36 18 Pent. 18 Ref.	I–IV	1200 mg 12 weeks	"walking ability" + other subjective parameters	mostly elderly patients, all stages, methods (walking distance) not described, 5 years age difference between the groups
Tonak	1977	placebo	2 × 55 27 Pent. 28 Ref.	II–III	600 mg 4 weeks	walking distance	two groups of 55 patients were evaluted separately
Weitgasser	1977	placebo	59	III–IV	1200 mg 6–8 weeks	rest pain, photographic documentation of ulcers	main criterium was photo documentation
Völker	1978	placebo	50 25 Pent. 25 Ref.	II	1200 mg 4 weeks	walking distance	33 patients had concomitant coronary disease
Accetto	1982	nylidrin	47 23 Pent. 24 Ref.	II and III	1200 mg 8 weeks	walking distance (treadmill) + plethysmography	improvement significantly greater on Pent., difference between groups 25 m, treadmill test in stage III!
Porter	1982	placebo	128 67 Pent. 61 Ref.	II	increasing from 600 to 1200 mg 24 weeks	standardized walking distance	careful multicenter study, showing clear benefit of Pent.
Di Perri	1983	placebo	24 24 Pent. 24 Ref.	II	1200 mg 8 weeks	walking distance	unusually little placebo effect, cross over study
Strano	1984	placebo	18 18 Pent. [illegible]	II	800 mg 90 days	walking distance	cross over

An equally large number of workers have found clinical improvement in controlled trials on subjective and objective parameters in peripheral [171] (Table 12.4) as well as cerebral vascular disease [172]. Relevant long term data on rheological and clinical parameters during treatment with Pentoxifylline are still scarce, but would seem essential for the evaluation of any hemorheological drug. Recently it has been shown that the drug's rheological action may be also brought about by changing the rheological behavior of white cells [173]. This finding seems important as white cell rheology is increasingly recognized to influence the microcirculation and casts new light on results obtained by whole blood or red cell filtration. Our own group recently demonstrated in an uncontrolled study on claudicants that white cell rheology markedly improved during oral Pentoxifylline medication [174].
In view of the wealth of information on this substance, the evidence for its clinical efficacy is clearly stronger than for other vasoactive drugs with hemorheological action. There are also some data suggesting that symptomatic improvement is indeed brought about by rheological mechanisms.

Buflomedil
Buflomedil is a vasodilator which acts by inhibiting alpha-adrenergic action on vascular smooth muscle. Its ability to normalize red cell filterability was shown in vitro under "calcium-stress" and ex vivo in a double-blind, cross-over study, where acute effects after intravenous administration were examined [175]. Given orally for 20 days, it also normalizes filterability, reduces blood viscosity, increases ankle pressures, and peripheral perfusion in claudicants [176]. Similar results were obtained in a placebo-controlled trial on diabetics [177]. Furthermore, buflomedil was shown to prevent the hemorheological alterations induced by ischemic exercise in claudicants [178]. Clinically buflomedil was demonstrated by controlled trials to be superior to placebo in terms of walking distance in claudicants [179,180] and in terms of psychometric assessment in cerebrovascular patients [181,182]. In an open, multicenter trial of 300 claudicants, intravenous buflomedil was shown to increase pain-free walking distance during 3 weeks of treatment. 60% of the patients doubled their performance [183]. Possibly the effects are related to a decrease in collateral resistance, as shown in animal models [184]. Recently it was demonstrated in a randomized double-blind study using vital microscopy that buflomedil (150 mg t.d.s.) significantly ameliorated the diseased microcirculation in vascular patients with ischemic skin necroses. There was no measureable difference in the arterial macrocirculation [185]. Whether buflomedil selectively promotes vasomotion, is still uncertain at present.

Cinnarizine, flunarizine
These two calcium-channel blocking substances, antihistamines of the piperazine group, have similar pharmacological properties; the relatively more powerful difluoro derivate is assessed in greater detail. A wide variety of further actions

have been described, such as effects on the vascular endothelium, platelet function, as well as vascular and muscular tone. Hemorheological action seems to concentrate mainly on the red cell, possibly by blocking calcium ions in the membrane [186]. Its effects on red cell filterability have been shown in vitro [187] and ex vivo [188]. Cinnarizine decreased blood viscosity given orally in an open study on claudicants [189]. Long term oral Flunarizine lowered blood viscosity and normalized red cell filterability as well as peripheral hemodynamics in the same disease [190]. In volunteers, both drugs prolonged reactive hyperemia after temporary arterial occlusion [191]. These uncontrolled experimental trials are paralleled by at least two controlled and numerous uncontrolled clinical studies suggesting symptomatic improvement in peripheral and cerebral vascular diseases [191,192].

Isoxsuprine
This substance is also a peripheral vasodilator acting by alpha-adrenergic blocking and beta-adrenergic mimetic properties. In vitro [194] and in vivo [195,196] it acutely lowers blood viscosity. This was partly contradicted by a study on diabetics, where after 3 months' medication only the viscosities of a highly concentrated red cell suspension and blood at low shear, but not those of plasma or blood at high shear were decreased [197]. Clinically there is ample evidence of its efficacy in circulatory disorders, employing parameters such as arterio-venous oxygen difference, rheography, plethysmography, thermography, oscillometry, and scintigraphy. In the aforementioned double-blind trial [195], claudicants also benefited in respect of walking distance. Similar results were described in another trial on peripheral vascular disease, where additional improvements in Doppler and thermographic readings were reported [198]. Furthermore, a double-blind study showed a decrease in frequency of transient ischemic attacks in cerebrovascular disease [199].

Bencyclane
Bencyclane is a spasmolytic, vasoactive drug possibly acting on the red cell by stabilizing the membrane [200]. In various stress models in vitro and in claudicants, it decreases blood viscosity and normalizes red cell filterability [201,202,203]. These uncontrolled data are supported by controlled studies demonstrating enhanced muscular xenon clearance [204], increased muscle pO_2 [205], and favourable changes in the pyruvate/lactate quotient [206]. When bencyclane was compared double-blind to placebo, there was a significant increase in walking distance with claudicants [207,208,209] and clinical improvement in geriatric cerebrovascular patients [209].

Eicosapentaenoic acid
The well known relatively low incidence of atherosclerosis in Eskimos may be (partly) related to their high nutritional intake in eicosapentaenoic acid (EPA).

For this reason the rheological effects of this compound seemed worth investigating. Uncontrolled data suggested that EPA may reduce blood viscosity [210]. In addition it could be demonstrated that supplementation of EPA resulted in the incorporation of EPA into the phospholipids of the red cells. This was paralleled by an increase in red cell deformability, which correlated positively with erythrocyte EPA [211]. Recently it could be shown in a controlled, double-blind trial with claudicants, that oral EPA supplementation reduced blood viscosity at high shear rates and lowered plasma triglyceride levels. Plasma viscosity, hematocrit, platelet count, cholesterol, and HDL did not change during 6 weeks of 1,8 g EPA daily [212]. Unfortunately this study was too small to evaluate clinical improvement. With additional effects on platelet function, blood lipids, and prostaglandin biosynthesis as well as blood pressure and white cell function [213], EPA might have considerable potential in the treatment of vascular disease.

Miscellaneous

The number of drugs which have been claimed to have some effect on red cell deformability or other hemorheological variables seems to increase daily. For most of them the hemorheological effects need to be confirmed and/or the proof of clinical efficacy in circulatory disorders awaits assessment in controlled trials. The following is a list of some of the medications that might possibly gain importance in the near future:

Naftidrofuryl
Rutosides
Vincamine
Ginkgo biloba extract
Piracetam
Nicerogolin

12.6.3. Evaluation

In spite of the vast amount of literature on this subject, there are many unanswered questions. Although the preceeding chapters have partly dealt with them in more detail, it seems worthwile to again briefly review and evaluate some of these.

Probably the most fundamental question concerns the role of hemorheology in human pathophysiology. Can a patient "suffer" from abnormal blood rheology, and if so, under what circumstances? Presently the link between theory and experimental evidence exists only fragmentarily. The problem of ascertaining a therapeutic benefit is closely related. There is evidence that malperfusion can be normalized on the macrocirculatory level by hemorheotherapy. But does that really mean that oxygen exchange can be enhanced in the microcirculation? And if so, is an increase in microcirculatory blood flow desirable in all cases? For instance, raising perfusion to atrophic brain tissue might be a wrong approach. In other cases it might be more promising to influence the metabolic state of tissues threatened by ischemia.

Presently we do not know the exact mechanism(s) causing an abnormality in blood cell rheology. Neither do we know to what extent it is the cause or the consequence (or both) of hypoxia. From this point of view it seems premature to employ drugs to normalize this property - particularly as the drugs' precise rheological mode of actions are obscure. There is an unfortunate lack of clinical studies showing a parallel improvement in both blood rheology and symptoms on a patient-to-patient basis. (By no means is this a specific drawback for hemorheology, in contrary, it seems to be a general problem in medicine). Thus it is difficult, if not impossible, to establish an effect - effectiveness relationship. In this field there is a clear demand for more basic research.

Steal phenomena are still a controversial issue. Vasodilators were widely used in therapy of circulatory disorders until they were thought to harm rather than to benefit the diseased tissue. The vasculature in hypoxia is maximally dilated. Hence dilators only increase the calibre in non-hypoxic areas, thus stealing "from the poor and giving to the rich". Clearly the reverse, the "Robin Hood steal", would be desirable. This phenomenon was claimed to be a feature of hemorheotherapy. In poststenotic areas blood fluidification theoretically yields its strongest effects in terms of blood flow, while perfusion remains largely unaffected in vascular beds with normal driving forces. Thus the poor might gain from the rich. However, looking at the list of drugs claiming such effects, one cannot but hesitate. Most of them are in fact vasodilators. Is hemorheological therapy only a "renaissance of dilators"? Are we indeed dealing with the "Robin Hood phenomenon" or with the "wishful thinking syndrome"? Of course, the situation might change when drugs become available that are actually designed for hemorheological therapy and do not stem from the "rheological renaissance of vasodilators".

With regard to methodology: since it is still not fully established what is exactly measured by most techniques to quantify red cell deformability, it seems problematic to state that a certain drug can definitively normalize this factor in a certain disease. Yet another aspect concerns statistical evaluations. Apart from the demand for placebo-controlled, randomized double-blind studies investigating simultaneously blood rheology and relevant clinical endpoints, there may be, in certain cases, a discrepancy between clinical relevance and statistical significance. An average increase of 25 m in walking distance within a group of claudicants can be significant, but is it relevant? On the other hand, it may be possible to observe statistically non-significant changes which can still bear clinical relevance.

The number of unanswered questions seems only to be exceeded by the number of studies published in this field. This is perhaps not surprising when one considers the complexity of the problems involved and the relative youth of hemorheology. What, then, is a reasonable attitude towards hemorheological medications? The most effective way to normalize hypoperfusion is to increase the driving forces acting in vivo. In case of an arterial stenosis, this should be done by disobliterating the vessel using biochemical lysis, with or without mechanical manipulations, or by vascular surgery - whatever may be indicated. In other instances the driving forces may be increased by optimizing the pumping function of the heart in hypotensive states. All these treatments can cause blood to flow in its most fluid state. Frequently re-establishment of vessel patency may not be possible or insufficient or short lived. In this large group of patients lies the true domain of hemorheological therapy. The aim of such a therapy is to improve blood flow under driving forces that previously caused it to stagnate. The potential of hemorheological drugs is to fluidify blood in order to provide a nearly normal perfusion in blood vessels that are functionally or organically altered beyond repair. Treatment and prevention of atherosclerosis being still one of medicine's major aims for years to come, effective hemorheological therapy is an important challenge of the present days. In this respect we have taken some first decisive steps but with a long way still ahead of us.

12.6.4. Drugs with "hemorheological side-effects"

There are several drugs with sufficiently defined (non-rheological) actions, established efficacy, and indications, *also* exerting some rheological effects. In some cases these "hemorheological side-effects" might contribute to the therapeutic usefulness of the particular medication. Unlike the previously mentioned substances, these drugs will be prescribed not for their effects on blood fluidity, but for other, well accepted reasons.

Beta blockers
Alprenolol has been shown to reduce blood viscosity in hypertensives and patients with ischemic heart disease [214]. Oral metoprolol given during 2 weeks to volunteers reduced blood and plasma viscosity and increased red cell filterability [215]. Although some investigators fail to confirm such effects and though the mechanisms of hemorheological actions are speculative at present (for a review see [216]), these results might bear some relevance to the cardioprotective effect of beta blockers after myocardial infarction [217,218]. Furthermore they might play a role in abandoning the relative contraindication of cardioselective beta blockers in peripheral vascular disease [216].

Ketanserin
This serotonin antagonist and vasodilator is a new antihypertensive drug [219]. It also seems to be effective in peripheral vascular disease [220]. The drug was

documented to have effects on blood viscosity and red cell filterability [221]. Thus Ketanserin could decrease viscous resistance by rheological mechanisms, which could account partly for its clinical effects [222].

Nifedipine

The anti-anginal effects of calcium-antagonists are not fully understood. Employing both filtration and centrifugation for quantifying red cell deformability, nifedipine was shown in a placebo-controlled study with angina patients to have favourable influence on this parameter [223]. Similar results were obtained in an open study in ischemic heart disease using whole blood filtration [224]. But another trial failed to observe this effect [225]. It has been postulated that the rheological effects of calcium-antagonists contribute to their efficacy in angina pectoris [223]. Several controlled trials report good clinical effects in Raynaud's phenomenon, possibly aided by its rheological actions [226,227,228].

Prazosin

Blood viscosity is abnormal in essential hypertension [229]. Theoretically a decrease in viscous resistance could counteract arterial hypertension [229]. Prazosin, an antihypertensive drug of the piperazine group, decreases hematocrit and blood viscosity in patients with essential hypertension [230]. A possible mechanism of this effect is plasma volume expansion.

Nitroglycerin

Nitroglycerin exerts its powerful anti-anginal effects by acute vasodilatation. Recently it has been described to reduce blood viscosity [231]. This was confirmed in a placebo-controlled, double-blind trial in volunteers with both sublingual and transdermal application [232]. Subsequent to acute or long-term nitroglycerin, a pronounced intravascular auto-hemodilution takes place, an effect that persists for hours after the acute treatment. Most likely this is secondary to vasodilation, nevertheless it could theoretically contribute to the anti-ischemic effect and might furthermore be a way of monitoring the drugs effects on the venous system [232].

Heparin

In addition to their well known effects on the coagulation system, some of the most widely used anticoagulants may induce hemorheological alterations. Subcutaneous heparin (5000 I.U.) was shown to have effects on blood viscosity as determined in a Couette [233] viscometer. In postoperative patients low dose heparin was followed by a reduction in blood viscosity which was more pronounced at low shear rate [233]. The mechanism of these alterations is unclear. It is not induced by quantitative changes in fibrinogen or plasma lipids, nor by a reduction in hematocrit. A recent study re-investigated the problem, confirmed the previous findings, and speculated that cell-cell and protein-cell-interactions might be the cause [234]. Other workers, however, using less sensitive techniques of measurement, did not find any viscosity changes with heparin [235]. It seems that only methods controlling the shear history of the sample are sensitive enough for quantifying the discrete changes.

Coumarin
The oral vitamin K antagonist was shown to decrease hematocrit, as well as plasma and blood viscosity (capillary viscometer) in volunteers and patients with ischemic heart disease. Interestingly, this was paralleled by symptomatic improvement of angina in patients [236]. In dogs, heparinization and indirect anticoagulation lead to increased coronary perfusion not explainable by vasodilatation or altered hemodynamics [237]. Using a cone-and-plate viscometer, another group demonstrated relatively lower blood viscosity at middle and high shear rates in a mixed patients group as compared to a similar non-anticoagulated group [238].

Oral heparinoids
Na-pentosan polysulphate (SP-54) is a synthetic heparinoid for oral administration. Among others, it induces fibrinolytic and antilipemic effects. It has been shown to reduce plasma lipids, fibrinogen levels, as well as plasma and blood viscosity in two studies - one on 54 arteriosclerotic patients [239] and the other on 16 patients with primary hyperlipoproteinemias [240]. Heparinoids may have a number of beneficial effects on various body systems and induce little adverse effects.

Prostaglandins
The literature is controversial concerning the effects of prostaglandins (PG) on red cell filterability. Infusion of PG I2 and PG E1 was shown to improve filterability in Raynaud's phenomenon and systemic sclerosis patients using a 3 μm filter system [242]. Others [243] have failed to see such effects after infusion of PG E1 in a placebo-controlled trial with Raynaud patients using 5 μm filters. In vitro results do not help to resolve this discrepancy. Incubation of red cells with PG E1 was reported to increase [244,245], decrease [246] and not alter [247,248] red cell filterability. One clue to the problem might be a dose dependency, as low doses were followed by improvement and high ones not. Other explanations could lie in the methodology applied and/or duration of treatment. Owing to the potential importance of prostaglandin E as a potent dilator in vascular disease, the controversies demand to be solved by further experimental work.

Miscellaneous
Insulin was shown to have a normalizing effect on red cell rheology both in vitro and ex vivo on diabetic red cells [241]. This aspect is dealt with in more detail in Chapter 10.

Two extensive intervention trials have demonstrated an increase in mortality when subgroups of patients were treated with oral, long-term hydrochlorthiazide [249]. One of the many possible explanations is that this may be linked to adverse rheological effects (hemoconcentration) which can also be seen in volunteers [250].

The adverse effects of oral contraceptives are discussed in detail in Chapter 9. Our group tested two low dose contraceptive pills and found no marked influences on the flow properties of blood (unpublished results)

The aspect of "hemorheological side-effects" of non-rheological drugs has so far gained little attention in the literature. In some cases, however, it may have considerable clinical relevance, which merits to be studied in more detail.

12.7. Non-pharmacological approach

Today's doctors sometimes forget that pharmacotherapy is not the only form of non-surgical treatment. For obvious reasons (i.e. the lack of commercial impetus for such clinical research) this field has been widely neglected. However, several types of non-pharmacological modifications of blood rheology have been demonstrated recently.

12.7.1. Physical fitness

Two groups have reported that volunteers involved in regular exercise yield lower values of plasma and blood viscosity compared to a sedentary control group [251,252]. This has been confirmed recently in an investigation comparing soccer players to sedentary volunteers; in this study it was reported that there was an additional relative increase in red cell filterability in athletes [253]. Blood fluidification could be a part of a physiological adaptation in prolonged regular exercise. Its principal mechanism might be an expansion of the normal plasma volume [254]. By analogy to a dose-effect-relationship a correlation between blood rheology factors and maximal work capacity was shown in a group of healthy volunteers with varying degrees of fitness [255]. It was also reported that blood fluidification can be achieved intraindividually by regular training in healthy volunteers [256] and claudicants [257]. Recent unpublished data suggests that a relatively minor degree of regular exercise (around one hour per day) may be sufficient to induce this effect.

These findings include a variety of aspects with clinical potential, of which only the therapeutical one will be mentioned here. Regular exercise is accepted as the treatment of choice in intermittent claudication. Its working principle seems multifactorial and is not entirely understood at present [258]. The above findings suggest that blood rheology is involved together with other factors.

12.7.2. *Physical therapy*

Physical therapy entails a number of possible alternatives to drug treatment. In many cases its efficacy has been established only empirically and it frequently defies placebo-controlled blind trials. Several approaches of physical therapy have recently been shown to induce acute blood fluidification in volunteers and patients. Such treatments are balneotherapeutic interventions [259], certain types of hyperthermia [260] and mechanical manipulations [261]. The data available at present support the hypothesis that physiological stimuli may increase fluidity, while unphysiological ones could limit the flow properties of blood. Whether or not hemorheological responses to such manoeuvers are linked with the therapeutic success in patients, cannot be decided at present.

12.7.3. *Diet*

According to a Chinese saying, three tenth of all diseases can be cured by medicines, the rest by diets. The influence of diets on hemorheology is a field which at present is relatively unexplored. Our group has shown that pathological blood cell filterability in grossly obese individuals returns back to normal during total fasting for 10 days [262]. We could also demonstrate that blood rheology is better than "normal" in vegetarians [263]. Thus diets may have some unrecognized potential in favourably changing blood fluidity which could be integrated into the hemorheological repertoire. (For the effects of fish oil see Section 12.6.2.) Treatments other than drugs may therefore modify blood rheology. This seems hardly surprising and might have advantages over pharmacological therapy. However, data are still far too fragmentary to allow therapeutic conclusions. Although information is similarly fragmentary, it seems perfectly reasonable to recommend regular exercise and to abandon life habits representing a risk factor. (For discussions on the association of cardiovascular risk factors and blood rheology, see [264] and Chapter 7). This concept is firmly established in medicine, yet it is new from the hemorheologist's point of view. It may sound like a common place to many but this does not neccessarily mean that it is without value.

12.8. Conclusions

Amelioration of blood fluidity as a mean of enhancing blood flow can be achieved by hemodilution, defibrinogenation, apheresis, oral medications, physical stimuli, and diet. The true aim of any therapy is, of course, to help the patient. Does hemorheological therapy indeed ease sufferings or cure diseases? Clearly this is also the criterium by which a relatively novel field like hemorheology will be judged by clinicians unfortunately conclusive evidence on precisely this point is still scarce and contradictions are plenty. So at present, enthusiasts, fascinated by the intriguing possibilities of this new approach, are confronted with disillusioned clinicians who see how disappointingly little can be achieved in practice. This should be a strong challenge for hemorheologists to provide the necessary data and fill the large gaps between the theory and its application. Hopefully we will then one day be able to state that for a specific condition a certain hemorheological treatment may be useful, while it is superfluous or even harmful in another disease.

"Experience teaches slowly and at the cost of mistakes" (J.A. Froude).

12.9. References

1. Hamblin T. 1984: Where now for therapeutic apheresis? Brit. Med. J. 289, 779.
2. Bauer J. 1966: Die Geschichte der Aderlässe. (Reprint) W. Fritsch, München.
3. Gelin L.E. 1956: Studies in anemia of injury. Acta Chir. Scand. Suppl. 210, 1.
4. Koga G. 1913: Zur Therapie der Spontangangrän an den Extremitäten. Dtsch. Zschr. Chir. 121, 371.
5. Gelin L., Ingelmann B. 1961: Rheomacrodex - a new dextran solution for rheological treatment of impaired capillary flow. Acta Chir. Scand. 122, 294-302.
6. Thomas D.J., Du Boulay G.H., Marshall J. 1977: Cerebral blood flow in polycythemia. Lancet 2, 161-163.
7. Messmer K. 1975: Hemodilution. Surg. Clins. N. Am. 55, 659-678.
8. Guyton A.C., Richardson T.Q. 1961: Effect of hematocrit on venous return. Circ. Res. 9, 157.
9. Jan K.M., Chien S. 1977: Effect of hematocrit variations on coronary hemodynamics and oxygen utilization. Am. J. Physiol. 233, H 107-113.
10. Geha A.S. 1976: Coronary and cardiovascular dynamics and oxygen availability during acute normovolemic anemia. Surgery 80, 47-53.
11. Race C., Dedichen H., Schenck W.G. 1967: Regional blood flow during dextran induced normovolemic hemodilution in the dog. J. Thor. Cardiovasc. Surg. 53, 578.
12. Schmid-Schoenbein H., Messmer K., Rieger H. (eds) 1981: Hemodilution and flow improvement. S. Karger, Basel.
13. Guyton A.C., Jones C.E., Coleman T.G. 1973: Circulatory physiology: Cardiac output and its regulation. W.B. Saunders.
14. Gottstein U. 1984: Evaluation of isovolemic hemodilution. Clin. Hemorheol 4, 133-139.
15. Gilbert J.P., Mc Peek B., Mosteller F. 1977: Statistics and ethics in surgery and anaesthesia. Science 198, 684-689.
16. Gilroy J., Barnhart M.J., Meyer J.S. 1969: Treatment of acute stroke with dextran 40. JAMA 210, 293.
17. Walz A. G. 1966: Experimental cerebral infarction: The microvasculature of the cortex. Effects of occlusion of the middle cerebral artery and administration of hemodiluting agents. In: Sickert R.G., Whisnant J.P. (eds): Cerebral Vascular Diseases. 5th Conf. New York, Grune Stratton pp. 177-183.
18. Matthews W.B., Oxbury J.M., Grainger K.M.R., Greenhall R.C.D. 1976: A blind controlled trial of dextran 40 in the treatment of ischemic stroke. Brain, 99, 193-206.
19. Asplund K., Eriksson S., Hägg E., Lithner F., Strand T., Wester P.O. 1983: Ischemic stroke treated by hemodilution. An interim report of a randomized trial. In: Cerebral Vascular Disease. Meyer J.S., Leckher H., Reivich M. (eds). Excerpta Medica, Amsterdam pp. 148-150.

20. Herrschaft H. 1984: Die Therapie cerebraler Durchblutungsstoerungen. In: Beiträge zur Anaesthesiologie und Intensivmedizin. Band 3, O. Mayrhofer, K. Steinbreitner, H. Bergmann (eds), Mandrich, Wien, München, Bern, pp. 106-125.
21. Gottstein U., Sedlmeyer I., Schoettler M., Gülk V. 1970: Der Effekt von niedermolekularem Dextran auf die Unterschenkeldurchblutung von Gesunden und Kranken mit peripheren arteriellen Zirkulationsstoerungen. Dtsch. Med. Wschr. 95, 1955-1959.
22. Yates C.J.P., Berent A., Andrews V., Dormandy J.A. 1979: Increase in leg blood flow by normovolemic hemodilution in intermittent claudication. Lancet, i, 166.
23. Rudofsky G., Strohmenger H.G., Trexler S., Brock F.E. 1981: Isovolämische Hämodilution bei Patienten mit arterieller Verschlußkrankheit im Stadium II. In: Bredding K. (ed), Thrombose und Atherogenese. Witzstock, Baden Baden.
24. Willison J.R., Thomas D.J., Du Boulay G.H., Marshall J., Paul E.A., Pearson T.C., Russell R.W., Symon L., Wetherley-Mein G. 1980: Effect of hematocrit on alertness. Lancet 1, 846-848.
25. Ernst E., Magyarosy I., Paulsen H.F., Kleinschmidt Th., Drexel H. 1984: Hämorheologische Parameter bei Apoplektikern in der Rehabilitationsphase. In: Therapie mit hämorheologisch aktiven Substanzen. A.M. Ehrly ed. Zuckschwerdt München, pp. 115-121.
26. Ernst E., Matrai A., Kollar L.: A randomized, double-blind, placebo-controlled, cross-over trial on isovolemic hemodilution in claudicants - preliminary results. Clin. Hemorheol. 6, 297-302.
27. Linden L. 1964: Lägmolikylär dextranbehandling vid hjärt- infarkt. Svensk. Läk. Tidn. 61, 2300-23-5.
28. Langsjoen P.H., Falconer H.S., Sanchez S.A., Lynch D.J. 1963: Observations in treatment of acute myocardial infarction with low molecular weight dextran. Angiology 14, 465-469.
29. Bassenge E., Schmid-Schoenbein H., von Restorff W., Volger E. 1974: Effect of hemodilution on coronary hemodynamics in conscious dogs. In: Messmer K., Schmid-Schoenbein H. (eds). Hemodilution. Karger, Basel, p. 174.
30. Tucher W. Z., Beam J., Vanderanter S., Cohn L.H. 1980: The effect of hemodilution on experimental myocardial infarct size. Eur. Surg. Res. 12, 1.
31. Borchgrevink C. F., Euger E. 1966: Low molecular weight dextran in acute myocardial infarction. Brit. Med. J. 1235.
32. Linden L. 1967: Rheomakrodex - behandling vid hjardinfarkt. Nord. Med. 78, 957.
33. Reuter F.W., Mazzoni S., Wegmann T. 1968: Die Behandlung des akuten Myokardinfarktes mit niedermolekularem Dextran. Schweiz. Med. Wschr. 98, 1218.
34. Langsjoen P.H., Sanchez S.A., Lynch D.J., Inmont T.W. 1968: The treatment of myocardial infarction with low molecular weight dextran. Am Heart J. 76, 28.
35. Ditzel J., Bang H.O., Thorsen N. 1969: The effect of dextran 40 on hemorheological factors during the course of acute myocardial infarction. In: Bibl. anat. Vol. 10, Karger, Basel, pp. 132-136.
36. Noerregaad S. 1969: In: Low molecular weight dextran in acute myocardial infarction. Borchgrevink C.F. (ed). Geriatrics 24.
37. Mymin D. 1969: In: Low molecular weight dextran in acute myocardial infarction. Borchgrevink C.F. (ed). Geriatrics 24.
38. Messmer K. 1981: Compensatory mechanisms for acute dilutional anemia. Biblthca. hematol. 47, Karger, Basel, pp. 31-42.
39. Roche J.K., Stengle J.M. 1973: Open heart surgery and the demand for blood. JAMA 225, 1516-1521.
40. Lockey E., McIntyre N., Ross D.N. et al 1967: Jaundice after open heart surgery. Thorax 22, 165.
41. Eiseman B., Spencer F.C. 1962: Effect of hyperthermia on the flow characteristics of blood. Surgery 52, 532.
42. Gelin L.E., Jansen H. 1975: Moderate preoperative hemodilution, mortality and thrombus formation in general surgery. Bibl. Haematol. 41, 239-247.

43. Sunder Plasman L., Messmer K. 1979: Akute präoperative Hämodilution. Chirurg 50, 410-416.
44. Parker M.C. 1983: Pre-operative normavolaemic hemodilution - a clinical trial. Clin. Hemorheol. 3, 277.
45. Kinsely M.H., Ellion T.S., Block E.H. 1945: Sluged blood in traumatic shock: microscopic observations and precipitation and agglutination of blood flowing through vessels in crushed tissues. Arch. Surg. 51, 220.
46. Landgraf H. 1983: Klinische Hämorheologie und Schock. In: Klinische Hämorheologie - Eine Bestandsaufnahme. Ehrly A.M. (ed), W. Zuckschwerdt Verlag München, pp. 29-37.
47. Neuhof H. 1979: Kreislaufinsuffizienz, Schock. In: Innere Medizin und Chirurgie. Voßschulte, Rasch, Heinrich (eds), p. 154.
48. Gersmeyer E.F., Yasargil E.C. 1978: Schock und hypotone Kreislaufstörungen. Thieme, Stuttgart.
49. Ehrly A.M. 1978: Zur Frage der Erythrozytenaggregation und des Verhaltens der Blutviskosität im hämorheologischen Schock. Anaesthesist 17, 327.
50. Yao S.T., Shoemaker W.C. 1966: Plasma and whole blood viscosity changes in shock and after dextran infusion. Ann. Surg. 164, 973-984.
51. Chien S., Dellenback R.J., Usami S., Gregersen M.J. 1965: Hematocrit changes in endotoxin shock. Proc. Soc. Exp. Biol. Med. 118, 1182.
52. Gelin L.E. 1961: Disturbance of the flow properties of blood and its counteraction in surgery. Acta chir. scand. 122, 287.
53. Braasch D., Gössling G. 1966: Erythrozytendeformierung und Quellung durch Plasmafaktoren nach schweren Verbrennungen. Pflügers Archiv. 289, 1.
54. Heilmann L., Genz G.J., Ludwig H. 1982: Schwere geburtshilfliche Hämostasedefekte: Diagnostik und therapeutisches Vorgehen. Geburtsh. und Frauenheil. 42, 853-856.
55. Abel J.J., Rowntree L.G., Turner B.B. 1914: Plasma removal with return of the corpuscles. J. Pharmacol. Exp. Ther. 5, 625-641.
56. Soloman A., Fahey J.L. 1963: Plasmapheresis therapy in macroglobulinaemia. Ann. Int. Med. 58, 789-800.
57. Russell J.A., Toy J.L., Powles R.L. 1977: Plasma exchange in malignant paraproteinaemias. Exp. Haematol. 5, 100.
58. Brown M.M., Marshall J. 1982: Effect of plasma exchange on blood viscosity and cerebral blood flow. Brit. Med. J. 284, 1733-1736.
59. Buskard N.A. 1981: Blood flow studies in the hyperviscosity syndrome before and after plasma exchange. In: Plasma Exchange Therapy. H. Borberg, P. Reuter, Thieme, Stuttgart, pp. 89-94.
60. Postiglione A., Soricelli A., Scarpato N. et al 1982: Increased cerebral blood flow after plasma exchange in patients with familial hypercholesterolemia. Clin. Hemorheol. 2, 195.
61. Kilpatrick D., Fleming J., Clyne C., Thompson G.R. 1979: Reduction of blood viscosity following plasma exchange. Atherosclerosis 32, 301-306.
62. Postiglione A., Rubba P., Scarpato N., Tannuzzi A., Mancini M. 1982: Increased blood flow to lower limbs in patients with familial hypercholesterolemia after plasma exchange. Atherosclerosis 41, 421-425.
63. Walker R.T., Matrai A., Dormandy J.A., Flute P.T. 1985: Hemorheological and functional changes in intermittent claudication following plasmapheresis with Haemacell. Clin. Hemorheol. 5, 99-106.
64. Strauer B.E., Fateh-Moghadam A., Kment A., Samtleben W., Volger E. 1981: Use of plasmapheresis and immunosuppressive therapy in coronary microangiopathies. Biblthca. haemat. 47, 213-227, Karger, Basel.
65. Sentinella K., Thompson R., Hunt D., Simpson L., Marshall C.E. 1982: Erythrocytapheresis (red cell exchange) therapeutic apheresis and plasma perfusion. Prog. Clin. Biol. Res. 106, 425-435.
66. Newland A.C., Wedzicha J.A. 1984: Isovolemic hemodilution (erythrapheresis) in polycythemia. Apheresis Bulletin 2, 24.

67. Wedzicha J.A., Rudd R.M., Apps M.C.P., Cotter F.E., Newland A.C., Empey D.N. 1983: Erythrapheresis in patients with polycythemia secondary to hypoxic lung disease. Brit. Med. J. 286, 511-514.
68. Lichtmann M.A., Rowe J.M. 1982: Hyperleucocytic leukemias: rheological, clinical and therapeutic considerations. Blood 60, 279-283.
69. Schmidt B., Lysaght M.J., Henne W., Gurland H.J. 1983: Quantitative evaluation of secondary filters for closed loop membrane plasmapheresis. 2nd Int. Symp. Plasmapheresis. Cleveland.
70. Ray P.K., Idiculla A., Rhados J.E., Besa E., Bassett I.G., Cooper D.R. 1980: Immunoadsorption of IgG molecules from the plasma of multiple myeloma and autoimmune hemolytic anemia patients. Plasma Ther. 1, 11.
71. Samtleben W., Lysaght M.J., Blumenstein M., Gurland H.J. 1984: Therapeutic plasmapheresis in rheological disorders: Indications and limitations. Clin. Hemorheol. 4, 35.
72. Gelin L.E. 1970: Reaction of the body as a whole to injury. J. Traum 10, 932.
73. Meiselman H.J., Merrill E.W., Salzman E.W., Gilliand E.R., Pelletier G.A. 1967: Effect of dextran on rheology of human blood: low shear viscosity. J. Appl. Physiol. 22, 480.
74. Corry W.D., Jackson L.J., Seaman G.V.F. 1983: Action of hydroxyethyl starch on the flow properties of human erythrocyte suspensions. Biorheology 20, 705.
75. Köhler H., Zschiedrich H., Clasen R., Linfante A., Gamm H. 1982: Blutvolumen, kolloidosmotischer Druck und Nierenfunktion von Probanden nach Infusion mittelmolekularer 10% Hydroxyaethylstärke 200/0.5 und 10% Dextran 40. Anaestesist 31, 61-67.
76. Harke H., Pieper C., Meredig J., Rahman S., Rüssler P. 1980: Rheologische und gerinnungsphysiologische Untersuchungen nach Infusion von HAS 200/0.5 und Dextran 40. Anaesthesist 29, 71-77.
77. Harke H. 1982: Indikation und Abgrenzung der kolloidalen Plasmaersatzmittel. In: Blutkomponenten und Plasmaersatzmittel, J.R. Kalden, U.D. Koenig (eds). Springer, Berlin, pp. 1-13.
78. Köhler H. 1979: Unerwünschte Nebenwirkungen kolloidaler Plasmaersatzmittel. Klinikarzt 8, 616.
79. Messmer K., Jesch F. 1978: Volumenersatz und Hämodilution durch Hydroxyäthylstärke. Infusionsther. Klin. Ernähr. 5, 169-177.
80. De Venuto F., Busse K.R., Zegna A.I. 1981: Viscosity of human blood hemodiluted with crystalline hemoglobin solution. Transfusion 21, 752-756.
81. Cerny L.C., Cerny E.L., Cerny M.E., Baldwin J.E., Gill B. 1983: Mixtures of whole blood and hydroxyethylstarch - hemoglobin polymers. Critical Care Med. 11, 739-743.
82. Reid H.A. 1963: Clinical effects of bites by the Malayan Viper. Lancet 1, 617.
83. Esnouf M.P., Tunnak G.W. 1967: The isolation and properties of the thrombin like activity from Aghistrodon rhodostoma. Brit. J. Haematol. 13, 581.
84. Collen D., Verstraete M. 1978: Activation of the fibrinolytic system during reptilase therapy and following strenuous exercise in man. In: Progress in Chemical Fibrinolysis and Thrombolysis. J.F. Davidson, R.M. Rowan, M.M. Samama, P.C. Desnoyers (eds) New York, Raven Press, pp. 155-157.
85. Vinazzer H. 1971: Zur Wirkung von Arvin auf die Blutgerinnung. Wien. Inn. Med. 52, 378-392.
86. Prentice C.R.M., Hassnein A.A., Turpic A.G.G., Mc Nicol G.P., Douglas A.S. 1969: Changes in platelet behaviour during arvin therapy. Lancet 1, 644.
87. Vinazzer H. 1975: Clinical experience with arvin. Folia Angiol. 23, 402.
88. Kwaan H.C. 1973: Status of arvin and reptilase therapy in thromboembolism. In: Moser K.M., Stein M. (eds). Pulmonary embolism. Year book of medical publishers, pp. 299-312.
89. Pizzo S.V., Schwartz M.L., Hill R.L., McKee P.A. 1972: Mechanism of Ancrod anticoagulation. A direct proteolytic effect on fibrin. J. Clin. Invest. 51, 2841-2850.
90. Ehrly A.M. 1973: Influence of arvin on the flow properties of blood. Biorheology 10, 453-456.
91. Ehrly A.M. 1976: Improvement of the flow properties of blood: A new therapeutical approach in occlusive arterial disease. Angiology 27, 118-198.

92. Ernst E., Dormandy J. 1981: The effects of arvin and surgery on red cell filterability. Scand. J. Clin. Lab. Invest. 41, suppl. 156, 317-319.
93. Hauck G. 1975: Tierexperimentelle Untersuchungen über die Wirkung von Arwin auf die Mikrozirkulation. Folia Angiol. 23, 381-385.
94. Heidrich H. 1978: Thrombotische arterien- und Venenverschlüsse unter Ancrod-Therapie. Med. Klin. 73, 798-800.
95. Lowe G.D.O. 1984: Defibrination, blood flow and blood rheology. Clin. Hemorheol. 4, 15.
96. Douglas A.S., Bennett B., Ogston D. 1984: Antithrombotic therapy. In: Human Blood Coagulation, Hemostasis and Thrombosis, Blackwell, p. 514.
97. Barrie W.W., Schenk W.G. 1975: Improvement in blood flow through a critical arterial stenosis by defibrination with ancrod. Archiv. Surg. 111, 561-563.
98. Awad A.M., White R.J., Lowe G.D.O., Forbes C.D. 1983: The effect of blood viscosity on blood flow in the experimental saphenous flap model. Brit. J. Plast. Surg. 36, 383.
99. Ehringer H., Dudczek R., Lechner K. 1974: A new approach in the treatment of peripheral vascular occlusions. Defibrination with Arvin. Angiology 25, 279-283.
100. Ehrly A.M. 1974: Langzeitergebnisse der Therapie chronischer arterieller Verschlußkrankheiten mit Arwin. Jahrestagung Dtsch. Ges. Angiol.
101. Wolf G.K. 1976: Arvin in peripheral arterial circulatory disorders: Controlled multicentre trials. Europ. J. Clin. Pharmacol. 9, 387-392.
102. Bericht über eine kontrollierte Studie mit Arwin in subcutaner Anwendung im Vergleich zur Ronical-Therapie 1974. Med. Forschung, Knoll AG.
103. Martin M., Hirdes E., Auel H. 1976: Defibrinogenation treatment in patients suffering from severe intermittent claudication: a controlled study. Throm. Res. 9, 47.
104. Tonnesen K.H., Sager P., Gormesen J. 1978: Treatment of severe foot ischemia by defibrination with ancrod: a randomized blind study. Scand. J. Clin. Lab. Invest. 38, 431-435.
105. Lowe G.D.O., Dunlop D.J., Lawson D.H., Pollock J.G., Watt J.K., Forbes C.D., Prentic C.R., Drummond M.M. 1982: Double blind controlled clinical trial of ancrod in the relief of ischemic rest pain of the leg. Angiology 33, 46-50.
106. Ernst E. 1983: Therapeutische Defibrinogenierung als konservative Therapie der peripheren arteriellen Verschlußkrankheit - Eine kritischen Analyse. Münch. Med. Wschr. 125, 796-798.
107. Neugebauer G. 1976: Verbesserung der Fließeigenschaften mit Arwin beim akuten experimentellen Infarkt. Z. Kardiol. 65, 1010-1021.
108. Goslinga H. 1984: Blood viscosity and shock. Springer, Berlin.
109. Fedor E.J., Broady H.D., Wiemeler L.H., Hwang K. 1971: Effect of Abbott 38414 (ancrod) on renal blood flow and clearance, coronary sinus flow and PO2 and femoral arterial flow. Fed. Proc. 30, 1269.
110. Leube G., Sondern W. 1975: Klinische Anwendung von Arwin bei schwerer Angina pectoris. Folia Angiol. 23, 411.
111. Spöttl F., Pimmingstorfer E., Froschauer J. 1978: Defibrinierende Therapie der instabilen Angina pectoris bei Hyperfibrinogenämie durch Arwin. Wien. Klin. Wschr. 90, 792-796.
112. Barrie W.W., Wood E.H., Crumlish P., Forbes C.D., Prentice C.R.M. 1974: Low-dosage Ancrod for prevention of thrombotic complications after surgery for fractured neck of femur. Brit. Med. J. 4, 130-133.
113. Lowe G.D.O., Campbell A.F., Meek D.R., Forbes C.D., Prentice C.R.M., Cummings S.W. 1979: Subcutaneous ancrod in prevention of deep vein thrombosis (after operation for fractured neck of femur). Lancet 1, 51-52.
114. Belch J.J.F., Meek D.R., Lowe G.D.O., Campbell A.F., Young A.B., Forbes C.D., Prentice C.R.M. 1982: Subcutaneous ancrod in prevention of deep vein thrombosis after hip replacement surgery. Thrombos. Res. 25, 23-31.
115. Meissner A.G., O'Sullivan G., Macbeth R.A. 1976: The effect of defibrinogenation on pulmonary embolism in dogs. Thromb. Haemostas. 36, 140-149.

116. Bowell R.E., Marmion V.J., Mc Carthy C.F. 1970: Treatment of central retinal thrombosis with ancrod. Lancet 1, 173.
117. Gent A., Ingram G., Arocha-Pinango C.L., Fenton P., Buckley R.J. 1979: Central retinal vein thrombosis: serial treatment with defibrination, aspirin and plasminotropic drugs. Thrombos. Res. 14, 61-66.
118. Davies J.A., Merrick M.V., Sharp A.A., Holt J.M. 1972: Controlled trial of ancrod and heparin in treatment of deep vein thrombosis of lower limb. Lancet i, 113-115.
119. Ernst E. 1984: Hämorheologische Aspekte der tiefen Venenthrombose. Münch. Med. Wschr. 20, 652.
120. Dormandy J., Reid H.L. 1978: Controlled defibrination in the treatment of peripheral vascular disease. Angiology 29, 80-88.
121. Browse N., Clemenson G. 1978: Vein surgery during defibrinogenation. Brit. J. Surg. 65, 452-455.
122. Naish P., Evans D.J., Peters D.K. 1975: The effects of defibrination with ancrod in experimental allergic glomerular injury. Clin. Exp. Immunol. 20, 303-309.
123. Pollak V.E., Glueck H.J., Weiss M.A., Lebron-Berges A., Miller M.A. 1982: Defibrination with ancrod in glomerulonephritis: effects on clinical and histologic findings and on blood coagulation. Am. J. Nephrol. 2, 195.
124. Dosekun A.K., First M.R., Chandran P.K.G., Kant K.S., Glas-Greenwalt P., Weiss M.A., Alexander J.W., Pollak V.E. 1982: Successful treatment by defibrination with ancrod in a patient with hyperacute renal allograft failure and a deficiency of plasma prostacyclin stimulating factor. Clin. Nephrol. 18, 101-105.
125. Bell W.R., Pitney W.R. 1969: Management of priapism by therapeutic defibrination. N. Engl. J. Med. 280, 649.
126. Mann J.R., Deeble T.J., Breeze G.R., Stuart J. 1972: Ancrod in sickle cell crisis. Lancet i, 934-937.
127. Williams J.R.B., Maughan E. 1972: Treatment of tumor metastases by defibrination. Brit. Med. J. 3, 174-175.
128. Aluken N., Tiejeon J.U. 1973: Defibrination therapy in progressive scleroderma. Phlebologie 32, 79.
129. Kollar L., Kiss T., Matrai A. 1983: Treatment of Bürger's disease with Arvin. Clin. Hemorheol. 3, 308.
130. Dosekun A.K., Pollak V.E., Glas-Greenwalt P. et al 1982: Ancrod in systemic lupus erythematosus with thrombosis. Arch. Int. Med. 144, 37.
131. Sueishi K., Nanno S., Tanaka K. 1981: Permeability enhancing and chemotactic activities of lower molecular weight degradation products of human fibrinogen. Thromb. Haemost. 45, 90-94.
132. Budzynski A.Z., Pandya B.V., Rubin R.N., Brizuela B.S., Soszka T., Stewart G.J. 1984: Fibrinogenolytic afibrinogenemia after envenomation by western diamond back rattlesnake (Crotalus atrox). Blood 63, 1-14.
133. Schmid-Schönbein H., Rieger H., Hess H. 1977: Quantitative Erfassung der Effekte fibrinolytischer Therapie auf das Fließverhalten des Blutes. Klin. Wschr. 55, 111-119.
134. Ehrly A.M. 1971: Rheological changes due to fibrinolytic therapy. Int. Symp. Hemodil. Rottach-Egern, pp. 289-297.
135. European Collaborative Study Group for streptokinase treatment in acute myocardial infarction 1979. N. Engl. J. Med. 301, 797.
136. Ernst E. 1984: Sind "Rheologika" therapeutisch von Nutzen? ZfA 60, 192-200.
137. Srivastava S.C., Smith M.J., Dewar H.A. 1963: The effect of astromid on fibrinolytic activity of patients with ischemic heart disease and hypercholesterinemia. J. Atheroscler. Res. 3, 640.
138. Green K.G. 1984: Interpretation of Clofibrate trial. Lancet 2, 1095.
139. Dormandy J.A., Gutteridge J.M.C., Hoare E., Dormandy T.L. 1974: Effect of clofibrate on blood viscosity in intermittant claudication. Brit. Med. J. 4, 259-262.

140. Postlethwaite J.C., Dormandy J.A. 1975: Results of ankle systolic pressure measurements in patients with intermittent claudication being treated with clofibrate. Ann. Surg. 181, 799-802.
141. Thomas D.J., Du Boulay G.H., Marshall J., Pearson T.C., Ross Russell R.W., Symon L., Wetherley-Mein G., Willison J.R., Zilkha E. 1979: Prevention of stroke - the viscosity factor. In: Cerebral Vascular Disease. 2. J.S. Meyer, H. Lechner, M. Reivich (eds), Excerpa Medica, Amsterdam, pp. 211-215.
142. Report of the Committee of Principal Investigators 1984. WHO Cooperative trial on primary prevention on ischemic heart disease with clofibrate to lower serum cholesterol. Final mortality follow up. Lancet 2, 600.
143. Spöttl F., Froschauer J. 1976: Influence of Etofibrate on plasma fibrinogen and plasminogen concentrations in patients with different forms of primary hyperlipoproteinemia. Atherosclerosis 25, 293-301.
144. Pfeiffer M., Tilsner V. 1978: Einfluß von Etofibrat auf die Plasmaviskosität bei Hyperlipoproteinämien. Med. Klinik 73, 60.
145. Preston F.E., Burakowski B.K., Porters N.R., Malia R.G. 1981: The fibrinolytic response to stanozolol in normal subjects. Throm. Res. 22, 543-551.
146. Jarrett P.E.M., Morland M., Browse N.L. 1978: Treatment of Raynauds's phenomenon by fibrinolytic enhancement. Brit. Med. J. 2, 523-525.
147. Burns P., Small M., Blamey S.L., Lowe G.D.O., Forbes C.D. 1983: Effects of stanozolol on viscosity in volunteers and in surgical patients. Clin. Hemorheol. 3, 287.
148. Charkabarti R., Fearnley G.R. 1976: Phenphormin plus ethylestrenol in survivors of myocardial infarction. Lancet 2, 556.
149. Pickart L., Thaler M.M. 1980: Fatty acids, fibrinogen and blood flow: a general mechanism for hyperfibrinogenemia and its pathologic consequences. Med. Hypothesis 6, 545-557.
150. Katsumura T., Mishima Y., Kamiya K., Sakaguchi S., Tanabe T., Sakuma A. 1980: Therapeutic effect of Ticlopidine, a new inhibitor of platelet aggregation, on chronic arterial occlusive diseases - a double blind study with inactive placebo. Cardioangiology 7, 396-406.
151. Aukland A., Hurlow R.A., George A.J., Stuart J. 1982: Platelet inhibition with Ticlopidine in atherosclerotic intermittent claudication. J. Clin. Pathol. 35, 740-743.
152. Strano A., Avellone G., Davi G., Mandala V., Raneli G. 1983: Ticlopidine induced hemorheological changes in patients suffering from atherosclerosis obliterans of the lower limbs. Clin. Hemorheol. 3, 290.
153. Neumann V., Cove D.H., Shapiro L.M., George A.J., Kenny M.W., Meakin M., Stuart J. 1983: Effect of ticlopidine on platelet function and blood rheology in diabetes mellitus. Clin. Hemorheol. 3, 13.
154. Conrad J., Lecrubier C., Scarabin P.Y., Horellou M.H., Samama M., Bousser M.G. 1980: Effects of long term administration of Ticlopidine on platelet function and hemostatic variables. Thrombos. Res. 20, 143-148.
155. Van Stalle F., Lambelin G. 1981: Suloctidil: review of its effects on platelet survival time, platelet activation and blood viscosity. Clin. Hemorheol. 1, 90.
156. Jones N.A.G., De Haas H., Zahavi J., Kakkar V.V. 1982: A double-blind trial of suloctidil versus placebo in intermittent claudication. Brit. J. Surg. 69, 38-40.
157. Roncucci R., De Hertogh R., Dormandy J.A., Doumont J., Gurewich V., Lambelin G., Lansen J., Rottiers R., Souridis E., Van Stalle F., Versee L. 1979: Effects of long term treatment with suloctidil on blood viscosity, erythrocyte deformability and total fibrinogen plasma levels in diabetic patients. Arzneimittel Forschung 29, 682-684.
158. Barras J.P., Graf C. 1980: Behandlung der Hyperviskosität bei diabetischer Retinopathie mit Doxium. VASA 9, 161-164.
159. Ernst E., Marshall M. 1984: Verbesserung der reduzierten Erythrozyten-Flexibilität durch Calciumdobesilat. Ergebnisse einer Pilotstudie. Münch. Med. Wschr. 126, 125-126.
160. Ernst E., Marshall M.: unpublished results.

161. Vojnikovic B. 1985: Verminderung der Vollblut-, Plasma- und Kammerwasserhyperviskosität bei Diabetikern mit Retinopathie und Glaukom durch Doxium (Calciumdobesilat): Eine doppelblind kontrollierte Studie. Opth. Res. 16, 150.
162. Carter A.E., Eban R. 1974: Prevention of post-operative deep vein thrombosis in legs by orally administered hydroxychloroquine sulphate. Brit. J. Med. 3, 94-95.
163. Ernst E., Rose M., Lee R. 1984: Modification of transoperative changes in blood fluidity by hydroxychloroquine: a possible explanation for the drug's antithrombotic effect. Pharamcotherapeutica 4, 48.
164. Stoltz J.F. 1982: Main determinants of red cell deformability. Clinical and pharmaceutical applications. Clin. Hemorheol. 2, 163.
165. Dormandy J. 1981: Drug modification of erythrocyte deformability. In: Clinical aspects of blood viscosity and cell deformability. G.D.O. Lowe, J.C., Barbanel, C.D. Forbes (eds), Springer, 251-265.
166. Müller R. 1981: Hemorheology and peripheral vascular diseases: A new therapeutic approach. J. Med. 12, 209-235.
167. Stefanovich V. 1978: The biochemical mechanism of action of pentoxifylline. Pharmacotherapeutica 2, suppl. 1, 5-16.
168. Le Devehat C., Lemoine A., Cirette B., Ramet M., Vimeux M. 1981: Kinetics of variations of erythrocyte filterability and 2.3 diphosphoplycerate in diabetic patients with arteriopathy of lower limbs treated by pentoxifylline. In: Hemorheology and Diseases. J.F. Stoltz, P. Drouin (eds). Doin, Paris, pp. 683-687.
169. Dormandy J., Ernst E., Flute P. 1981: Increase in red cell deformability after incubation with oxypentifylline. Curr. Med. Res. Opin. 7, 520-522.
170. Martin P., Vives P. 1979: Deformabilité des globules rouges et accidents vasculaires cérébraux. Intérèt de la pentoxifylline. Gaz. Med. France 86, 2586.
171. Porter J.M., Cutler B.S., Lee B.Y., Reich T., Reichle F.A., Scogin J.T., Strandness D.E. 1982: Pentoxifylline efficacy in the treatment of intermittent claudication: multicenter controlled double blind trial with objective assessment of chronic occlusive arterial disease patients. Am Heart J. 104, 66-72.
172. Takamatsu S. 1980: A two year follow up study on blood constituents in aged atherosclerotic patients treated with pentoxifylline. In: Pathophysiology and pharmacotherapy of cerebrovascular disorders. E. Betz, J. Grote, D. Heuser, R. Wüllenweber (eds). Witzstrock, Baden Baden, pp. 290-293.
173. Schmalzer E.A., Chien S. 1984: Filterability of subpopulations of leucocytes: Effect of pentoxifylline. Blood 64, 542-546.
174. Matrai A., Ernst E. 1986 Pentoxifylline improves white cell rheology in claudicants. Clin. Hemorheol. 5, 483–491.
175. Dormandy J., Ernst E. 1981: Effects of buflomedil on erythrocyte deformability. Angiology 32, 714-716.
176. Perego M.A., Sergio G., Espureo M., Francisci A., Artale F. 1982: Hemodynamic and hemorheological effects of buflomedil in patients with peripheral occlusive arterial disease. Curr. Med. Res. Opin. 8, 178-187.
177. Coccheri S., Palareti G., Poggi M., Tricarico M.G. 1982: Improvements in the rheologic properties of blood induced by medium-term treatment with buflomedil in diabetic patients. J. Int. Med. Res. 10, 394-398.
178. Guerrini M., Acciavatti A., Materazzi M., Del Bigo C., Forconi S., Di Perri T. 1982: Protective effect of buflomedil against exercise induced reduction in regional erythrocyte deformability of patients with peripheral arterial disease. J. Int. Med. Res. 10, 387-392.
179. Trübestein G.K., Balzer K., Bisler H., Klüken N., Mahfoud Y., Müller-Wiefel H., Unkel B., Ziegler W. 1982: Buflomedil bei arterieller Verschlußkrankheit. Dtsch. Med. Wschr. 107, 1957-1961.

180. Bisler H. 1983: Klinische Erfolge der Buflomediltherapie bei arterieller Verschlußkrankheit. Therapiewoche 33, 2204-2210.
181. Kugler J., Krauskopf R., Dersch J.E. 1981: Comparison of the effects of buflomedil and placebo on the EEG and psychometric test performance of patients with cerebrovascular insufficiency. In: Microcirculation and ischemic vascular disease. Proc. Congr. Rio de Janeiro, BMI, New York, pp. 157-169.
182. Schenk G.K., Olbrick H., Filler W., Zerbin D. 1981: Double blind comparisons between the effects of buflomedil and placebo on quantified EEG parameters and physiological variables. In: Microcirculation and ischemic vascular disease. Proc. Congr. Rio de Janeiro, BMI, New York, pp. 215-237.
183. Petry H., Zielke E. 1984: Erfahrungen mit Buflomedil bei der intravenösen Behandlung von arteriellen Durchblutungsstörungen. Therapiewoche 34, 6965.
184. Sunder Plasmann L. 1981: Resistance of collateral vessels in experimental occlusive disease. 2nd Int. Cong. Microcirc. Isch. Vasc. Disease, Rio de Janeiro.
185. Fagrell B., Hermanson J.L. 1985: Wirkung von Buflomedil auf die Mikrozirkulation der Haut bei Akralgangrän. Fortschr. Med. 103, 51.
186. De Clerck F., Beerens M., Thone F., Borgers M. 1981: Effect of flunarizine on the human red cell shape changes and calcium deposition induced by A 23187. Thromb. Res. 24, 1-12.
187. Scott C.K. 1980: The effects of flunarizine, a new calcium antagonist on human red cells in vitro. Angiology 31, 320.
188. De Cree J., De Cock W., Geukens H., De Clerck F., Beerens M., Verhaegen H. 1979: The rheological effects of cinnarizine and flunarizine in normal and pathological conditions. Angiology 30, 505-515.
189. Di Perri T.D., Forconi S., Guerrini M., Passini F.L., Del Cippola R., Rossi C., Agnusdei D. 1979: Action of cinnarizine on the hyperviscosity of blood in patients with peripheral obliterative arterial disease. Angiology 30, 13-20.
190. Guerrini M., Rossi C., Acciavatti A., Pieragalli D., Pecchi S., Cappelli R., Forconi S., Di Perri T. 1981: Possibility of treating vascular diseases from a rheological point of view. Study of the effects of Flunarizine and Cinnarizine. Clin. Hemorheol. 1, 5/6.
191. Jageneau A., Loots W., Brugmans J. 1974: Prolongation of an anoxia induced hyperemia in healthy middle-aged men treated with cinnarizine and flunarizine. Arzneimittel-Forschung 24, 1839-1841.
192. Straessen A.J. 1977: Treatment of circulatory disturbances with flunarizine and cinnarizine. A multicentre, double-blind and placebo-controlled evaluation. Vasa 6, 59.
193. Domschky K., Nelson M., Dammhayn B., Terjung E. 1977: Flunarizin bei Patienten mit zerebraler und peripherer Mangeldurchblutung. Multizentrische Doppelblindstudie. Med. Welt 28, 1062-1066.
194. Di Perri T.D., Forconi S., Guerrini M., Agnusdei D. 1977: In vitro activity of isoxuprine on blood, plasma and serum viscosity. Pharmacotherapeutica 1, 447-452.
195. Weber G., Kreisel T., Peter S., Künzel J. 1980: A double-blind placebo controlled cross-over study in patients with peripheral vascular diseases, using a new capillary viscometer. Angiol. 31, 1-5.
196. Matsuda T., Ogawara M., Miura R., Seki T. 1979: Effects of isoxuprine hydrochloride on blood viscosity. Biorheology 16, 493.
197. Bode W.A., Fonk E.A., Van der Veen E.A., Van der Meer 1982: Effects of long term treatment with isoxuprine on the blood viscosity profile in maturity onset diabetics. Clin. Hemorheol. 2, 189-193.
198. Kuypers P.H., Skotnicki S.H.: A double blind, placebo controlled study with isoxsuprine retard in peripheral vascular disease. (in press).
199. Ohrymiotis A.D., Whittier J.R. 1962: Effect of a vasodilator, isoxuprine, on cerebral ischemic episodes. Curr. Ther. Res. 4, 124.

200. Manyai S. 1974: Über die Wirkungen von Benzyclan auf Erythrozytenmembranen. Therapiewoche 24, 2877.
201. Heidrich H., Ott M., Schlichting K. 1974: Blutviskosität unter Fludilat. In-vitro- und in-vivo-Untersuchungen. Therapiewoche 25, 66-68.
202. Ehrly A.M., Bredin K. 1974: Untersuchungen zur Frage des Einflusses von Bencyclan auf die Fließeigenschaften des Blutes. Therapiewoche 25, 61-62.
203. Schmid-Schönbein H., Weiss J., Brandhuber M. 1974: Der Einfluß von Bencyclan auf das Fließverhalten von Erythrozyten und Vollblut. Therapiewoche 25, 63-65.
204. Kiss T. 1981: Die Wirkungen der Vasodilatoren Bencycln und Tolazolin auf die Muskeldurchblutung im pharmakologischen und klinischen Experiment. Therapiewoche 22, 2791.
205. Spaan G., Hild R. 1974: Veränderungen einiger Stoffwechselparameter in der ischämischen Extremität durch Fludilat. Therapiewoche 24, 2833.
206. König F.K. 1972: Zur Therapie peripherer Durchblutungsstörungen. Doppelblindstudie zur Überprüfung der Wirkung von Fludilat. Med. Welt (Stuttg.) 23, 763-768.
207. Battke K. 1974: Fludilat bei trainierten Patienten mit peripherer arterieller Verschlußkrankheit der Beine. Therapiewoche 24, 2838.
208. Spinella G., Roxas M., Lazzara N. 1981: The role of bencyclane in the treatment of claudicatio intermittens. Folia Angiol. suppl. 7, 72-77.
209. Van Flasselaer G., Vankulle G. 1981: Double blind study of bencyclane versus placebo in an older population with symptoms of cerebrovascular insufficiency. Folia Angiol. Suppl. 7, 97.
210. Kobayashi S., Kirai A., Terano T. et al 1981: Reduction in blood viscosity by eicosapentaenoic acid. Lancet 2, 197.
211. Terano T., Hirai A., Hamazaki T., Kobayahi S., Fujita T., Tamura Y., Kumagai A. 1983: Effect of oral administration of highly purified eicosapentaenoic acid on platelet function, blood viscosity and red cell deformability in healthy human subjects. Atherosclerosis 46, 321-331.
212. Woodcock B.E., Smith E., Lambert W.H., Jones W.M., Galloway J.H., Greaves M., Preston F.E. 1984: Beneficial effect of fish oil on blood viscosity in peripheral vascular disease. Brit. Med. J. 288, 592-594.
213. Dyerberg J., Bang H.O., Stoffersen E., Moncada S., Vane J.R. 1978: Eicosapentaenoic acid and prevention of thrombosis and atherosclerosis. Lancet 2, 117-119.
214. Dintenfass L., Lake R. 1976: Betablockers and blood viscosity. Lancet 1, 1026-1028.
215. Ernst E., Roloff Ch., Marshall M. 1984: Betablocker erhöht Blutfluidität. Herz Gefäße 4, 447.
216. Heilmann E., Kiesewetter H., Ernst E. (eds) 1984: Klinische Rheologie und Beta-1-Blockade. Zuckschwerdt Verlag.
217. Ernst E., Matrai A. 1984: Besserung der Claudicatio unter β-Blockern? JAMA-D 5, 302.
218. Ernst E., Matrai A. 1984: Effect of metoprolol on chest pain in acute myocardial infarction. Brit. Heart J. 52, 240.
219. Fagard R., Fiocchi R., Lijnen P., Staessen J., Amery A., Vanhees L., Moerman E. 1984: Ketanserin treatment in essential hypertension. Brit. Heart J. 51, 149-156.
220. De Cree J., Lempöls J., Geukens H., Verhaegen H. 1984: Placebo controlled double blind trial of ketanserin in treatment of intermittent claudication. Lancet 2, 775.
221. De Clerck F., Jagenau A., Dom J. 1982: Hemorheological effects of ketanserin, a selective 5-HT2 receptor antagonist, in aged, spontaneously hypertensive dogs. Arch. Int. Pharmacodyn. Ther. 258, 100-115.
222. Ernst E., Matrai A. 1984: Ketanserin treatment in essential hypertension. Brit. Heart J. 52, 359-360.
223. Waller D., Nicholson H., Roath S. 1983: The acute effects of Nifedipine on red cell deformability in angina pectoris. Clin. Hemorheol. 3, 294.
224. Slonim A., Cristal N., Erez R., Shainkin-Kestenbaum R. 1981: The effects of Nifedipine, a calcium antagonist on red blood cell filterability. Proc. 2nd Europ. Conf. Clin. Hemorheol. London.

225. Perret G., Garnier M., Modigliani E., Hanss M. 1984: Lack of effect of nifedipine on erythrocyte filterability and on erythrocyte membrane lipids in healthy volunteers: A double blind cross-over study. Clin. Hemorheol. 4, 401-408.
226. Smith C.D., Mc Kendry R. 1982: Controlled trial of nifedipine in the treatment of Raynaud's phenomenon. Lancet 2, 1299-1301.
227. Kahan A., Weber S., Amor B., Saporta L., Hodara M., Degeorges M. 1982: Controlled study of nifedipine in the treatment of Raynaud's phenomenon. Rev. Rhum. Mal. Osteoartic. 49, 337-343.
228. Sauza J., Kraus A., González-Amaro R., Alarcón-Segovia D. 1984: Effect of the calcium channel blocker nifedipine on Raynaud's phenomenon. A controlled double blind trial. J. Rheumatol. 11, 362-364.
229. Letcher R.L., Chien S., Pickering T.G., Sealey J.E., Laragh J.H. 1981: Direct relationship between blood pressure and blood viscosity in normal and hypertensive subjects. Role of fibrinogen and concentration. Am. J. Med. 70, 1195-1202.
230. Letcher R.L., Chien S., Laragh J.H. 1979: Changes in blood viscosity accompanying the response to Prazosin in patients with essential hypertension. J. Cardiovasc. Pharmacol. 1, S8-S20.
231. Hossmann V., Wegener H. 1983: Hämorheologische und hämodynamische Wirkungen von Isosorbiddinitrat bei essentieller Hypertonie und arterieller Verschlußkrankheit. In: Nitrate III - kardiovaskuläre Wirkungen. H.J. Engel, A. Schrey, P.R. Lichtlen (eds). Springer, pp. 287.
232. Ernst E., Matrai A.: Hämorheologische Effekte von Nitroglycerin 1986: Eine Placebo-kontrollierte Doppelblindstudie. Fortschr. Med. 104, 957–960.
233. Erdi A., Thomas D.P., Kakkar V.V., Lane D.A., Dormandy J.A. 1976: Effect of low dose subcutaneous heparin on whole blood viscosity. Lancet 2, 342-344.
234. Matrai A., Murray W.J.G., Melissary E., Dormandy J.A., Kakkar V.V. 1985: On the hemorheological effects of low molecular weight heparin. Lancet (in preparation).
235. Girolami A., Cella G. 1976: Effect of low dose subcutaneous heparin on whole blood viscosity. Lancet 2, 909.
236. Mayer G.A. 1964: Blood viscosity in healthy subjects and patients with coronary heart disease. Can. Med. Ass. J. 91, 951-954.
237. Gilbert N.C., Nalefski L.A. 1949: The effect of Heparin and dicumarol in increasing the coronary flow volume. J. Lab. Clin. Med. 34, 797.
238. Marshall M., Reiser R. 1983: Changes of blood viscosity by indirect anticoagulation. Clin. Hemorheol. 3, 244.
239. Matrai A., Fendler K., Horvath L. 1981: Hemorheological changes after heparinoid, SP 54, therapy. Proc. 2nd Europ. Conf. Clin. Hemorheol. London.
240. Fendler K., Horváth L. 1983: Effect of oral SP 54 treatment on the primary lipoproteinemias and on the viscosity of blood. Clin. Hemorheol. 3, 293.
241. Juhan J., Buonocore M., Jouve R., Vague Ph., Moulin J.P., Vialettes B. 1982: Abnormalities of erythrocyte deformability and platelet aggregation in insulin-dependent diabetics corrected by insulin in vivo and in vitro. Lancet 1, 535-537.
242. Dowd P.M., Kovacs I.B., Bland C.J.H., Kirby J.D.T. 1981: Effect of prostaglandins I2 and E1 on red cell deformability in patients with Raynaud's phenomenon and systemic sclerosis. Brit. Med. J. 283, 350.
243. Lucas G.S., Simms M.H., Caldwell N.M., Alexander S.J.C., Stuart J. 1984: Hemorheological effects of prostaglandin E1 infusion in Raynaud's syndrome. J. Clin. Pathol. 37, 870-873.
244. Rasmussen H., Lake W., Gasic G., Allen J. 1975: Vasoactive hormones and the human erythrocyte. In: Brewer G.J. (ed). Erzthrocyte structure and function. New York, Liss, 467-490.
245. Kury P.G., Ramwell B.W., Mc Connell H.M. 1974: The effect of prostaglandins E1 and E2 on the human erythrocyte as monitored by spin labels. Biochem. Biophys. Res. Commun. 56, 478-483.

246. Johnston C.C., Dowers S.L., Urbanski R.J. 1977: Examination of the filterability of oxygenated erythrocytes in the presence of L-epinephrine, DL-isoproterenol or prostaglandins (PG) A1, A2, E1, E2, F1 alpha or F2 alpha. Prostaglandins 13, 281-309.
247. Gerbstädt H., Hädelt M., Schuster R., Zunker E. 1978: Effects of prostaglandins E1, E2, suprarenin and isoprenaline on erythrocyte flexibility. Acta Biol. Med. Ger. 37, 907-908.
248. Jay A.W.L., Rowlands S., Skibo L. 1973: Red blood cell deformability and the prostaglandins. Prostaglandins 3, 871-877.
249. Holme J. 1984: Treatment of mild hypertension with diuretics. The importance of EEC abnormalities in the Oslo Trial and MRFIT, 252, 1298.
250. Ernst E., Matrai A. 1984: Increased mortality in hypertensives treated with diuretics - A hemorheological problem? Clin. Hemorheol. 4, 591.
251. Charm S.E., Paz H., Kurland G.S. 1979: Reduced plasma viscosity among joggers compared with non-joggers. Biorheology 16, 185-189.
252. Letcher R.L., Pickering T.G., Chien S., Laragh J.H. 1981: Effects of exercise on plasma viscosity in athletes and sedentary normal subjects. Clin. Cardiol. 4, 172-179.
253. Ernst E., Matrai A., Aschenbrenner E. 1985: Blood rheology in athletes. J. Sport Med. Phys. Fitness 25, 207–210.
254. Ernst E., Matrai A. 1984: Hematocrit and plasma volume in runners. Ann. Int. Med. 101, 571.
255. Ernst E, Matrai A, Aschenbrenner E, Will V. Schmidlechner Ch 1985: Relationship between fitness and blood rheology. Clin. Hemorheol. 5, 507–510.
256. Ernst E. 1985: Changes in blood rheology produced by exercise. JAMA 253, 2962.
257. Gallasch G., Diehm C., Dorfer Ch., Schmitt Th., Stage A., Mörl H. 1985: Einfluß von körperlichem Training auf die Blutfließeigenschaften bei Claudikatio intermittens-Patienten. Klin. Wschr. 63, 554.
258. Larsen O.A., Lassen N.A. 1966: Effect of daily muscular exercise in patients with intermittant claudication. Lancet 2, 1093.
259. Ernst E., Magyarosy I., Scherer A., Schmidlechner Ch. 1984: Einfluß physikalischer Reize auf die Blutfluidität. Z. Phys. Med. Baln. Med. Klim. 13, 359.
260. Ernst E., Scherer A. 1984: Cancer chemotherapy. Ann. Int. Med. 101, 399.
261. Ernst E. 1985: Hämorheologie: Methodische, klinische und therapeutische Aspekte unter Berücksichtigung der Physikalischen Medizin. Ph. D. Thesis, University of Munich.
262. Ernst E., . 1985: Hämorheologische Veränderungen bei Adipositas und unter Heilfasten. In: Naturheilweisen. J. Sonntag, Regensburg. pp 35–51
263. Pietsch L., Ernst E., Roloff Ch., Eisenberg J. 1985: Blutfluidität bei Vegetariern. Ernährungsumschau 32, 205.
264. Ernst E, Weihmayr T, Schmid M, Baumann M Matrai A 1986: Cardiovascular risk factors and hemorheology-physical fitness, stress, and obesity Atherosclerosis 59, 263–269

13. Summary, Conclusions and Perspectives

S. Chien, J. Dormandy, E. Ernst, A. Matrai

13.1. Brief summary

As pointed out in the Preface, an interdisciplinary approach is employed in this book to present the basic principles and clinical applications of the new science of hemorheology.

Following the Forward by A.L. Copley, who reviews the history of development of clinical hemorheology, four Chapters have been written to cover the basic aspects of rheology of blood and blood cells, including biophysical principles, in vitro rheology and the relevance of hemorheology to blood flow in vivo. These are followed by six Chapters on the clinical application of hemorheology in various disease states, and the book concludes with a Chapter on hemorheological therapy.

The aim of the four Chapters on basic hemorheology is to provide the readers, especially those with little or no prior exposure to this new field, with the background information needed to understand the roles of hemorheology in the pathophysiology and therapy of clinical disorders.

Chapter 2 on "Biorheology" (by A. Matrai, R.B. Whittington and R. Skalak) summarizes the basic principles of flow and deformation of blood and its constituents. The terms commonly used in rheology are defined. The principles and practical aspects of rheological methods are discussed; these include the methodologies for determining blood viscosity, the commercially available instruments, and the techniques for performing the blood filtration test, which is being increasingly utilized to study blood cell deformability in clinical conditions. The Chapter ends with a discussion on the rheological behavior of normal blood as a suspension, with emphasis on the various factors which affect blood viscosity. This Chapter provides the basic vocabulary and conceptual framework for the remainder of the book. An understanding of the basic principles set forth in this Chapter would allow the reader to appreciate the roles of blood rheology in flow regulation under physiological conditions and in flow disturbance under disease states.

Chapter 3 on "Rheology of Blood Cells" (by D.E. Brooks and E.A. Evans) provides in-depth discussions on two of the factors which govern the rheological behavior of blood as a suspension, viz. blood cell deformability and aggregation.

Both of these factors are manifestations of the biophysical and biochemical properties of individual blood cells, and the microrheological behavior on a cellular basis is the focus of the treatment in this Chapter. Current knowledge on the intrinsic deformability of red blood cells and white blood cells, the aggregation of red blood cells, and the adhesion of blood cells to vessel walls is reviewed and analyzed, and the implications of these cellular phenomena in blood rheology and blood flow are discussed. Therefore, this Chapter provides the cellular basis of the preceding Chapter on Biorheology, and together they summarize the essential knowledge on rheology of blood and blood cells in vitro and provide the background needed for the subsequent Chapters.

Chapter 4 on "Structural, Hemodynamic and Rheological Characteristics of Blood Flow in the Circulation" (by P. Gaehtgens, A.R. Pries and K. Ley) concentrates on several physiological aspects of the vascular system in relation to its vascular architecture. The aim is to provide a structure-function correlation such that the hemodynamics of blood flow can be analyzed in terms of blood rheology and vascular hindrance. Following a discussion of the vascular features of the four functional compartments in the circulatory system (conduit, resistance, exchange and capacity vessels), the rheology of blood cells (especially erythrocytes and leukocytes) is analyzed as a function of vascular dimension. The flow behavior of blood cells in the circulatory system is considered under conditions of bulk flow, single file flow, and a transition regime in between. This Chapter provides a summary of the rheological phenomena in individual blood vessels in vivo, taking into account the properties of the blood cells (Chapters 2 and 3) and the vascular system, as well as their interactions.

Chapter 5 on "Physiological Significance of Hemorheology (by S. Chien) discusses the relevance of rheological properties of blood and blood cells (Chapters 2 and 3) to their flow behavior in the vascular system in vivo, especially at the organ level. The influence of alterations in blood rheology on in vivo flow resistance is shown to depend on the concurrent behavior of the vasculature. The detrimental effect of abnormal blood rheology on blood flow can be offset by compensatory vasodilation when the vasculature is normal, but it is amplified and exacerbated in the presence of coexisting cardiovascular disorders. The level of optimal hematocrit for maximal oxygen delivery is affected by rheological factors; increase in plasma viscosity and cell aggregation or decreases in cell deformability and blood flow cause the optimal hematocrit to shift to lower levels. This Chapter and Chapter 4 serve as a link between the in vitro blood rheology and the in vivo hemodynamic and metabolic functions and provide a transition from the basic considerations to the clinical applications in the subsequent Chapters.

Chapter 6 on "Cardiovascular Diseases" (by J.A. Dormandy) deals with clinical hemorheology in myocardial ischemia, cerebral ischemia, hypertension and peripheral ischemia. The discussion begins with the criteria required for linking hemorheological abnormalities to circulatory diseases. Based on these criteria, there is good evidence that hemorheological factors are important in the coronary and cerebral circulations, both in terms of primary and secondary risks. The role of these factors in precipitating infarction requires further studies, and they may be related to thrombosis, which is considered in Chapter 7. Once the initial ischemic accident has taken place, the ensuing extent of damage and the clinical progress seem to be closely related to the degree of hemorheological changes observed immediately after myocardial or cerebral infarction. Hemorheological abnormalities may also play a role in the pathophysiology of hypertension and peripheral vascular diseases. The use of hemorheological treatments, e.g. normovolemic hemodilution, plasma exchange and hemorheologically active oral medications, is discussed; further discussions of this are found in Chapter 12.

Chapter 7 on "Thrombosis and Hemorheology" (by G.D.O. Lowe) reviews the contribution of hemorheology to thrombosis. Evidence is presented to show that shearing condition, hematocrit and fibrinogen concentration affect platelet adhesion, platelet aggregation, coagulation and fibrinolysis; platelet adhesion and aggregation are also affected by red cell size and deformability. The role of hemorheology in thrombosis in vivo is considered in various parts of the cardiovascular system. Several rheological factors have been shown to play a role in venous thromboembolism (leg and retinal veins); these include local flow conditions, hematocrit and fibrinogen concentration. The possible roles of these and other rheological factors are also considered in other forms of thromboembolic conditions, including cardiac thromboembolism, arterial thrombosis and atherogenesis, the no-reflow phenomena, thrombosis of arterial shunts and grafts, disseminated intravascular coagulation, and leukostasis. Controlled trials of defibrination with ancrod and hemodilution with dextran have been found to reduce the postoperative incidence and extent of deep vein thrombosis in patients with hip fracture.

Chapter 8 on "Hemorheology and Blood Diseases" (by P. Leblond) reviews hemorheology in hematological disorders. Blood diseases may cause hemorheological disturbances by affecting the major determinants of blood viscosity outlined in Chapter 2. The clinical conditions discussed are erythrocytosis, leukemia, sickle cell disease, hemolysis, paraproteinemias, and the hematological stress syndrome which accompanies several chronic disorders. In each of these disease states, specific abnormalities found in hemorheological measurements made in vitro provides a rational explanation for the clinical manifestations. Studies on hemorheology in hematological diseases have led to useful concepts on patient management, especially with regards to the appropriate use and monitoring of blood transfusions and plasmapharesis. It is pointed out, however, that an understanding of the complex blood rheology in the living circulation necessitates simultaneous measurements of in vivo hemodynamic functions in addition to in vitro rheological tests.

Chapter 9 on "Gynecology, Obstetrics and Neonatalogy" (by P.C. Buchan) reviews the current state of knowledge of hemorheology in these three fields. In normal pregnancy, maternal blood viscosity decreases to a nadir at 30-34 weeks, followed by a rise towards term; this may account for the lowering of peripheral resistance and increase in cardiac output. Normal fetal blood has an elevated viscosity because of high hematocrit and reduced cell deformability, but this is partially offset by a low fibrinogen concentration. Elevated maternal blood viscosity found in pathological pregnancy, e.g. maternal smoking, pre-eclampsia and diabetes mellitus, is associated with an increase in peripheral resistance and may contribute to the decrease in intervillous blood flow and fetal hypoxia. The consequent stimulation of fetal erythropoiesis would exaggerate the fetal hyperviscosity and compromize the vulnerable fetal microcirculation. Neonatal hyperviscosity syndrome is also found in newborns with cardiorespiratory failure, hyperbilirubinemia, convulsions, neurological damage, and low birth weight for gestational age. Hyperviscosity infants with hematocrit above 65% should be treated by partial exchange hemodilution. The Chapter closes with a discussion on the rheological sequelae of oral contraception. Both estrogen, which raises plasma fibrinogen and hematocrit, and progestogens, which raise hematocrit and reduce red cell deformability, can cause hyperviscosity and contribute to thromboembolic complications.

Chapter 10 on "Diabetes" (by A. Barnes and E. Willars) reviews rheological abnormalities in diabetes mellitus in the context of the overall pathology. Diabetic patients have an elevated blood viscosity, particularly at low shear rates and during episodes of poor metabolic control. The in vivo significance of this moderate degree of hyperviscosity of blood ex vivo may be enhanced when there is significant pathology of the blood vessels (see Chapter 5), e.g. vascular narrowing in lower limbs or disturbed autoregulation in cerebral and coronary circulations. Further studies are needed to evaluate the role of such rheological abnormalities in promoting intravascular thrombosis and the efficacy of hemorheological therapy. The possible roles of reduced red cell deformability and increased plasma viscosity in contributing to microcirculatory derangement in diabetes are discussed. It is pointed out that improvements of methodologies of determining erythrocyte deformability and in vivo hemodynamics are needed to further elucidate the rheological abnormalities in diabetes. It is suggested that prospective, longitudinal studies be carried out to evaluate the relative importance of various risk factors in diabetes, including blood rheology and abnormalities of platelet aggregation and fibrinolysis.

Chapter 11 on "Other Syndromes Associated with Impaired Blood Flow and Rheology" (by S. Forconi, D. Pieragalli and E. Ernst) discusses the hemorheological findings and their possible pathophysiological significance in several diseases not covered in the preceding Chapters. These include shock, surgery and anesthesia, rheumatic disease, renal diseases, neoplastic diseases, and several other conditions. It is concluded that the hemorheological deficits in these conditions usually develop as a consequence of ischemia or other primary disturbances. Such secondary hemorheological changes probably do not play a major pathophysiological role in the disease process, except in the case of shock, where hemorheological factors could play a key part in the evolution, perpetuation and irreversibility of microcirculatory failure.

Chapter 12 on "Hemorheological Treatment" (by E. Ernst) discusses the use of methods to improve the fluidity of blood or its components as an alternative medical intervention to prevent or improve ischemia. Hemorheological therapies aimed at correcting abnormalities in various components of blood viscosity (Chapter 2) include hemodilution, apheresis, defibrinogenation, oral medications to lower plasma fibrinogen levels, and drugs to increase blood cell deformability. The modes of action and the clinical efficacies of these treatment modalities are discussed for the various disease states covered in Chapters 6-11. The available evidence is sometimes contradictory, and conclusions cannot yet be drawn as to the therapeutic effectiveness of hemorheological treatments in many clinical conditions. There exists a stronger challenge for investigators in the field of hemorheology to fill the gaps between the theory and its application and to provide a definitive answer regarding the intriguing possibilities of this new therapeutic approach.

13.2. Conclusions

Hemorheology is a new, interdisciplinary field in which basic knowledge on the biophysical behavior of the constituents of blood and their interactions with the vascular system has been applied to elucidate the pathophysiology of clinical disorders and to provide a rational basis for therapy. The development of this frontier of science and medicine requires an understanding of the molecular and cellular bases of the flow properties of blood, knowledge on the interactions between rheological and physiological factors in controlling hemodynamic and metabolic functions, elucidation of pathophysiological roles of these factors in disease states, and critical evaluation of the utility of rheological manipulations as a therapeutic modality.

In many cardiovascular, hematological and other disorders, there is laboratory evidence that the rheological properties of blood are abnormal. In cases where a systematic analysis has been made, these abnormalities can be understood on the basis of fundamental factors governing blood rheology. There is a need for standardizing the methodology and the interpretations of hemorheological tests so that the results obtained from different laboratories can be compared for the derivation of meaningful conclusions.

In several clinical and experimental conditions, alterations in hemorheology determined in vitro can be correlated with disturbances in blood flow and metabolism simultaneously in vivo. The critical questions that need be addressed are whether the rheological abnormalities are sufficient to be a major factor in causing the pathophysiological disturbance and that whether they are the cause, the result, or coexisting phenomena. In some cases, especially in hematological diseases, there is sufficient reason to believe that rheological abnormalities contribute significantly to the functional derangements of the patients; in other cases, however, further studies are needed to provide a definitive answer. Vascular compensation can occur to minimize the detrimental effect of abnormal blood rheology on blood flow, and the importance of rheological abnormalities is magnified when there is coexistent vascular derangement. The importance of simultaneous in vivo physiological measurements in interpretating the role of blood rheology in various clinical conditions cannot be overemphasized.

Although hemorheological therapy is beneficial in conditions where rheological abnormalities are clearly primary in nature, e.g. in some hematological disorders, the available evidence does not allow definitive conclusions to be drawn regarding the applicability of such treatment to other conditions. It is extremely important in the design of clinical investigations, especially in evaluating therapeutic effectiveness, to use objective protocols based on the scientific methods of clinical trials. Anecdotal observations, or even open studies, are of limited value and can be misleading.

Additional investigations are needed in various disease states to determine the specific hemorheological factors which are responsible for the pathophysiological disturbance and to assess whether hemorheological therapy would lead to clinical improvements.

13.3. Perspectives

Clinical hemorheology is a new field which has made rapid advances during the last few years. This progress has been made possible by the developments in methodology and theory of blood rheology and by the interests of clinicians and investigators in studying the role of hemorheology in disease. Based on the findings emerging from such investigations, there is sufficient reason to suspect that hemorheological disturbance may play a role in many clinical disorders, but the proof of such postulations requires the systematic pursuit by clinicians and researchers. The fact that the exact role of hemorheology has not been conclusively established in many of the clinical disorders surveyed in this book reflects the newness of the development of the field and underscores the need for further investigations.

Efforts should be made to develop and standardize hemorheological methods for making reliable clinical tests on flow properties of blood and to increase our understanding of the relationship between the functional characteristics of blood components and the tests used. These require the cooperation among instrument manufactures, research scientists, laboratory personnel and clinicians. The aim is to develop a practical set of hemorheological tests which would allow the systematic characterization and analysis of abnormalities of components of blood rheology in disease states.

There is increasing evidence that the flow properties of blood in the microcirculation is affected by the rheology of leukocytes as well as erythrocytes and that blood rheology may have a significant influence in thrombosis and hemostasis. The rheological role of leukocytes and the interrelationship between blood rheology and thromboembolism in various disease states deserve further studies.

In order to elucidate the pathophysiological roles of abnormal blood rheology in various clinical conditions, in vitro hemorheological determinations must be combined with in vivo hemodynamic and metabolic measurements. The latter include systemic hemodynamic functions, regional blood flows, microvascular functions (e.g. nailfold intravital microscopy), and metabolic status (e.g. oxygen consumption, local oxygen tension, etc.).

While it is necessary to study a sufficiently large number of patients and apply statistical methods to assess the significance of hemorheological and related data, attention should be paid to individual variations, especially among clinical patients. The proper interpretation of clinical hemorheological findings necessitates considerations of the clinical conditions of the patients, as well as the results of other concurrent tests. Prospective, longitudinal studies would be valuable in providing data on the relevance of hemorheology to the pathophysiology and clinical evolution of disease. In order to objectively assess the efficacy of hemorheological therapy in various diseases, especially those with secondary hemorheological changes, it is necessary to conduct clinical trials, with a double-blind, placebo-controlled protocol.

There has been a rapid expansion of scientific information in clinical hemorheology, and it is reasonable to expect this to accelerate in the next few years. It is vital to establish a successful transfer of such information to the clinicians who are direct contact with the patients. This book is written with this as a primary aim, i.e. to bridge the gap between scientific investigations and clinical practice. Other avenues of approach, e.g. audiovisual teaching materials or symposia or workshops at various clinical meetings, would also be valuable.

Clinical hemorheology is an interdisciplinary field. Its future progress requires the collaborative efforts of clinicians, rheologists, bioengineers, physiologists, pharmacologists and biochemists, as well as scientists in other disciplines, e.g. epidemiologists, cell biologists and molecular biologists. As a result of their collaborations, and with the use of rigorous scientific methodologies, clinical hemorheology will be able to develop into a full-fledged branch of clinical science in which basic knowledge on the flow properties of blood can be applied by physicians and surgeons to treat appropriate clinical disorders and to lessen the suffering of patients.

Acknowledgements:

The editors gratefully appreciate the work of Mrs. D. Ernst as librarian for this book. The art work was done by Mr. A. Pazmany, Pecs, Hungary.

INDEX

GPSR Compliance

The European Union's (EU) General Product Safety Regulation (GPSR) is a set of rules that requires consumer products to be safe and our obligations to ensure this.

If you have any concerns about our products, you can contact us on ProductSafety@springernature.com

In case Publisher is established outside the EU, the EU authorized representative is:

Springer Nature Customer Service Center GmbH
Europaplatz 3
69115 Heidelberg, Germany

Batch number: 10607220

Printed by Printforce, the Netherlands